CONTENTS

S0-BRP-501

EMT-Intermediate Review Manual for National Certification

American Academy of Orthopaedic Surgeons and Stephen J. Rahm, NREMT-P
ISBN: 0-7637-1830-0
154 pages

The *EMT-Intermediate Review Manual for National Certification* is designed to prepare you to sit for the National Certification Exam, based on the 1999 EMT-Intermediate curriculum, by including the same type of skill-based and multiple-choice questions that you are likely to see on the exam. The review manual will also evaluate your mastery of the material presented in your EMT-Intermediate training program. The *EMT-Intermediate Review Manual for National Certification* includes:

- Practice questions with answers and model exam
- Step-by-step walkthrough of skills including helpful tips, commonly made errors, and sample scenarios
- Self-scoring guide and winning test taking tips
- Covers of the entire 1999 Department of Transportation EMT-Intermediate National Standard Curriculum.

To order:
Call 1-800-832-0034
Visit www.EMSzone.com

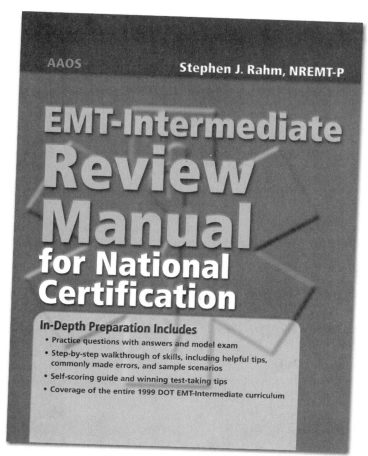

AAOS   **Stephen J. Rahm, NREMT-P**

EMT-Intermediate
Review
Manual
for National
Certification

In-Depth Preparation Includes
- Practice questions with answers and model exam
- Step-by-step walkthrough of skills, including helpful tips, commonly made errors, and sample scenarios
- Self-scoring guide and winning test-taking tips
- Coverage of the entire 1999 DOT EMT-Intermediate curriculum

Workbook Activities

The following activities have been designed to help you. Your instructor may require you to complete some or all of these activities as a regular part of your EMT-I training program. You are encouraged to complete any activity that your instructor does not assign as a way to enhance your learning in the classroom.

Chapter Review

The following exercises provide an opportunity to refresh your knowledge of this chapter.

Matching

Match each of the items in the left column to the appropriate definition in the right column.

_____ 1. ALS	**A.** EMS professional trained in ALS	
_____ 2. BLS	**B.** a system of internal reviews and audits	
_____ 3. EMT-B	**C.** a system to provide prehospital care to the sick and injured	
_____ 4. EMT-I	**D.** the physician who authorizes the EMT to perform in the field	
_____ 5. EMT-P	**E.** responsibility of medical director to ensure appropriate care is delivered by EMT	
_____ 6. Medical control	**F.** basic lifesaving interventions, such as CPR	
_____ 7. CQI	**G.** EMS professional trained in some ALS interventions	
_____ 8. EMS	**H.** advanced procedures such as drug administration	
_____ 9. Continuing education	**I.** designated area for which the EMS service is responsible	
_____ 10. Quality control	**J.** protects disabled individuals from discrimination	
_____ 11. Primary service area	**K.** physician instructions to EMS team	
_____ 12. Medical director	**L.** training required to maintain skills	
_____ 13. Americans with Disabilities Act	**M.** EMS professional trained in BLS	

Multiple Choice

Read each item carefully, then select the best response.

_____ 1. Control of external bleeding, provision of oxygen, and CPR are included in the "scope of practice" of the:

    A. EMT-P.

    B. EMT-B.

    C. EMT-I.

    D. EMT-D.

Introduction to Emergency Medical Care

_____ **2.** EMS is regulated by:
- **A.** NHTSA.
- **B.** NREMT.
- **C.** US DOT.
- **D.** the state in which you are certified.

_____ **3.** _____ is direction given over the phone or radio.
- **A.** Online medical control
- **B.** Off-line medical control
- **C.** Protocol
- **D.** A standing order

_____ **4.** All of the following are examples of off-line medical control EXCEPT:
- **A.** supervision authorized by medical control.
- **B.** standing orders.
- **C.** directions over the phone.
- **D.** training.

_____ **5.** All of the following are true of medical control EXCEPT:
- **A.** it is determined by the dispatcher.
- **B.** it may be written or "standing orders."
- **C.** it may require online radio or phone consultation.
- **D.** it describes the care authorized by the medical director.

_____ **6.** All of the following are components of continuous quality control EXCEPT:
- **A.** periodic run reviews.
- **B.** remedial training.
- **C.** internal reviews and audits.
- **D.** public seminars and meetings.

_____ **7.** The major goal of quality improvement is to ensure that:
- **A.** quarterly audits of the EMS system are done.
- **B.** EMTs have received BLS/CPR training.
- **C.** the public receives the highest standard of care.
- **D.** the proper information is received in the billing department.

_____ **8.** Your main concern while responding to a call should be the:

A. safety of the crew and yourself.

B. number of potential patients.

C. request for mutual assistance.

D. type of call.

_____ **9.** The first phase of the emergency care continuum consists of:

A. recognition of the emergency by the public.

B. patient assessment, stabilization, packaging, and transport.

C. safe delivery of the patient to definitive care.

D. accurate relay of information by the dispatcher.

_____ **10.** Care for burns, delivery of a baby, and management of patients with behavioral problems are conditions covered in which category of the EMT-I's training?

A. Care of life-threatening problems

B. Care of problems not life threatening

C. Important nonmedical problems

D. These are outside the EMT-I's scope of practice

_____ **11.** Understanding legal and ethical issues, learning defensive driving, and stocking the ambulance are covered in which category of the EMT-I's training?

A. Care of life-threatening problems

B. Care of problems not life threatening

C. Important nonmedical problems

D. These are not the concern of the EMT-I

_____ **12.** Which of the following groups is responsible for the national standard curriculum for the EMT-I?

A. American Academy of Orthopaedic Surgeons

B. Department of Transportation

C. American Heart Association

D. National Association of Emergency Medical Technicians

_____ **13.** AEDs are one of the most dramatic recent developments in prehospital emergency care. All of the following are true of the AED EXCEPT:

A. some are no larger than a cell phone.

B. they require extensive training.

C. they detect treatable life-threatening cardiac arrhythmias.

D. they are included in every level of prehospital emergency training.

Vocabulary EMT-I vocab explorer web

Define the following terms in the space provided.

1. Emergency medical services (EMS):

_____

_____

_____

2. First responder:

_____

_____

_____

3. Primary service area (PSA):

_____

_____

_____

4. Emergency medical technician (EMT):

_____

_____

_____

Fill-in
Read each item carefully, then complete the statement by filling in the missing word(s).

1. _____ is the recognition by one state of another state's certification, allowing a health

care professional to practice in a new state.

2. Identifying the exact geographic coordinates of the cellular phone at the time a call is made is possible

with _____ technology.

3. A system in which dispatchers are provided with training and scripts to help them relay relevant

instructions to the caller is called _____.

4. Certification of the EMT-I is a _____ function.

5. In most of the country, a communications center can be reached easily by the public by dialing

_____.

6. The appropriate care for injury or illness as described by the medical director, either by radio or in

written form, is _____.

True/False
If you believe the statement to be more true than false, write the letter "T" in the space provided. If you believe the statement to be more false than true, write the letter "F".

_____ **1.** EMT-I personnel are the highest qualified members of the prehospital care team.

_____ **2.** Medical control is either off-line or online, as authorized by the medical director.

_____ **3.** Medical direction can be transferred by the physician's designee; it does not have to be transferred by the physician himself or herself.

_____ **4.** The purpose of continuous quality improvement (CQI) is to support discipline of personnel.

_____ **5.** A professional appearance and manner by the EMT-I will help a patient build confidence.

_____ **6.** Essential keys to being a good EMT-I include compassion, commitment, and professionalism.

_____ **7.** Direct transport from the scene to a specialty center should never be considered because transport time is usually longer.

Short Answer

Complete this section with short written answers in the space provided.

1. Describe the EMT-I's role in the EMS system.

_____

_____

_____

2. What role has the US Department of Transportation played in the development of EMS?

_____

_____

_____

3. List five roles and/or responsibilities of an EMT-I.

_____

_____

_____

4. Describe the two basic types of medical direction that help the EMT-I provide care.

_____

_____

_____

Word Fun EMT-I vocab explorer web

The following crossword puzzle is an activity provided to reinforce correct spelling and understanding of medical terminology associated with emergency care and the EMT-I. Use the clues in the column to complete the puzzle.

Across

2. Designed to protect individuals with disabilities
3. BLS intervention in cardiac arrest
4. Advanced lifesaving procedures, ie, defibrillation
6. A type of 9-1-1 system that displays the caller's address
8. Simple lifesaving interventions, ie, CPR
9. A circular system of reviews and changes in an EMS system
10. Medical or quality _____

Down

1. An EMT with extensive training in advanced life support
5. Section of the US DOT that created programs to improve EMS
6. An individual trained to provide emergency care
7. System that provides prehospital emergency care
8. An EMT with training in BLS/CPR

Ambulance Calls

The following real case scenarios provide an opportunity to explore the concerns associated with patient management. Read each scenario, then answer each question in detail.

1. While responding to a call for a "man down" at a local restaurant, you encounter a motor vehicle collision between a delivery van and a station wagon. There appear to be injuries among several of the occupants of the vehicles. The restaurant is several blocks away.

   How would you best manage this situation?

   _____

   _____

   _____

   _____

   _____

   _____

   _____

   _____

2. You are dispatched to a private residence. Several neighbors are gathered on the front lawn. There appears to be an argument taking place between two of them. A teenage boy is sitting on the doorstep, bleeding profusely from a cut above his left eye.

How would you best manage this situation?

_____

_____

_____

_____

_____

_____

_____

3. You have been called by the local fire service to transport a heart attack patient to an area hospital outside their primary service area. The paramedics have established an IV line and administered medication to the patient, who is now pain-free. It will be a 15-minute transport to the hospital. The paramedics state that they will not be accompanying the patient but have contacted the hospital, which has accepted the patient.

How would you best manage this situation?

_____

_____

_____

_____

_____

_____

_____

4. You are called to a residence for a 36-year-old female patient with a decreased LOC. Family members tell you that she was recently diagnosed as diabetic. She is conscious but somewhat confused.

How would you best manage this situation?

_____

_____

_____

_____

_____

_____

_____

_____

Workbook Activities

The following activities have been designed to help you. Your instructor may require you to complete some or all of these activities as a regular part of your EMT-I training program. You are encouraged to complete any activity that your instructor does not assign as a way to enhance your learning in the classroom.

Chapter Review

The following exercises provide an opportunity to refresh your knowledge of this chapter.

Matching

Match each of the terms in the left column to the appropriate definition in the right column.

_____ 1. Cover

_____ 2. Burnout

_____ 3. Occupational Safety and Health Administration

_____ 4. Posttraumatic stress disorder

_____ 5. Body substance isolation

_____ 6. Pathogen

_____ 7. Transmission

_____ 8. Tuberculosis

_____ 9. Virulence

_____ 10. Hepatitis

_____ 11. Exposure

_____ 12. Infection control

_____ 13. Meningitis

_____ 14. Host

_____ 15. Contamination

A. chronic fatigue and frustration

B. approach that assumes all body fluids are potentially infected

C. regulatory compliance agency

D. concealment for protection

E. capable of causing disease in a susceptible host

F. delayed stress reaction

G. the organism or individual that is attacked by the infecting agent

H. chronic bacterial disease that usually affects the lungs

I. an inflammation of the meningeal coverings of the brain

J. an infection of the liver

K. contact with blood, body fluids, tissues, or airborne particles

L. the presence of infectious organisms in or on objects or a patient's body

M. the strength or ability of a pathogen to produce disease

N. the way in which an infectious agent is spread

O. procedures to reduce transmission of infection among patients and health care personnel

Multiple Choice

Read each item carefully, then select the best response.

_____ 1. Self-control is developed through all of the following EXCEPT:

A. proper training.

B. medication.

C. a dedication to serve humanity.

D. ongoing experience in dealing with all types of physical and mental distress.

C H A P T E R 2

The Well-Being of the EMT-I

_____ **2.** From the age of 1 to the age of 34, _____ is the leading cause of death.

 A. cardiac arrest

 B. congenital disease

 C. trauma

 D. AIDS

_____ **3.** Presumptive signs of death would not be adequate in cases of sudden death due to:

 A. hypothermia.

 B. acute poisoning.

 C. cardiac arrest.

 D. all of the above.

_____ **4.** Definitive or conclusive signs of death that are obvious and clear to even nonmedical persons include all of the following EXCEPT:

 A. profound cyanosis.

 B. dependent lividity.

 C. rigor mortis.

 D. putrefaction.

_____ **5.** Medical examiner's cases include:

 A. violent death.

 B. suicide.

 C. suspicion of a criminal act.

 D. all of the above.

_____ **6.** Records taken on medical examiner's cases should include documentation of:

 A. the position the patient was found in.

 B. any weapons.

 C. anything witnessed by the EMT-I relating to the scene.

 D. all of the above.

_____ **7.** The stage of the grieving process where an attempt is made to secure a prize for good behavior or a promise to change lifestyle is known as:

 A. denial.

 B. acceptance.

 C. bargaining.

 D. depression.

_____ **8.** The stage of the grieving process that involves refusal to accept a diagnosis or care is known as:

    A. denial.

    B. acceptance.

    C. bargaining.

    D. depression.

_____ **9.** The stage of the grieving process that involves an open expression of grief, internalized anger, hopelessness, and/or the desire to die is:

    A. denial.

    B. acceptance.

    C. bargaining.

    D. depression.

_____ **10.** The stage of grieving where the person is ready to die is known as:

    A. denial.

    B. acceptance.

    C. bargaining.

    D. depression.

_____ **11.** When providing support for a grieving person, it is okay to say:

    A. "I'm sorry."

    B. "Give it time."

    C. "I know how you feel."

    D. "You have to keep on going."

_____ **12.** When grieving, family members may express:

    A. rage.

    B. anger.

    C. despair.

    D. all of the above.

_____ **13.** _____ is a response to the anticipation of danger.

    A. Rage

    B. Anger

    C. Anxiety

    D. Despair

_____ **14.** Signs of anxiety include all of the following EXCEPT:

    A. diaphoresis.

    B. comfort.

    C. hyperventilation.

    D. tachycardia.

_____ **15.** Fear may be expressed as:

    A. anger.

    B. bad dreams.

    C. restlessness.

    D. all of the above.

_____ **16.** If you find that you are the target of the patient's anger, make sure that you:

    A. are safe.

    B. do not take the anger or insults personally.

    C. are tolerant and do not become defensive.

    D. all of the above.

_____ **17.** All of the following are common characteristics of mental health problems EXCEPT:

    A. confusion.

    B. exhilaration.

    C. distortion of perception.

    D. abnormal mental content.

_____ **18.** When caring for critically ill or injured patients, _____ will be decreased if you can keep the patient informed at the scene.

    A. confusion

    B. anxiety

    C. feelings of helplessness

    D. all of the above

_____ **19.** When acknowledging the death of a child, reactions vary, but _____ is/are common.

    A. shock

    B. disbelief

    C. denial

    D. all of the above

_____ **20.** Factors influencing how a patient reacts to the stress of an EMS incident include all of the following EXCEPT:

    A. family history.

    B. age.

    C. fear of medical personnel.

    D. socioeconomic background.

_____ **21.** Negative forms of stress include all of the following EXCEPT:

    A. long hours.

    B. exercise.

    C. shift work.

    D. the frustration of losing a patient.

_____ **22.** _____ stressors include situations or conditions that may cause a variety of physiologic, physical, and psychological responses.

    A. Emotional

    B. Physical

    C. Environmental

    D. All of the above

_____ **23.** Physical symptoms of stress include all of the following EXCEPT:

    A. fatigue.

    B. changes in appetite.

    C. increased blood pressure.

    D. headaches.

_____ **24.** Prolonged or excessive stress has been proven to be a strong contributor to:

    A. heart disease.

    B. hypertension.

    C. cancer.

    D. all of the above.

_____ **25.** _____ occur(s) when insignificant stressors accumulate, forming a larger stress-related problem.

    A. Negative stress

    B. Cumulative stress

    C. Psychological stress

    D. Severe stressors

_____ **26.** Events that can trigger critical incident stress include:

  A. mass-casualty incidents.

  B. serious injury or traumatic death of a child.

  C. death or serious injury of a coworker in the line of duty.

  D. all of the above.

_____ **27.** The quickest source of energy is _____; however, this supply will last less than a day and is consumed in greater quantities during stress.

  A. glucose

  B. carbohydrate

  C. protein

  D. fat

_____ **28.** The body conserves water during periods of stress through retaining _____ by exchanging and losing potassium from the kidneys.

  A. water-soluble B vitamins

  B. sodium

  C. calcium

  D. water-soluble C vitamins

_____ **29.** Stress management strategies include:

  A. changing work hours.

  B. changing your attitude.

  C. changing partners.

  D. all of the above.

_____ **30.** _____ is a condition of chronic fatigue and frustration that results from mounting stress over time.

  A. Posttraumatic stress disorder

  B. Cumulative stress

  C. Critical incident stress

  D. Burnout

_____ **31.** The safest, most reliable sources for long-term energy production are:

  A. sugars.

  B. carbohydrates.

  C. fats.

  D. proteins.

_____ **32.** A _____ is any event that causes anxiety and mental stress to emergency workers.

  A. disaster

  B. mass-casualty incident

  C. critical incident

  D. stressor

_____ **33.** A CISD meeting is an opportunity to discuss your:

  A. feelings.

  B. fears.

  C. reactions to the event.

  D. all of the above.

_____ **34.** Components of the CISM system include:

  A. preincident stress education.

  B. defusings.

  C. spouse and family support.

  D. all of the above.

_____ **35.** Sexual harrassment is defined as:

   A. any unwelcome sexual advance.

   B. unwelcome requests for sexual favors.

   C. unwelcome verbal or physical conduct of a sexual nature.

   D. all of the above.

_____ **36.** Drug and alcohol use in the workplace can result in all of the following EXCEPT:

   A. absence from work more often.

   B. enhanced treatment decisions.

   C. an increase in accidents and tension among workers.

   D. lessened ability to render emergency medical care because of mental or physical impairment.

_____ **37.** You should begin protecting yourself:

   A. as soon as you arrive on the scene.

   B. before you leave the scene.

   C. as soon as you are dispatched.

   D. before any patient contact.

_____ **38.** _____ is the way an infectious agent is spread.

   A. The route

   B. The mechanism

   C. Transmission

   D. Exposure

_____ **39.** _____ is/are contact with blood, body fluids, tissues, or airborne droplets by direct or indirect contact.

   A. Transmission

   B. Exposure

   C. Handling

   D. All of the above

_____ **40.** Modes of transmission for infectious diseases include:

   A. blood or fluid splash.

   B. surface contamination.

   C. needlestick exposure.

   D. all of the above.

_____ **41.** The spread of HIV and hepatitis in the health care setting can usually be traced to:

   A. careless handling of sharps.

   B. improper use of BSI precautions.

   C. not wearing PPE.

   D. sexual interaction with infected persons.

_____ **42.** _____ is equipment that blocks entry of an organism into the body.

   A. Vaccination

   B. Body substance isolation

   C. Personal protective equipment

   D. Immunization

_____ **43.** _____ is a major factor in determining which hosts become ill from which germs.

   A. Immunization

   B. Immunity

   C. Vaccination

   D. A pathogen

_____ **44.** Recommended immunizations include:

   A. MMR vaccine.

   B. hepatitis B vaccine.

   C. influenza vaccine.

   D. all of the above.

_____ **45.** _____ is the presence of an infectious organism on or in an object.

   A. Virulence

   B. Contamination

   C. Immunity

   D. Transmission

_____ **46.** Why isn't tuberculosis more common?

   A. Absolute protection from infection with the tubercle bacillus does not exist.

   B. Everyone who breathes is at risk.

   C. The vaccine for tuberculosis is widely used in the United States.

   D. Infected air is easily diluted with uninfected air.

_____ **47.** A virus that has caused significant concern of late is SARS, which stands for:

   A. sudden acute respiratory sickness.

   B. severe acute respiratory syndrome.

   C. severe adult respiratory symptoms.

   D. sudden adult respiratory syndrome.

_____ **48.** You can use a bleach and water solution at a dilution of _____ to clean the unit.

   A. 1:1

   B. 1:10

   C. 1:100

   D. 1:1000

_____ **49.** Hazardous materials are classified according to _____, which dictate(s) the level of protection required.

   A. danger zones

   B. flammability

   C. toxicity levels

   D. all of the above

_____ **50.** Breathing concentrations of carbon dioxide above _____ will result in death within a few minutes.

   A. 5% to 8%

   B. 10% to 12%

   C. 13% to 15%

   D. 18% to 20%

_____ **51.** Factors to take into consideration for potential violence include:

   A. poor impulse control.

   B. substance abuse.

   C. depression.

   D. all of the above.

_____ **52.** You should recognize signs and symptoms of _____ to ensure your safety.

   A. exposure to hazardous materials

   B. temperature extremes

   C. communicable diseases

   D. all of the above

Vocabulary EMT-I [vocab explorer web]

Define the following terms in the space provided.

1. Critical incident stress management (CISM):

_____

_____

_____

2. Posttraumatic stress disorder (PTSD):

_____

_____

_____

3. Critical incident stress debriefing (CISD):

_____

_____

_____

4. Concealment:

_____

_____

_____

_____

Fill-in

Read each item carefully, then complete the statement by filling in the missing word(s).

1. The personal health, safety, and _____ of all EMT-Is are vital to an EMS operation.

2. The struggle to remain calm in the face of horrible circumstances contributes to the

_____ of the job.

3. Sixty percent of all deaths today are attributed to _____.

4. Determination of the cause of death is the medical responsibility of a _____.

5. In cases of hypothermia, the patient should not be considered dead until the patient is

_____ and dead.

6. In most states, when trauma is a factor or the death involves suspected criminal or unusual situations

such as hanging or poisoning, the _____ _____ must be notified.

7. _____ is generally thought of in relation to oncoming pain and the outcome of the damage.

8. You must also realize that the most _____ symptoms may be early signs of severe illness or injury.

9. EMS is a _____ job.

10. _____ is a serious, potentially life-threatening viral infection caused by a recently discovered family of viruses best known as the second most common cause of the common cold.

11. _____ is the impact of stressors on your physical well-being. _____ include emotional, physical, and environmental situations or conditions that may cause a variety of physiologic, physical and psychological responses.

True/False

If you believe the statement to be more true than false, write the letter "T" in the space provided. If you believe the statement to be more false than true, write the letter "F."

_____ 1. Developing self-control is aided by proper training.
_____ 2. A low or decreased body temperature is sufficient evidence of death.
_____ 3. Rigor mortis is a softening of body muscles shortly after death.
_____ 4. Putrefaction is the decomposition of body tissues.
_____ 5. Denial is generally the first step in the grieving process.
_____ 6. Body fluids are generally not considered infectious substances.
_____ 7. Most EMT-Is never suffer from stress.
_____ 8. Physical conditioning and nutrition are two factors the EMT-I can control in helping reduce stress.

Short Answer

Complete this section with short written answers in the space provided.

1. Describe the basic concept of body substance isolation (BSI).

_____

_____

_____

2. List five of the presumptive signs of death.

_____

_____

_____

3. List the four definitive signs of death?

_____

_____

_____

4. List the five stages of the grieving process.

_____

_____

_____

5. List five warning signs of stress.

_____

_____

_____

6. List two strategies for managing stress.

_____

_____

_____

7. Describe the process for proper handwashing.

_____

_____

_____

8. Complete the following table on the toxicity of hazardous materials.

Level	Hazard	Protection Needed
0	_____	_____
1	_____	_____
2	_____	_____
3	_____	_____
4	_____	_____

9. List the three layers of clothing recommended for cold weather.

_____

_____

_____

10. List the four principal determinants of violence.

_____

_____

_____

11. List the components of negligence:

_____

_____

_____

Word Fun EMT-I vocab explorer web

The following crossword puzzle is an activity provided to reinforce correct spelling and understanding of medical terminology associated with emergency care and the EMT-I. Use the clues in the column to complete the puzzle.

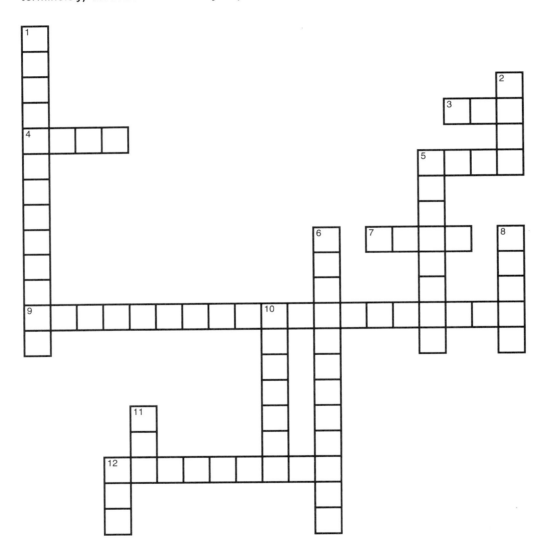

Across

3. Infection control process

4. Confronts responses and defuses them

5. Delayed reaction to past incident

7. Federal workplace safety agency

9. Disease spread from person to person

12. Infection of the liver

Down

1. Exposure by physical touching

2. Confidential discussion group

5. Capable of causing disease

6. Disease of the lungs

8. Impenetrable barrier for tactical use

10. Chronic fatigue and frustration

11. Blocks entry of an organism into the body

12. May progress to AIDS

Ambulance Calls

The following real case scenarios provide an opportunity to explore the concerns associated with patient management. Read each scenario, then answer each question in detail.

1. You are dispatched to a residence for a "person not breathing." Upon arrival, you find a 78-year-old female with a cardiac history who is apneic and pulseless. She also shows signs of rigor mortis and dependent lividity. The family is extremely upset and asking you and your partner to do something. How would you best manage this situation?

_____

_____

_____

_____

_____

_____

_____

2. You are on the scene of a motor vehicle crash where the driver, a 27-year-old female, is breathing shallowly and has blood in her airway. She is unresponsive and you can see obvious fractures of her lower legs. Her 3-year-old son is restrained in a car seat in the back and is screaming and covered in blood. There is no damage to the vehicle where he is sitting and from a quick check you determine that the blood probably belongs to his mother.

How would you best manage these patients?

_____

_____

_____

_____

_____

_____

_____

3. In the process of working a motor vehicle crash, your arm is gashed open and you are exposed to the blood of a patient who tells you that he is HIV positive. You have no water supply in which to wash. Your patient is stable and you are able to control his bleeding with direct pressure.

How would you best manage this situation?

_____

_____

_____

_____

_____

_____

_____

_____

Skill Drills

Skill Drill 2-1: Proper Glove Removal Technique

Test your knowledge of skill drills by placing the photos below in the correct order. Number the first step with a "1," the second step with a "2," etc.

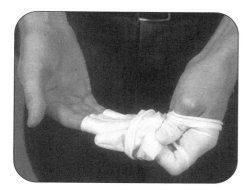

Pull the second glove inside out toward the fingertips.

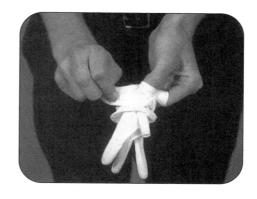

Grasp both gloves with your free hand touching only the clean, interior surfaces.

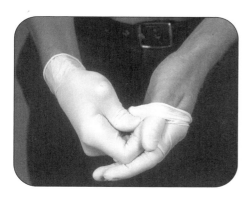

Partially remove the first glove by pinching at the wrist. Be careful to touch only the outside of the glove.

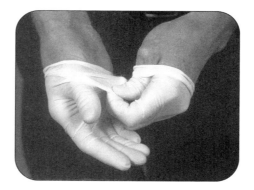

Remove the second glove by pinching the exterior with the partially gloved hand.

Workbook Activities

The following activities have been designed to help you. Your instructor may require you to complete some or all of these activities as a regular part of your EMT-I training program. You are encouraged to complete any activity that your instructor does not assign as a way to enhance your learning in the classroom.

Chapter Review

The following exercises provide an opportunity to refresh your knowledge of this chapter.

Matching

Match each of the terms in the left column to the appropriate definition in the right column.

_____ **1.** Assault

_____ **2.** Abandonment

_____ **3.** Advance directive

_____ **4.** Battery

_____ **5.** Certification

_____ **6.** Competent

_____ **7.** Consent

_____ **8.** Duty to act

_____ **9.** Expressed consent

_____ **10.** Forcible restraint

_____ **11.** Implied consent

_____ **12.** Medicolegal

_____ **13.** Negligence

_____ **14.** Standard of care

A. able to make decisions

B. specific authorization to provide care expressed by the patient

C. confining a person from mental or physical action

D. permission granted

E. touching without consent

F. legal responsibility to provide care

G. written documentation that specifies treatment

H. unlawfully placing a patient in fear of bodily harm

I. unilateral termination of care

J. failure to provide standard of care

K. accepted level of care consistent with training

L. process that recognizes that a person has met set standards

M. legal assumption that treatment was desired

N. relating to law or forensic medicine

Multiple Choice

Read each item carefully, then select the best response.

_____ **1.** The care the EMT-I is able to provide as most commonly defined by state law is:

    A. duty to act.

    B. competency.

    C. scope of practice.

    D. certification.

_____ **2.** How the EMT-I is required to act or behave is called the:

    A. standard of care.

    B. competency.

    C. scope of practice.

    D. certification.

Medical, Legal, and Ethical Issues

_____ **3.** The process by which an individual, institution, or program is evaluated and recognized as meeting certain standards is called:

  A. standard of care.

  B. competency.

  C. scope of practice.

  D. certification.

_____ **4.** Legislative laws are products of:

  A. Congress.

  B. city councils.

  C. general assemblies.

  D. all of the above.

_____ **5.** _____ law is an area of law dealing with private complaints.

  A. Criminal

  B. Civil

  C. Legislative

  D. Administrative

_____ **6.** Murder is an example of a violation of a _____ law.

  A. criminal

  B. civil

  C. legislative

  D. administrative

_____ **7.** The best protection against claims of negligence includes:

  A. appropriate education and training.

  B. accurate, thorough documentation.

  C. a professional attitude and demeanor.

  D. all of the above.

_____ **8.** Negligence is based on the EMT-I's duty to act, proximate cause, breach of duty, and:

  A. expressed consent.

  B. termination of care.

  C. mode of transport.

  D. real or perceived damages.

_____ **9.** Which of the following forms of consent applies when the patient is considered mentally incompetent and the guardian is not readily available?

    A. Protective custody

    B. Informed

    C. Expressed

    D. Implied

_____ **10.** While treating a patient with a suspected head injury, he becomes verbally abusive and tells you to "leave him alone." If you stop treating him, you may be guilty of:

    A. neglect.

    B. battery.

    C. abandonment.

    D. slander.

_____ **11.** Good Samaritan laws generally are designed to offer protection to persons who render care in good faith. They do not offer protection from:

    A. properly performed CPR.

    B. acts of negligence.

    C. improvising splinting materials.

    D. providing supportive BLS to a DNR patient.

_____ **12.** Which of the following is generally NOT considered confidential?

    A. Assessment findings

    B. Patient's mental condition

    C. Patient's medical history

    D. Location of the emergency

_____ **13.** _____ is making false statements in writing.

    A. Slander

    B. Defamation

    C. Libel

    D. Confidentiality

_____ **14.** _____ is making false verbal statements.

    A. Slander

    B. Defamation

    C. Libel

    D. Confidentiality

_____ **15.** _____ is making an untrue statement about someone's character or reputation without legal privilege or consent of the individual.

    A. Slander

    B. Defamation

    C. Libel

    D. Confidentiality

_____ **16.** An important safeguard against legal implication is:

    A. responding to every call with lights and siren.

    B. checking ambulance equipment once a month.

    C. transporting every patient to an emergency department.

    D. a complete and accurate incident report.

Vocabulary EMT-I vocab explorer web

Define the following terms in the space provided.

1. Abandonment:

_____

_____

_____

2. Advance directive:

_____

_____

_____

3. Assault:

_____

_____

_____

4. Battery:

_____

_____

_____

5. DNR order:

_____

_____

_____

6. Certification:

_____

_____

_____

7. Duty to act:

_____

_____

_____

8. Expressed consent:

_____

_____

_____

9. Good Samaritan laws:

_____

_____

_____

10. Implied consent:

_____

_____

_____

11. Negligence:

_____

_____

_____

12. Standard of care:

_____

_____

_____

13. Criminal law:

_____

_____

_____

14. Civil law:

_____

_____

_____

15. Ethics:

_____

_____

_____

16. Licensure:

_____

_____

_____

17. Protocols:

_____

_____

_____

18. Standing orders:

_____

_____

_____

Fill-in

Read each item carefully, then complete the statement by filling in the missing word(s).

1. The _____ of _____ outlines the care you are able to provide.

2. The practice of medicine is defined as the _____ and _____ of disease or illness.

3. The _____ of _____ is the manner in which the EMT-I must act when treating patients.

4. The legal responsibility to provide care is called the _____ to _____.

5. The determination of _____ is based on duty, breach of duty, damages, and proximate cause.

6. Abandonment is the _____ of care without transfer to someone of equal or higher training.

7. _____ consent is given directly by an informed patient; _____ consent is assumed in the unconscious patient.

8. Unlawfully placing a person in fear of immediate harm is _____; _____ is unlawfully touching a person without his or her consent.

9. A(n) _____ is a written document that specifies authorized treatment in case a patient becomes unable to make decisions. A written document that authorizes the EMT-I not to attempt resuscitation efforts is a(n) _____ order.

10. As an EMT-I, you have a _____ _____ to make sure that you are knowledgeable in all areas of emergency care and to care for patients to the best of your ability.

11. Most personal health information is _____ and should not be released without the

patient's permission.

12. Mentally competent patients have the right to _____ _____.

13. Incidents involving child abuse, animal bites, childbirth, and assault have _____

_____ requirements in many states.

True/False

If you believe the statement to be more true than false, write the letter "T" in the space provided. If you believe the statement to be more false than true, write the letter "F".

_____ **1.** When unsure of proper care, you should contact medical control for orders.
_____ **2.** Failure to provide care to a patient once you have been called to the scene is considered negligence.
_____ **3.** For expressed consent to be valid, the patient must be a minor.
_____ **4.** If a patient is unconscious and a true emergency exists, the doctrine of implied consent applies.
_____ **5.** It is important to closely monitor the restrained patient for any signs of breathing difficulty.
_____ **6.** Purchasing liability insurance prevents you from being sued.
_____ **7.** The EMT-I can legally restrain patients against their will if the patients pose a threat to themselves or others.
_____ **8.** The best defense against legal action for the EMT is to always provide care in a manner consistent with ethical and moral standards.

Short Answer

Complete this section with short written answers in the space provided.

1. In many states, certain conditions allow a minor to be treated as an adult for the purpose of consenting to medical treatment. List three of these conditions.

_____

_____

_____

2. When does your responsibility for patient care end?

_____

_____

_____

3. There will be some instances when you will not be able to persuade a patient or the guardian, conservator, or parent of a minor child or mentally incompetent patient to proceed with treatment. List the five steps you should take to protect all parties involved.

_____

_____

_____

4. List the two rules of thumb courts consider regarding reports and records.

_____

_____

_____

5. List the four steps to take when you are called to the scene involving a potential organ donor.

_____

_____

_____

Word Fun EMT-I

The following crossword puzzle is an activity provided to reinforce correct spelling and understanding of medical terminology associated with emergency care and the EMT-I.

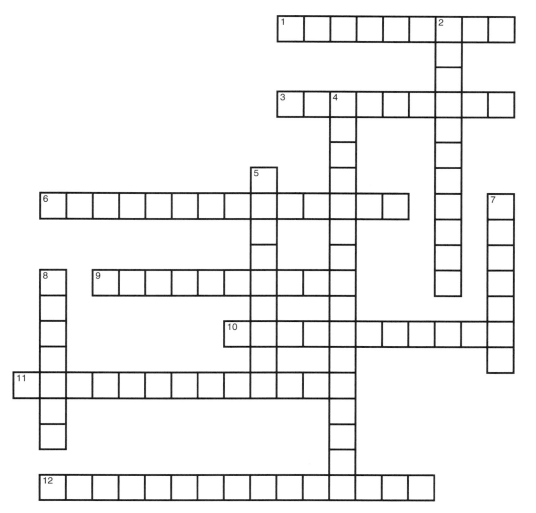

Across

1. Responsibility to provide care

3. A serious situation, such as an injury or illness

6. Assumed permission to provide care

9. Failure to provide standard of care

10. Relating to medical law

11. Evaluation and recognition of meeting standards

12. Care that the EMT-I is authorized to provide

Down

2. Unilateral termination of care

4. Direct permission to provide care

5. Able to make rational decisions

7. Placing one in fear of bodily harm

8. Touching another person without their expressed consent

Ambulance Calls

The following real case scenarios provide an opportunity to explore the concerns associated with patient management. Read each scenario, then answer each question in detail.

1. You and your partner have arrived on the scene of a domestic dispute where the wife has stabbed the husband while "defending" herself. The husband has a minor cut to his left forearm. Law enforcement officers have not yet arrived.

   What actions are necessary in the management of this situation?

   _____

   _____

   _____

   _____

   _____

   _____

   _____

   _____

2. You are flagged down by a teenager at a local playground. She tells you there is a small boy injured on one of the baseball diamonds. You arrive to find a 10-year-old boy complaining of a twisted ankle. There is obvious deformity to his right ankle with a noted loss of function. He says he came to the park to play with his friends while his mother went shopping. There are no adults immediately available.

   What actions are necessary in the management of this situation?

   _____

   _____

   _____

   _____

   _____

   _____

   _____

   _____

3. It is late in the night when police summon you to an auto crash. On arrival the officer directs you to the back of his patrol car. Sitting there is your patient, snoring loudly with blood covering his face. The officer states that the patient was involved in a drunk driving accident in which he hit his head on the rear-view mirror. The patient initially refused care at the scene. You were called because his wound continues to bleed. Assessment reveals a sleeping 56-year-old male with a deep, gaping wound over the right eye with moderate venous bleeding. During assessment the patient wakes suddenly and pushes you away. He tells you to leave him alone.

What actions are necessary in the management of this situation?

_____

_____

_____

_____

_____

_____

_____

Workbook Activities

The following activities have been designed to help you. Your instructor may require you to complete some or all of these activities as a regular part of your EMT-I training program. You are encouraged to complete any activity that your instructor does not assign as a way to enhance your learning in the classroom.

Chapter Review

The following exercises provide an opportunity to refresh your knowledge of this chapter.

Matching

Match each of the prefixes in the left column to the appropriate definition in the right column.

_____	**1.** angio-	**A.** below
_____	**2.** olig(o)-	**B.** false
_____	**3.** eu-	**C.** under, deficient
_____	**4.** infra-	**D.** easy, good, normal
_____	**5.** pseudo-	**E.** within
_____	**6.** dys-	**F.** above
_____	**7.** intra-	**G.** vessel
_____	**8.** hypo-	**H.** little
_____	**9.** supra-	**I.** difficult, painful, abnormal

Match each of the suffixes in the left column to the appropriate definition in the right column.

_____	**1.** -algia	**A.** cell
_____	**2.** -oma	**B.** pertaining to eating or swallowing
_____	**3.** -phasia	**C.** enlargement of
_____	**4.** -phagia	**D.** pertaining to pain
_____	**5.** -lysis	**E.** tumor
_____	**6.** -megaly	**F.** paralysis
_____	**7.** -cyte	**G.** pertaining to speech
_____	**8.** -plegia	**H.** decline, disintegration, or destruction

Medical Terminology

Match each of the root words in the left column to the appropriate definition in the right column.

_____	**1.** cleid(o)-	**A.** pouch or sac
_____	**2.** erythr-	**B.** disease
_____	**3.** acou-	**C.** rib, side
_____	**4.** path-	**D.** white
_____	**5.** bursa-	**E.** hear
_____	**6.** tact-	**F.** clavicle
_____	**7.** pleur-	**G.** fall
_____	**8.** leuk-	**H.** red
_____	**9.** pto-	**I.** touch

Match each of the abbreviations in the left column to the appropriate definition in the right column.

_____	**1.** ASA	**A.** above knee amputation
_____	**2.** BSA	**B.** coronary artery bypass graft
_____	**3.** ETOH	**C.** biopsy
_____	**4.** NS	**D.** intraosseous
_____	**5.** AKA	**E.** body surface area
_____	**6.** IO	**F.** aspirin
_____	**7.** bx	**G.** normal saline
_____	**8.** CABG	**H.** endotrachael tube
_____	**9.** q	**I.** family history
_____	**10.** NSR	**J.** every
_____	**11.** ET	**K.** ethyl alcohol
_____	**12.** FHx	**L.** normal sinus rhythm

Multiple Choice

Read each item carefully, then select the best response.

_____ 1. In medical terminology, a _____ usually indicates a procedure, condition, disease, or part of speech.
   A. prefix
   B. suffix
   C. root word
   D. abbreviation

_____ 2. A(n) _____ conveys the essential meaning of a word.
   A. prefix
   B. suffix
   C. root word
   D. abbreviation

_____ 3. The prefix _____ means "pertaining to blood."
   A. hepat(o)-
   B. hyst(o)-
   C. hypo-
   D. hemat(o)-

_____ 4. _____ is the prefix used to mean "within."
   A. Ect(o)-
   B. Electro-
   C. End(o)-
   D. Enter(o)-

_____ 5. A prefix used to pertain to the eyelid is:
   A. blast(o)-.
   B. blephar(o)-.
   C. ect(o)-.
   D. end(o)-.

_____ 6. _____ means "before" or "forward."
   A. Acr(o)-
   B. Ante-
   C. Bi(o)-
   D. Chole-

_____ 7. _____ means "to straighten" or "normal."
   A. Ortho-
   B. Oste(o)-
   C. Ot(o)-
   D. Scler(o)-

_____ 8. _____ means "under" or "moderately."
   A. Sub-
   B. Pseud(o)-
   C. Supra-
   D. Semi-

_____ 9. _____ means "by the side of."
   A. Iso-
   B. My(o)-
   C. Para-
   D. Uni-

_____ **10.** _____ means "surgical removal of."

    A. -ology

    B. -oma

    C. -ectomy

    D. -ostomy

_____ **11.** When referring to the time after surgery, use the prefix:

    A. poly-.

    B. post-.

    C. pre-.

    D. pro-.

_____ **12.** _____ is the suffix meaning a surgical creation of an opening.

    A. -ology

    B. -oma

    C. -osis

    D. -ostomy

_____ **13.** The suffix used to mean plastic surgery is:

    A. -phasia.

    B. -plasty.

    C. -plegia.

    D. -ptosis.

_____ **14.** A commonly used suffix is "-itis," which means:

    A. inflammation.

    B. pain.

    C. procedure.

    D. paralysis.

_____ **15.** A patient with cardiomegaly would have a(n):

    A. inflamed heart.

    B. enlarged heart.

    C. heart pain.

    D. heart tumor.

_____ **16.** _____ is the root word meaning "joint."

    A. Aden-

    B. Adip-

    C. Alges-

    D. Arthr-

_____ **17.** The root word meaning "abnormal" is:

    A. mal-.

    B. medi-.

    C. mega-.

    D. men-.

_____ **18.** "Vas" is the root word meaning:

    A. vessel.

    B. male.

    C. dry.

    D. hair.

_____ **19.** "-rrhaphy" means:

   A. abnormal or excessive flow or discharge.

   B. enlargement of.

   C. suture of; repair of.

   D. order; arrangement of.

_____ **20.** "Cyst-" means:

   A. blue.

   B. circle.

   C. bladder.

   D. cell.

_____ **21.** "Carcin-" refers to:

   A. cancer.

   B. heart.

   C. great arteries of the neck.

   D. wrist.

_____ **22.** The root word _____ is used to mean "large."

   A. mal-

   B. medi-

   C. mega-

   D. melan-

_____ **23.** _____ is the root word meaning "blood."

   A. Angi-

   B. Erythr-

   C. Melan-

   D. Sangui(n)-

_____ **24.** _____ is the root word that means "dry."

   A. Derm(at)-

   B. Leuk-

   C. Pyr-

   D. Xer-

_____ **25.** The term "biopsy" is abbreviated:

   A. bi.

   B. bx.

   C. BP.

   D. bid.

_____ **26.** "D" in the abbreviation "DON" refers to:

   A. dead.

   B. dyspnea.

   C. director.

   D. dry.

_____ **27.** In all of the following abbreviations, the "L" refers to left EXCEPT:

   A. LAC.

   B. LLL.

   C. LLQ.

   D. LUQ.

_____ **28.** The abbreviation "hs" is a tricky one. It means:

    A. history.

    B. hernia.

    C. at bedtime.

    D. without.

_____ **29.** The abbreviation CABG stands for:

    A. cerebral artery bypass graft.

    B. coronary artery bypass graft.

    C. coronary artery blood gauge.

    D. coronary angina blockage gauge.

_____ **30.** NPO means "nil per os," or:

    A. no pills orally.

    B. negative pressure object.

    C. nothing by mouth.

    D. none of the above.

Vocabulary EMT-I vocab explorer web

Define the following terms in the space provided.

1. Prefix:

_____

_____

_____

2. Suffix:

_____

_____

_____

3. Root word:

_____

_____

_____

Fill-in

Read each item carefully, then complete the statement by filling in the missing word(s).

1. The language of medicine is primarily derived from _____ and _____.

2. A _____ generally describes location and intensity.

3. A _____ usually indicates a procedure, condition, disease, or part of speech.

4. A _____ conveys the essential meaning of the word.

5. Three commonly confused prefixes are _____, meaning below; _____, meaning between; and _____, meaning within.

6. _____ is the suffix meaning surgical removal of, while _____ means surgical creation of an opening.

7. The order to take a medication twice daily would be indicated _____.

8. _____ refers to the left eye, _____ refers to the right eye, and _____ refers to both eyes.

9. _____ is the prefix that refers to the neck.

10. _____ means under or deficient.

11. _____ means fast.

12. The suffix _____ refers to a cell.

13. _____ is the clear portion of body fluids, including blood.

True/False

If you believe the statement to be more true than false, write the letter "T" in the space provided. If you believe the statement to be more false than true, write the letter "F."

_____ 1. The prefix "contra-" means "against."

_____ 2. "Intra-" means "between."

_____ 3. "Rhino-" means "pertaining to the nose."

_____ 5. "Vas(o)-" means "vessel."

_____ 6. The suffix meaning "arrangement of" is -taxis.

Short Answer

Complete this section with short written answers in the space provided.

1. Why is it important for the EMT-I to know correct medical terminology?

_____

_____

_____

2. What potential effects can incorrect medical terminology have on the patient?

_____

_____

_____

Word Fun EMT-I

The following crossword puzzle is an activity provided to reinforce correct spelling and understanding of medical terminology associated with emergency care and the EMT-I. Use the clues in the column to complete the puzzle.

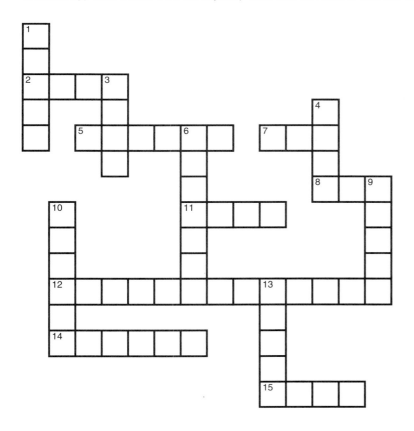

Across

2. Sudden infant death syndrome

5. Stomach

7. Aspirin

8. Liters per minute

11. To hear

12. Languages from which medical terminology is derived

14. Artery

15. Eye

Down

1. Decline, disintegration or destruction

3. Immediately

4. Sodium chloride

6. Abnormal flow or discharge

9. Black

10. Paralysis

13. Pertaining to anything white

Ambulance Calls

The following real case scenarios provide an opportunity to explore the concerns associated with patient management. Read each scenario, then answer each question in detail.

1. Your patient has a known history of non–insulin-dependent diabetes mellitus. He complains of nausea and vomiting for 4 days. His vital signs are within normal limits. Using medical terminology, abbreviate this as much as possible.

_____

_____

_____

_____

_____

_____

_____

2. You are transferring a patient from hospital to hospital. The medical information you are given is as follows. 64 y/o pt with hx AMI. Presented to ER c/o CP x 2 hr, DOE, and N/V. Was given ASA po and NTG SL. IV NaCl TKO. ECG and CXR normal. Translate fully.

_____

_____

_____

_____

_____

_____

_____

3. You respond to a motor vehicle crash and find a 20-year-old male patient who responds to pain only. He has several minor lacerations and abrasions to his forehead, and the windshield is spider webbed. You remove him from the vehicle onto a long spine board. You place him on oxygen at 15 liters per minute via nonrebreathing mask. You establish IV access with an 18-gauge catheter in his right forearm and run normal saline at a to-keep-open rate. The ECG monitor is placed, and the rhythm is sinus tachycardia. Using abbreviations, rewrite this scenario.

_____

_____

_____

_____

_____

_____

_____

_____

Workbook Activities

The following activities have been designed to help you. Your instructor may require you to complete some or all of these activities as a regular part of your EMT-I training program. You are encouraged to complete any activity that your instructor does not assign as a way to enhance your learning in the classroom.

Chapter Review

The following exercises provide an opportunity to refresh your knowledge of this chapter.

Matching

Match each of the terms in the left column to the appropriate definition in the right column.

_____ **1.** Anterior

_____ **2.** Anatomy

_____ **3.** Anatomic position

_____ **4.** Aerobic metabolism

_____ **5.** Anaerobic metabolism

_____ **6.** Superior

_____ **7.** Median

_____ **8.** Physiology

_____ **9.** Diffusion

_____ **10.** Osmosis

_____ **11.** Medial

_____ **12.** Inferior

_____ **13.** Endocytosis

_____ **14.** Crenation

_____ **15.** Cell

_____ **16.** Proximal

_____ **17.** Tissue

_____ **18.** Facilitated diffusion

_____ **19.** Selective permeability

_____ **20.** Distal

_____ **21.** Midaxillary

_____ **22.** Lysis

_____ **23.** Exocytosis

_____ **24.** Organ

A. closer to the midline

B. study of the function of an organism

C. most basic component of an organism

D. farther from midline

E. different types of tissues working together to perform a common function

F. allows normal differences in concentrations between intracellular and extracellular environment to be maintained

G. farther from the head; lower

H. similar cells working together to perform a common function

I. carrier molecule moves substances in or out of cells from areas of high concentration to areas of lower concentration

J. standing, facing forward, palms facing forward

K. movement of a solvent from areas of low solute concentration to areas of high concentration

L. passes longitudinally through the middle of the body

M. study of the structure of an organism

N. cells swell and burst

O. front surface of the body

P. movement of solutes from areas of high concentration to areas of low concentration

Q. cellular respiration in the presence of oxygen

R. closer to the head; higher

S. uptake of material through the cell membrane

T. energy molecules that fuel all of the body's functions

The Human Body

_____ **25.** Adenosine triphosphate
_____ **26.** Posterior

U. imaginary vertical line that descends from the middle of the armpit to the ankle

V. cellular respiration that produces less energy and produces wastes

W. release of secretions from the cells

X. back or dorsal surface of the body

Y. cells shrink

Z. closer to the trunk of the body

Multiple Choice

Read each item carefully, then select the best response.

_____ **1.** _____ allows normal differences in concentrations between intracellular and extracellular environments to be maintained.

A. Selective permeability

B. Diffusion

C. Osmosis

D. Filtration

_____ **2.** Cellular respiration is called normal _____ because it normally occurs in the presence of oxygen.

A. anaerobic metabolism

B. aerobic metabolism

C. glycolysis

D. the Krebs cycle

_____ **3.** _____ is/are a type of connective tissue.

A. Bone

B. Cartilage

C. Adipose

D. All of the above

_____ **4.** _____ typically conduct electrical impulses away from the cell body.

A. Dendrites

B. Axons

C. Neuroglia

D. Neurons

_____ **5.** The major organ responsible for regulation of body temperature is the:

    A. brain.

    B. skin.

    C. liver.

    D. heart.

_____ **6.** The _____ forms a prominent bony ridge in the center of the anterior fossa and is a point of attachment of the meninges.

    A. cribiform plate

    B. styloid process

    C. crista galli

    D. mastoid process

_____ **7.** The _____ "floats" in the superior aspect of the neck just below the mandible.

    A. sphenoid

    B. hyoid

    C. ethmoid

    D. carotid

_____ **8.** The firm cartilaginous ring that forms the inferior portion of the larynx is called the:

    A. thyroid cartilage.

    B. costal cartilage.

    C. cricoid cartilage.

    D. laryngo cartilage.

_____ **9.** The _____ lies at the level where the second rib is attached to the sternum.

    A. manubrium

    B. xiphoid process

    C. angle of Louis

    D. cliedosternal joint

_____ **10.** Most of the liver lies in the _____ of the abdomen.

    A. RUQ

    B. RLQ

    C. LUQ

    D. LLQ

_____ **11.** The spleen is located in the:

    A. RUQ.

    B. RLQ.

    C. LUQ.

    D. LLQ.

_____ **12.** An example of a hinge joint is the:

    A. hip.

    B. thumb.

    C. vertebrae.

    D. elbow.

_____ **13.** Which of the following is not a bone of the pelvis?

    A. Ilium

    B. Ischium

    C. Pubis

    D. Ileum

_____ **14.** A _____ is a tough white band of tissue that connects bones to other bones.
    A. tendon
    B. ligament
    C. cartilage
    D. periosteum

_____ **15.** _____ help(s) to maintain good bone health and prevent osteoporosis.
    A. Calcium-rich foods
    B. Vitamin D
    C. Exercise
    D. All of the above

_____ **16.** A _____ is the area of skin supplied by a given pair of spinal sensory nerves.
    A. ventral root
    B. dorsal root
    C. dermatome
    D. plexus

_____ **17.** The "master" gland is the:
    A. thyroid.
    B. parathyroid.
    C. pituitary.
    D. pancreas.

_____ **18.** The _____ is located high in the right atrium and is the normal site of origin of electrical impulses in the heart.
    A. SA node
    B. AV node
    C. Bundle of His
    D. Purkinje network

_____ **19.** _____ is/are a thin, plasma-like fluid formed from interstitial or extracellular fluid that bathes the tissues of the body.
    A. CSF
    B. Lymph
    C. Blood
    D. All of the above

_____ **20.** Virtually all of the blood in the body transverses the _____, where it is filtered and worn out blood cells, foreign substances, and bacteria are removed.
    A. liver
    B. pancreas
    C. bile duct
    D. splenic tissue

_____ **21.** _____ is the amount of air inspired during normal respiration.
    A. Tidal volume
    B. Residual volume
    C. Inhaled volume
    D. Vital volume

Labeling

Label the following diagrams with the correct terms.

Directional Terms

A. _____

B. _____

C. _____

D. _____

E. _____

F. _____

G. _____

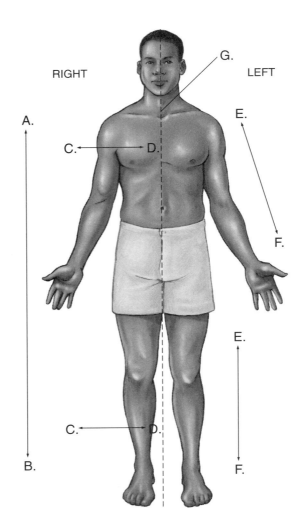

Abdominal Quadrants

A. _____

B. _____

C. _____

D. _____

E. _____

F. _____

G. _____

H. _____

I. _____

J. _____

K. _____

L. _____

M. _____

N. _____

O. _____

P. _____

Q. _____

R. _____

S. _____

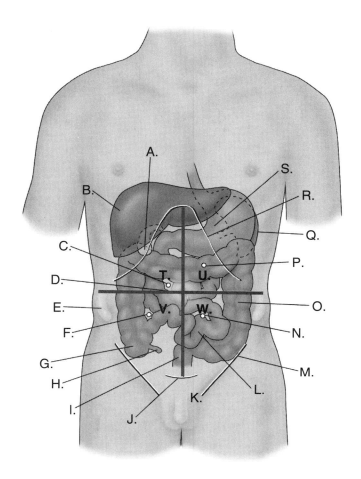

Anatomic Positions

A. _____

B. _____

C. _____

D. _____

E. _____

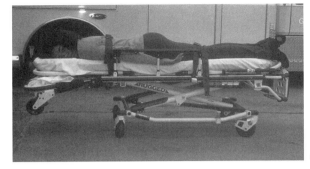

A.

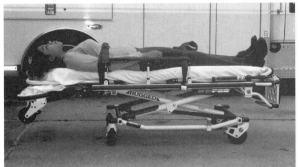

B.

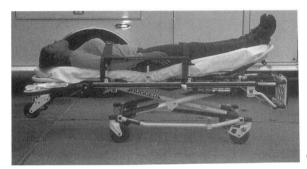

C.

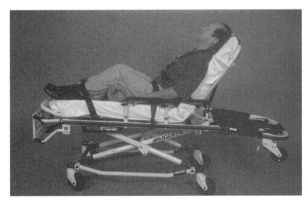

D.

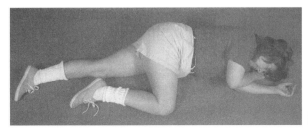

E.

The Neuron

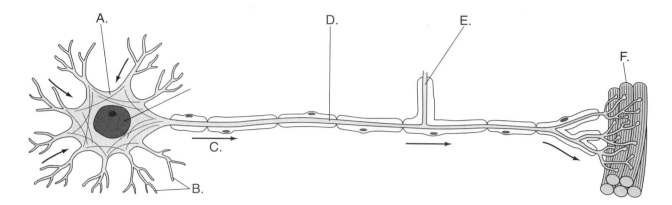

A. _____   D. _____

B. _____   E. _____

C. _____   F. _____

The Skin

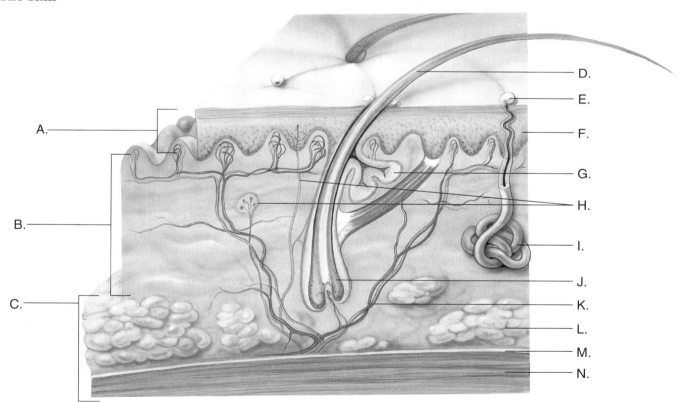

A. _____ D. _____ G. _____ J. _____ M. _____

B. _____ E. _____ H. _____ K. _____ N. _____

C. _____ F. _____ I. _____ L. _____

Skeletal System

A. _____

B. _____

C. _____

D. _____

E. _____

F. _____

G. _____

H. _____

I. _____

J. _____

K. _____

L. _____

M. _____

N. _____

O. _____

P. _____

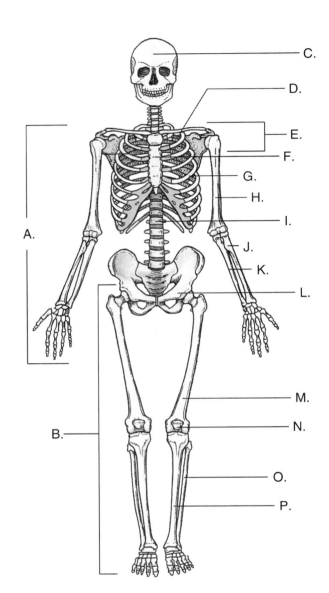

The Skull

A. _____

B. _____

C. _____

D. _____

E. _____

F. _____

G. _____

H. _____

I. _____

J. _____

K. _____

L. _____

M. _____

N. _____

O. _____

P. _____

Q. _____

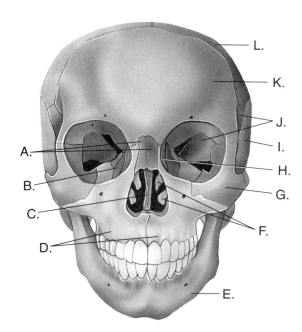

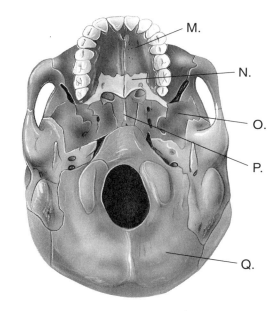

The Thorax

A. _____

B. _____

C. _____

D. _____

E. _____

F. _____

G. _____

H. _____

I. _____

J. _____

K. _____

L. _____

M. _____

N. _____

O. _____

P. _____

Q. _____

R. _____

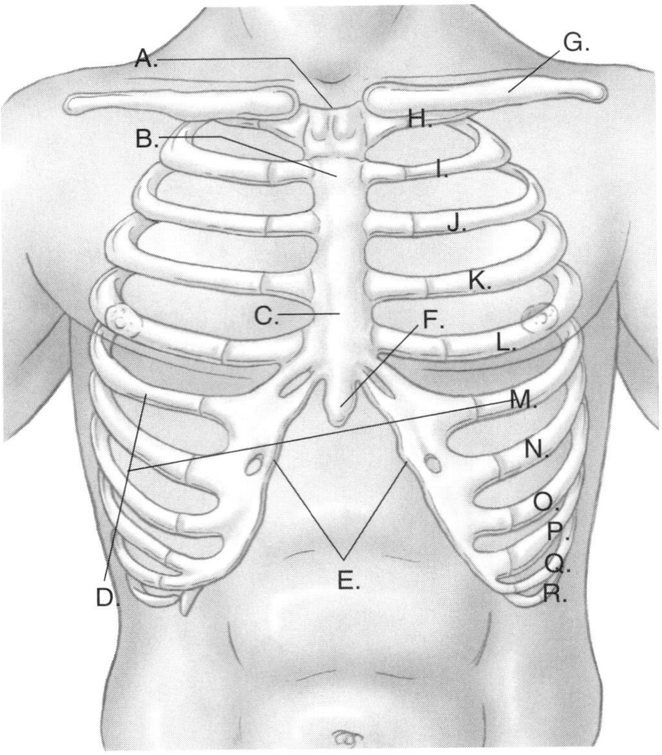

A. _____

B. _____

C. _____

D. _____

E. _____

F. _____

G. _____

H. _____

I. _____

J. _____

K. _____

L. _____

M. _____

N. _____

O. _____

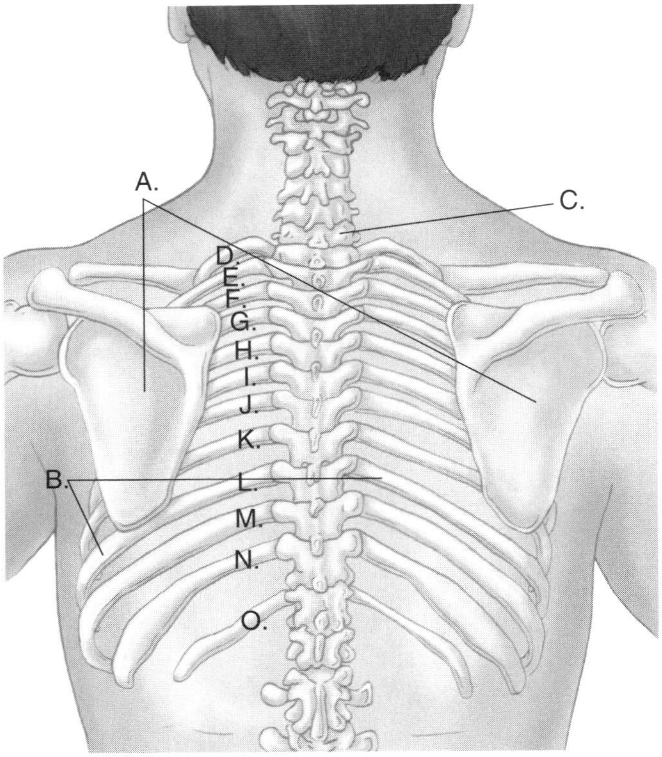

Shoulder Girdle

A. _____

B. _____

C. _____

D. _____

E. _____

F. _____

G. _____

H. _____

I. _____

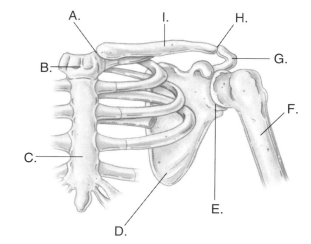

A. _____

B. _____

C. _____

D. _____

E. _____

F. _____

G. _____

H. _____

I. _____

J. _____

K. _____

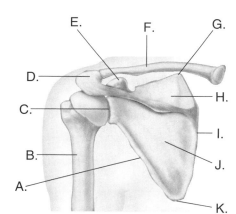

Upper Extremity

A. _____

B. _____

C. _____

D. _____

E. _____

F. _____

G. _____

H. _____

I. _____

J. _____

K. _____

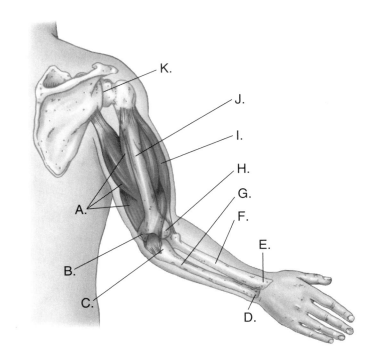

Wrist and Hand

A. _____

B. _____

C. _____

D. _____

E. _____

F. _____

G. _____

H. _____

I. _____

J. _____

K. _____

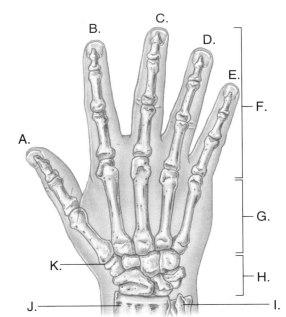

Pelvic Girdle

A. _____

B. _____

C. _____

D. _____

E. _____

F. _____

G. _____

H. _____

I. _____

J. _____

K. _____

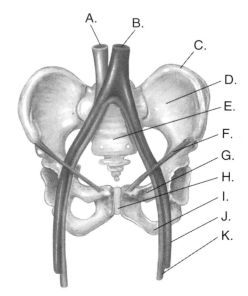

Hip Joint

A. _____

B. _____

C. _____

D. _____

E. _____

F. _____

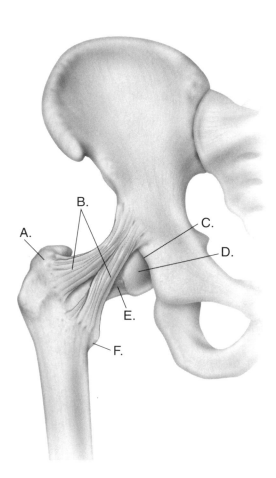

Lower Extremity

A. _____

B. _____

C. _____

D. _____

E. _____

F. _____

G. _____

H. _____

I. _____

J. _____

K. _____

L. _____

M. _____

N. _____

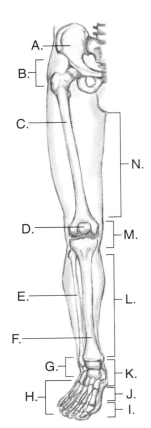

The Knee

A. _____

B. _____

C. _____

D. _____

E. _____

F. _____

G. _____

H. _____

I. _____

J. _____

K. _____

L. _____

M. _____

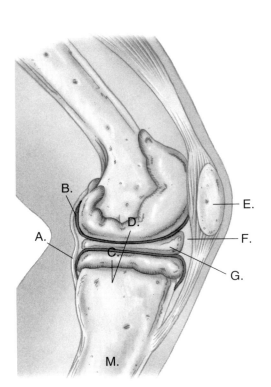

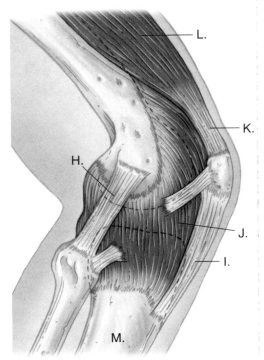

The Brain

A. _____

B. _____

C. _____

D. _____

E. _____

F. _____

G. _____

H. _____

I. _____

J. _____

K. _____

L. _____

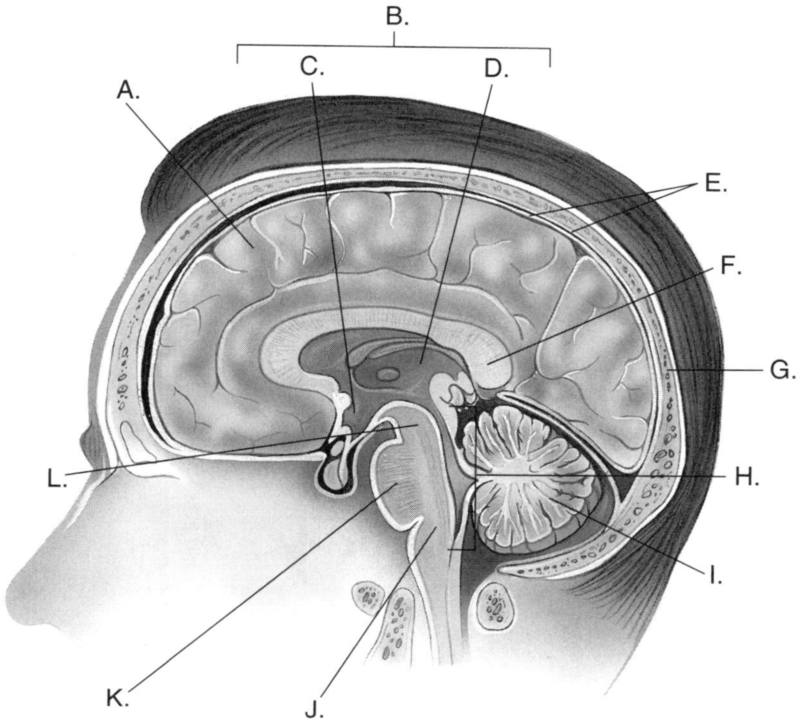

Spinal Cord

A. _____

B. _____

C. _____

D. _____

E. _____

F. _____

G. _____

H. _____

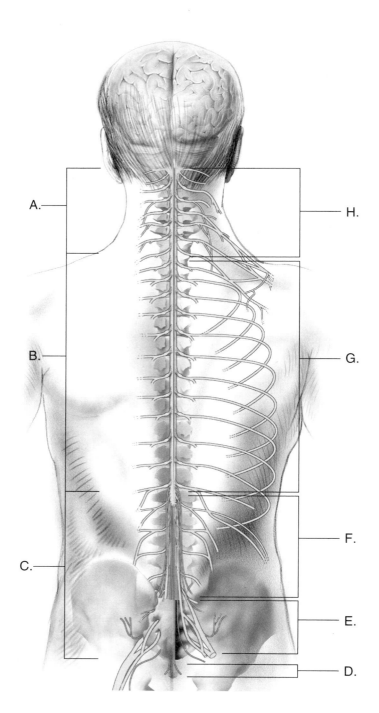

Cardiac Conduction System

A. _____

B. _____

C. _____

D. _____

E. _____

F. _____

G. _____

H. _____

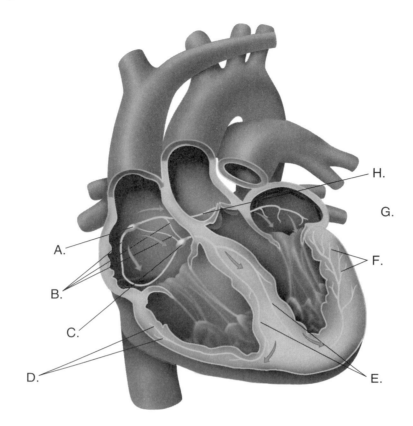

Coronary Arteries

A. _____

B. _____

C. _____

D. _____

E. _____

F. _____

G. _____

H. _____

I. _____

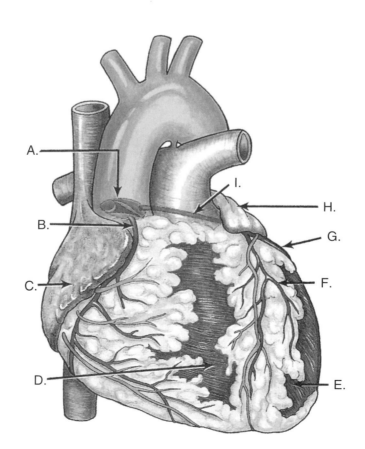

Cardiovascular System

A. _____

B. _____

C. _____

D. _____

E. _____

F. _____

G. _____

H. _____

I. _____

J. _____

K. _____

L. _____

M. _____

N. _____

O. _____

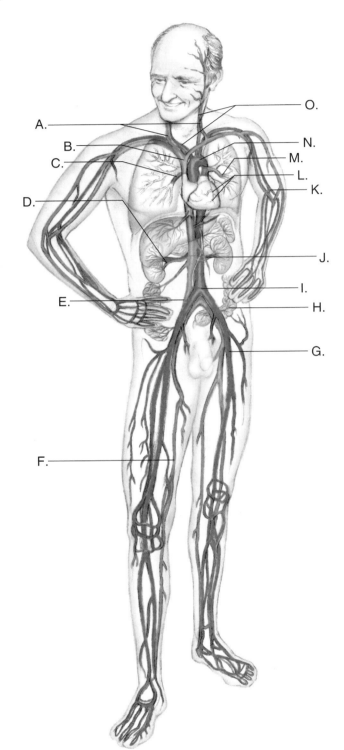

Veins of the Head and Neck

A. _____

B. _____

C. _____

D. _____

E. _____

F. _____

G. _____

H. _____

I. _____

J. _____

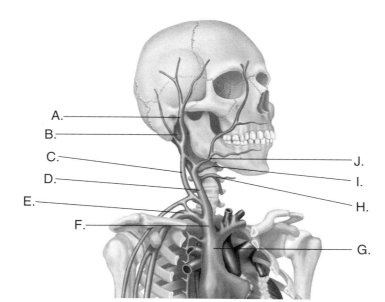

Hepatic Portal System

A. _____

B. _____

C. _____

D. _____

E. _____

F. _____

G. _____

H. _____

I. _____

J. _____

K. _____

L. _____

M. _____

N. _____

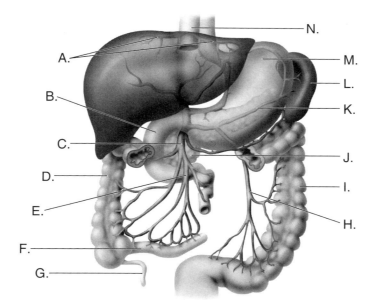

Male Reproductive System

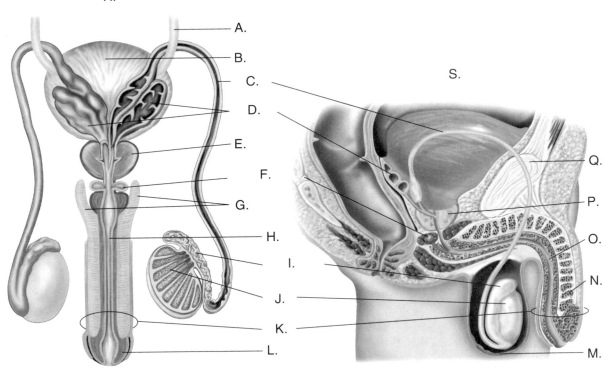

A. _____ F. _____ K. _____ P. _____

B. _____ G. _____ L. _____ Q. _____

C. _____ H. _____ M. _____ R. _____

D. _____ I. _____ N. _____ S. _____

E. _____ J. _____ O. _____

Female Reproductive System

F.   B.   G.

C.

A.

D.

E.

A. _____

B. _____

C. _____

D. _____

E. _____

F. _____

G. _____

Vocabulary EMT-I vocab explorer web

Define the following terms in the space provided.

1. Perfusion:

_____

_____

_____

2. Aerobic metabolism:

_____

_____

_____

3. Autonomic nervous system:

_____

_____

_____

4. Pleural space:

_____

_____

_____

5. Homeostasis:

_____

_____

_____

6. pH:

_____

_____

_____

7. Solutes:

_____

_____

_____

8. Endocrine system:

_____

_____

_____

9. Peripheral nervous system:

_____

_____

_____

10. Epiglottis:

_____

_____

_____

11. Metabolism:

_____

_____

_____

12. Brain stem:

_____

_____

_____

Fill-in

Read each item carefully, then complete the statement by filling in the missing word(s).

1. Typically, we have no conscious control over the function of _____ muscles.

2. _____ are the main conducting cells of nerve tissue. Two projections extending from

nerve cells are _____, which receive impulses and conduct them toward the cell body,

and _____, which conduct impulses away from the cell body.

3. The kidneys are called _____ organs because they lie behind the abdominal cavity.

4. The _____ is a ball-and-socket joint in which the head of the humerus articulates with

the _____ _____, which is part of the scapula.

5. Cells called _____ produce bone tissue, while _____ are large

multinucleated cells that dissolve bone tissue.

6. Glands secrete proteins called _____ that regulate many body functions, including

growth, reproduction, temperature, metabolism, and blood pressure.

7. _____ _____ and _____ are two hormones released by

the posterior pituitary gland.

8. Cardiac cells possess an ability to generate an impulse to contract even when there is no external nerve

stimulus, a process called intrinsic _____.

9. _____ _____ is the amount of blood pumped through the circulatory

system in one minute.

10. _____ is a wavelike contraction of smooth muscle.

11. A(n) _____ is a substance that increases the concentration of hydrogen ions in a water

solution, while a _____ is a substance that decreases the concentration of hydrogen ions.

True/False

If you believe the statement to be more true than false, write the letter "T" in the space provided. If you believe the statement to be more false than true, write the letter "F".

_____ **1.** Extension is the motion associated with the return of a body part from a flexed position to the anatomic position.

_____ **2.** Facilitated diffusion is the process in which a carrier molecule moves substances in or out of cells from areas of low concentration to areas of high concentration.

_____ **3.** Sweat glands, sebaceous glands, hair follicles, blood vessels, and nerve ends are found in the epidermis.

_____ **4.** The pituitary gland resides in the sella turcica of the sphenoid bone.

_____ **5.** The spinal column is composed of 39 bones.

_____ **6.** The diaphragm separates the thoracic and abdominal cavities.

_____ **7.** Neurotransmitters are contained within synaptic vesicles and are released into a synaptic cleft.

_____ **8.** Insulin is secreted from the alpha cells of the islets of Langerhans in the pancreas.

_____ **9.** The sinoatrial node is located high in the right atria and is the normal site of origin of the electrical impulse.

_____ **10.** During exhalation, the diaphragm contracts and negative pressure is created in the chest cavity.

Short Answer

Complete this section with short written answers in the space provided.

1. List the four components of blood and each of their functions.

_____

_____

_____

2. Describe each of the following:

Intracellular fluid:

_____

_____

_____

Extracellular fluid:

_____

_____

_____

Intravascular fluid:

_____

_____

_____

Interstitial fluid:

_____

_____

3. List four hormones released from the anterior pituitary lobe and the primary function of each.

_____

_____

_____

4. List the cranial nerves and their functions.

_____

_____

_____

Word Fun EMT-I

The following crossword puzzle is an activity provided to reinforce correct spelling and understanding of medical terminology associated with emergency care and the EMT-I. Use the clues in the column to complete the puzzle.

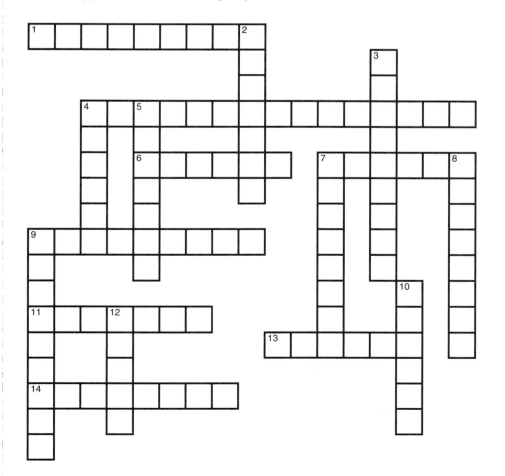

Across

1. Appears on both sides
4. Behind the abdomen
6. Slow, dying respirations or pulse
7. Upper chamber of the heart
9. Back surface of the body
11. Sitting up with knees bent
13. Inner layer of skin
14. Nearer to the feet

Down

2. Away from the midline; sides
3. Lower chamber of heart
4. Bone on thumb side of forearm
5. Windpipe
7. Front surface of the body
8. Lower jawbone
9. Adequate circulation of blood
10. Nearer the end
12. Large solid organ in RUQ

Ambulance Calls

The following real case scenarios provide an opportunity to explore the concerns associated with patient management. Read each scenario, then answer each question in detail.

1. You are dispatched to the scene of a bar fight. A 34-year-old male has been stabbed in the right upper quadrant of the abdomen with a knife. Using medical terminology, indicate which organ(s) might be affected.

How would you describe this patient's injuries?

_____

_____

_____

_____

_____

_____

_____

_____

2. You are dispatched to a school playground to find an 8-year-old who has fallen from the monkey bars and is complaining of pain to his left forearm just above his wrist. You see it sticking out at an odd angle.

Using medical terminology, how would you describe this patient's injuries?

_____

_____

_____

_____

_____

_____

_____

3. You are dispatched to a scene where a 14-year-old male was hit by a car. Upon arrival, you find the patient's left lower leg to be deformed and swollen.

Using medical terminology, how would you describe this patient's injuries?

_____

_____

_____

_____

_____

_____

_____

3. You are dispatched to a construction accident where a patient fell 20 feet. He has deformity to the back of the head, swelling and deformity to the right forearm, and the bone in his right upper leg is broken and sticking through the skin.

Using medical terminology, how would you describe this patient's injuries?

_____

_____

_____

_____

_____

_____

_____

Workbook Activities

The following activities have been designed to help you. Your instructor may require you to complete some or all of these activities as a regular part of your EMT-I training program. You are encouraged to complete any activity that your instructor does not assign as a way to enhance your learning in the classroom.

Chapter Review

The following exercises provide an opportunity to refresh your knowledge of this chapter.

Matching

Match each of the terms in the left column to the appropriate definition in the right column.

_____ 1. Absorption

_____ 2. Capsule

_____ 3. Metered-dose inhaler

_____ 4. Gel

_____ 5. Contraindication

_____ 6. Topical medication

_____ 7. Enteral

_____ 8. Side effect

_____ 9. Sympathomimetics

_____ 10. Trade name

_____ 11. Gases

_____ 12. Adsorption

_____ 13. Theraputic index

_____ 14. Solution

_____ 15. Theraputic threshold

_____ 16. Dose

_____ 17. Suspension

_____ 18. Excretion

_____ 19. Indication

_____ 20. Transcutaneous

_____ 21. Biotransformation

_____ 22. Action

_____ 23. Sympatholytic

_____ 24. Parenteral

_____ 25. Pharmacology

_____ 26. Generic name

A. mimic effects of the sympathetic nervous system

B. administered through any route other than the GI tract

C. study of the properties and effects of drugs and medications

D. neither solid or liquid

E. original chemical name

F. effect a drug is expected to have

G. designed to be absorbed through the skin

H. fine particles evenly distributed throughout a liquid by shaking

I. to bind or stick to a surface

J. amount of medication given

K. difference between minimal effective dose and a toxic level

L. miniature spray canister used to direct substances from the mouth to the lungs

M. gelatin shells filled with powder or liquid

N. elimination of waste products

O. when a drug should not be given

P. chemical alteration a substance goes through in the body

Q. therapeutic use for a particular medication

R. lotions, creams, and ointments

S. minimum effective concentration

T. any action other than desired one

U. fights effects of sympathetic nervous system

V. administered along the GI tract

W. brand name

X. cannot be separated by filtering

Y. process by which medications travel through body tissues

Z. semi-liquid substance administered orally

6

Pharmacology

Multiple Choice

Read each item carefully, then select the best response.

_____ **1.** Medications have been identified or derived from:

    A. plants.

    B. animals and humans.

    C. minerals.

    D. all of the above.

_____ **2.** The proper dose of a medication depends on all of the following, except:

    A. the patient's age.

    B. the patient's size.

    C. generic substitutions.

    D. the desired action.

_____ **3.** Nitroglycerin relieves the squeezing or crushing pain associated with angina by:

    A. dilating the arteries to increase the oxygen supply to the heart muscle.

    B. causing the heart to contract harder and increase cardiac output.

    C. causing the heart to beat faster to supply more oxygen to the heart.

    D. all of the above.

_____ **4.** The brand name that a manufacturer gives to a medication is called the _____ name.

    A. trade

    B. generic

    C. chemical

    D. prescription

_____ **5.** The fastest way to deliver a chemical substance is by the _____ route.

    A. intravenous

    B. oral

    C. sublingual

    D. intramuscular

_____ **6.** Medications that have the prefix "depo" in their names form a _____ in the muscle after being injected.

    A. deposition

    B. depository

    C. depot

    D. deponent

_____ **7.** Insulin is a medication that is given by the _____ route.

    A. intravenous

    B. oral

    C. subcutaneous

    D. intramuscular

_____ **8.** The form the manufacturer chooses for a medication ensures:

    A. the proper route of the medication.

    B. the timing of its release into the bloodstream.

    C. its effects on target organs or body systems.

    D. all of the above.

_____ **9.** Solutions may be given:

    A. orally.

    B. intramuscularly.

    C. rectally.

    D. all of the above.

_____ **10.** _____ separate if they stand or are filtered.

    A. Liquids

    B. Suspensions

    C. Gels

    D. Topicals

_____ **11.** When giving a drug ET, the dose should be:

    A. the same as IV.

    B. 2 to $2\frac{1}{2}$ times IV dose.

    C. $\frac{1}{2}$ of the IV dose.

    D. $1\frac{1}{2}$ times the IV dose.

_____ **12.** Which is true of subcutaneous injections?

    A. Medications are absorbed more slowly.

    B. Effects of the drug last longer.

    C. They would not be appropriate for patients with decreased peripheral perfusion.

    D. All of the above.

_____ **13.** The _____ is the primary organ for biotransformation.

    A. heart

    B. lungs

    C. liver

    D. spleen

_____ **14.** Organs of excretion include:

    A. kidneys.

    B. intestines.

    C. lungs.

    D. all of the above.

_____ **15.** An allergy to a drug occurring after previous exposure to the drug is:

    A. interaction.

    B. hypersensitivity.

    C. contraindication.

    D. tolerance.

_____ **16.** Morphine is a _____ drug as classified by the DEA.

    A. Schedule I

    B. Schedule II

    C. Schedule III

    D. Schedule IV

1999 _____ **17.** Adenosine is contraindicated in patients with:
  A. chest pain.
  B. tachycardia.
  C. 2nd or 3rd degree heart block.
  D. PSVT.

1999 _____ **18.** _____ is a side effect of atropine sulfate.
  A. Headache
  B. Tachycardia
  C. Dry mouth
  D. All of the above

1999 _____ **19.** Lidocaine HCl 2% is classified as a _____.
  A. narcotic analgesic
  B. antiarrhythmic
  C. sympathomimetic
  D. benzodiazepine

Vocabulary EMT-I vocab explorer web

Define the following terms using the space provided.

1. Trade name:

_____

_____

_____

2. Generic name:

_____

_____

_____

3. OTC:

_____

_____

_____

4. Solution:

_____

_____

_____

5. Suspension:

_____

_____

_____

6. Sublingual:

_____

_____

_____

7. Metered-dose inhaler (MDI):

_____

_____

_____

Fill-in

Read each item carefully, then complete the statement by filling in the missing word.

1. _____ are chemical agents used in the diagnosis, treatment, and prevention of disease.

2. All medications that are licensed for use in the United States are listed by their generic name in the

_____.

3. Nitroglycerin is usually taken _____.

4. As an EMT-I, you are _____, _____, and _____

responsible for each drug you administer.

5. When given by mouth, _____ may be absorbed from the stomach fairly quickly because

the medication is already dissolved.

6. The more _____ the drug, the faster it enters the circulatory system.

7. Drugs that bind to a receptor and create a response are known as _____ while drugs

that bind with a receptor site without creating a response but instead block other drugs from binding are

_____.

True/False

If you believe the statement to be more true than false, write the letter "T" in the space provided. If you believe the statement to be more false than true, write the letter "F."

_____ **1.** Street drugs are still pharmacologically active and will cause an effect.

_____ **2.** Before administering any medication to a female of childbearing age, the patient should be asked about the possibility of pregnancy.

_____ **3.** Drugs give new functions to tissues or organs.

_____ **4.** Nitroglycerin decreases blood pressure.

_____ **5.** Sublingual medications are rapidly absorbed into the digestive tract.

_____ **6.** Vital signs should be taken before and after a medication is given.

_____ **7.** Even though medications can react with each other, this is not a potentially harmful condition for the patient.

_____ **8.** Nitroglycerin should only be administered when the patient's systolic blood pressure is below 100 mm Hg.

Short Answer

Complete this section with short written answers using the space provided.

1. List seven routes of medication administration.

_____

_____

_____

2. Describe the general steps of administering medication.

_____

_____

_____

3. List four factors of drug absorption.

_____

_____

_____

1999 **4.** List the indications, contraindications, and dose for the following:

Epinephrine:

_____

_____

_____

Atropine sulfate:

_____

_____

_____

Lidocaine HCl:

_____

_____

_____

Morphine sulfate:

_____

_____

_____

Word Fun EMT-I vocab explorer web

The following crossword puzzle is a good way to reinforce correct spelling and understanding of medical terminology associated with emergency care and the EMT-I. Use the clues in the column to complete the puzzle.

Across

1. Raises heart rate and blood pressure
6. Binding to or sticking to a surface
8. Dilates arteries in angina patients
9. Through the skin

Down

2. Into the vein
3. Under the tongue
4. Process for medication to travel
5. Into the bone
7. Therapeutic use for medication

Ambulance Calls

The following real case scenarios provide an opportunity to explore the concerns associated with patient management. Read each scenario, then answer each question in detail.

1. You are dispatched to the home of a 56-year-old man with a history of angina. He is complaining of a "squeezing" chest pain that has lasted for approximately 20 minutes. You find out through your SAMPLE history that the patient takes nitroglycerin and has not taken any today. His blood pressure is 150/90 mm Hg. How would you best manage this patient?

_____

_____

_____

_____

_____

_____

_____

2. You respond to a residence for a 22-year-old female complaining of dyspnea and audible wheezing. The patient's mother tells you that the patient is an asthmatic and is also allergic to shellfish. The girl ate artificial crabmeat for lunch because she thought it was safe. She has an MDI and also an EpiPen for severe allergic reactions.

How would you best manage this patient?

_____

_____

_____

_____

_____

_____

_____

3. You are dispatched to the residence of a 68-year-old male who is complaining of a "crushing" chest pain radiating down his left arm for the past hour. He is pale, cool, diaphoretic, and is very nauseated. He tells you he had a heart attack several years ago and takes nitroglycerin as needed. He took two tablets prior to your arrival and reports no relief.

How would you best manage this patient?

_____

_____

_____

_____

_____

_____

_____

Workbook Activities

The following activities have been designed to help you. Your instructor may require you to complete some or all of these activities as a regular part of your EMT-I training program. You are encouraged to complete any activity that your instructor does not assign as a way to enhance your learning in the classroom.

Chapter Review

The following exercises provide an opportunity to refresh your knowledge of this chapter.

Matching

Match each of the items in the left column to the appropriate definition in the right column.

_____ 1. Sodium

_____ 2. Osmotic pressure

_____ 3. Molecule

_____ 4. Intravascular fluid

_____ 5. Bicarbonate

_____ 6. Crystalloid solution

_____ 7. Phosphorus

_____ 8. Electrolyte

_____ 9. Interstitial fluid

_____ 10. Edema

_____ 11. Potassium

_____ 12. Dehydration

_____ 13. Normal saline

_____ 14. Calcium

_____ 15. Chloride

_____ 16. Intracellular fluid

_____ 17. D₅W

_____ 18. Colloid

_____ 19. Homeostasis

_____ 20. Extracellular fluid

A. principle cation needed for bone growth

B. regulates pH of the stomach

C. charged atoms and compounds

D. water inside the cell

E. principle intracellular ion

F. depletion of body's total systemic fluid

G. two or more atoms bound together

H. pressures against the cell wall

I. principle buffer

J. contains molecules too large to pass out of capillary membranes

K. water outside the cell

L. principle extracellular cation

M. a normally balanced condition

N. important in the formation of ATP

O. 5% dextrose in water

P. dissolved crystals in water

Q. water portion of the circulatory system surrounding the blood cells

R. water outside the vascular system and between the cells

S. 0.9% sodium chloride

T. increased interstitial fluid levels

Intravenous Access

Multiple Choice

Read each item carefully, then select the best response.

_____ **1.** Electrolytes:
   A. help regulate water levels.
   B. are necessary for proper cardiac function.
   C. are needed for muscle contraction.
   D. all of the above.

_____ **2.** Hypocalcemia can lead to:
   A. hypertension.
   B. vasodilation.
   C. muscle cramps.
   D. skeletal muscle weakness.

_____ **3.** Signs and symptoms of dehydration include:
   A. edema.
   B. poor skin turgor.
   C. weight gain.
   D. polyuria.

_____ **4.** One of the causes of dehydration is:
   A. unmonitored IV lines.
   B. kidney failure.
   C. Hemorrhage.
   D. prolonged hypoventilation.

_____ **5.** Avoid attempts to insert an IV in an extremity if:
   A. there are signs of trauma, injury, or infection.
   B. there is an arteriovenous shunt for dialysis.
   C. it is on the same side a mastectomy was performed.
   D. all of the above.

_____ **6.** When drawing blood, fill the blood tubes in this order.
   A. Red, blue, green, lavender
   B. Blue, green, red, lavender
   C. Green, red, lavender, blue
   D. Red, blue, lavender, green

_____ **7.** _____ are used to maintain an active IV site without having to run fluids through a vein.

    A. Butterfly catheters

    B. Saline locks

    C. Over-the-needle catheters

    D. Intraosseous lines

_____ **8.** What can be infused through an intraosseous line?

    A. Fluid and blood only

    B. Fluid and medications only

    C. Fluid only

    D. Fluid, medications, and blood

1999 _____ **9.** IO lines are used in pediatric patients when immediate IV access is difficult or impossible. The rule of thumb is the inability to gain IV access in:

    A. 2 tries or 60 seconds.

    B. 3 tries or 90 seconds.

    C. 4 tries.

    D. several tries.

1999 _____ **10.** IO lines are contraindicated in:

    A. cardiac arrest.

    B. status epilepticus.

    C. tibias that are fractured.

    D. all of the above.

_____ **11.** A local reaction to IV therapy would be:

    A. allergic reaction.

    B. phlebitis.

    C. air embolism.

    D. catheter shear.

_____ **12.** All of the following are systemic complications of IV therapy EXCEPT:

    A. vasovagal reaction.

    B. allergic reaction.

    C. air embolus.

    D. infiltration.

Vocabulary EMT-I vocab explorer web

Define the following terms in the space provided.

    1. Cannulation:

_____

_____

_____

    2. Crystalloid solution:

_____

_____

_____

3. Colloid solution:

_____

_____

_____

4. Infiltration:

_____

_____

_____

5. Tonicity:

_____

_____

_____

6. Angiocath:

_____

_____

_____

7. Contaminated stick:

_____

_____

_____

8. Drip chamber:

_____

_____

_____

9. Intraosseous:

_____

_____

_____

10. "Piggyback" administration:

_____

_____

_____

Fill-in

Read each item carefully, then complete the statement by filling in the missing word(s).

1. _____ is one of the most invasive procedures an EMT-I learns.

2. _____ is the principle extracellular cation needed to regulate the distribution of water throughout the body in the intravascular and interstitial fluid compartments.

3. _____ is a type of diffusion, commonly used by the kidneys to clean blood.

4. The cell uses sodium outside the cell and potassium inside the cell for an important cellular function called _____.

5. The effect of osmotic pressure on a cell is referred to as the _____ of the solution.

6. When choosing an IV site; choose _____ and work _____.

7. The _____ the catheter, the more fluid can flow through it.

8. _____ is the escape of fluid into the surrounding tissues, while _____ is the physical blockage of a vein or catheter.

9. An IV site choice around a _____ increases the risk for perforation of tendons, ligaments, and nerves.

10. Veins of the geriatric patient are easily _____.

True/False

If you believe the statement to be more true than false, write the letter "T" in the space provided. If you believe the statement to be more false than true, write the letter "F."

_____ 1. When the body's total systemic fluid volume increases, overhydration occurs.

_____ 2. Isotonic solutions can be dangerous to use because they can cause a sudden fluid shift from the intravascular space to the cells.

_____ 3. A blood set is a special type of microdrip set designed to facilitate rapid fluid replacement by manual infusion of multiple IV bags or IV/blood combinations.

_____ 4. Large protruding arm veins can be deceiving in terms of their ease of cannulation.

_____ 5. The larger the diameter of the catheter, the smaller the gauge.

_____ 6. Blood tubes should be gently turned back and forth to mix anticoagulants and blood evenly.

_____ 7. The red-topped tube should be shaken if the blood clots.

_____ 8. An IO needle should be stabilized like an impaled object.

———— **9.** Signs and symptoms of air embolus include cyanosis, loss of consciousness, respiratory arrest, and signs and symptoms of shock.

———— **10.** Patients with a suspected air embolus should be transported with their heads elevated.

1999 ———— **11.** When cannulating the external jugular vein, the catheter is inserted midway between the angle of the jaw and the midclavicular line, with the catheter pointing toward the head.

Short Answer

Complete this section with short written answers in the space provided.

1. Describe the cell membrane.

_____

_____

_____

2. Tonicity is related to the concentration of sodium in a solution and the movement of water in relation to the sodium levels inside and outside the cell. Discuss:

Isotonic solutions:

_____

_____

_____

Hypertonic solutions:

_____

_____

_____

Hypotonic solutions:

_____

_____

_____

3. List the steps in assembling IV equipment.

_____

_____

_____

4. List the steps in performing IV therapy.

_____

_____

_____

5. You have an order for 300 mL/90 minutes. You are using a microdrip set. Figure the drip rate.

_____

_____

_____

6. To document an IV, what do you need to include?

_____

_____

_____

Word Fun EMT-I vocab explorer web

The following crossword puzzle is an activity provided to reinforce correct spelling and understanding of medical terminology associated with emergency care and the EMT-I. Use the clues in the column to complete the puzzle.

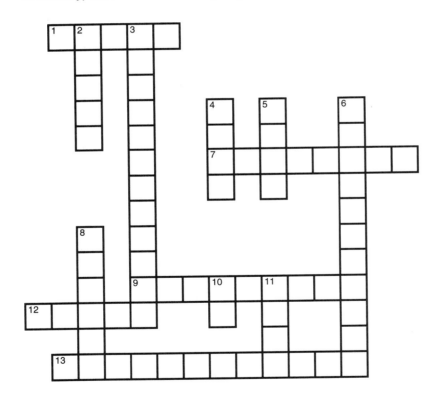

Across

1. Liquid
7. Flexible, hollow structure that delivers fluid
9. Blockage
12. Overall negative charge
13. Within a bone

Down

2. Rupture of a cell
3. Escape of fluid
4. Normal saline
5. Speed of flow
6. Within a vein
8. Overall positive charge
10. Lactated Ringer's
11. Area of cannulation

Ambulance Calls

The following real case scenarios provide an opportunity to explore the concerns associated with patient management. Read each scenario, then answer each question in detail.

1. You are called to the scene of a single-vehicle MVC. The driver was ejected and you suspect multiple system trauma with significant blood loss.

   What kind of IV would you choose for this patient (solution, catheter, rate, etc.)?

   _____

   _____

   _____

   _____

   _____

   _____

   _____

   _____

1999 2. You care called to care for a 5-month-old infant with severe dehydration. On arrival, the patient is limp and lifeless with a very weak and rapid pulse.

   How would you manage the circulatory status of this patient?

   _____

   _____

   _____

   _____

   _____

   _____

   _____

   _____

Skill Drills

Skill Drill 7-1: Spiking the Bag

Test your knowledge by placing the photos below in the correct order. Number the first step with a "1," the second step with a "2," etc.

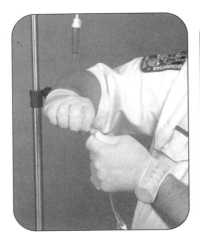

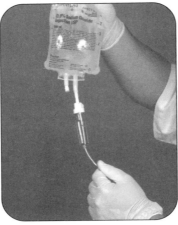

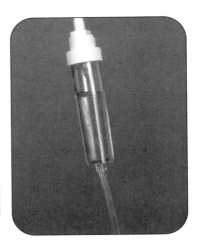

_____

Twist the protective cover on the opposite end of the IV tubing to allow air to escape. Do not remove this cover yet. Let the fluid flow until air bubbles are removed from the line before turning the roller clamp wheel to stop the flow.

_____

Allow the solution to run freely through the drip chamber and into the tubing to prime the line and flush the air out of the tubing.

_____

Slide the spike into the IV bag port until you see fluid enter the drip chamber.

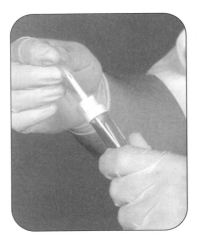

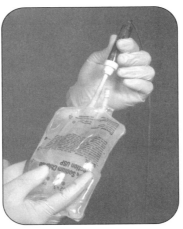

_____

Pull on the rubber pigtail on the end of the IV bag to remove it.

Remove the protective cover from the piercing spike.

_____

Check the drip chamber; it should be only half filled. If the fluid level is too low, squeeze the chamber until it fills; if the chamber is too full, invert the bag and the chamber and squeeze the chamber to empty the fluid back into the bag.

Hang the bag in an appropriate location.

Skill Drill 7-2: IV Therapy
Test your knowledge by placing the photos below in the correct order. Number the first step with a "1," the second step with a "2," etc.

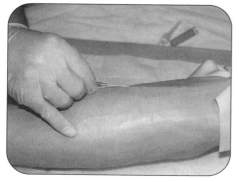

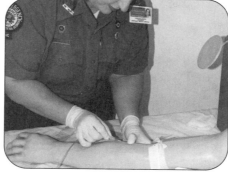

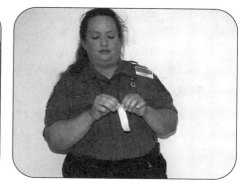

Insert the catheter at approximately 45° with the bevel up while applying distal traction with the other hand.

Attach the prepared IV line.

Tear tape prior to venipuncture or have a commercial device available.

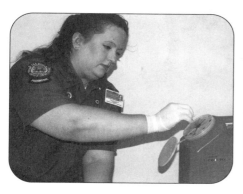

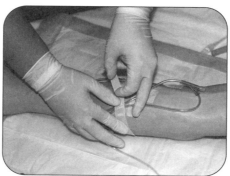

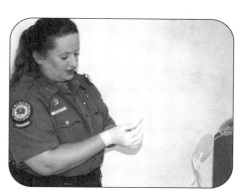

Immediately dispose of all sharps in the proper container.

Secure IV tubing and adjust the flow rate while monitoring the patient.

Choose the appropriate sized catheter and examine it for any imperfections.

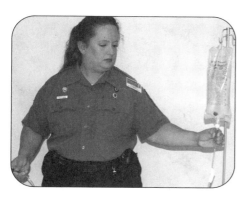

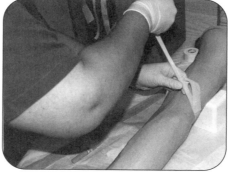

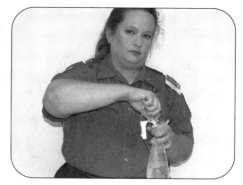

Fill the drip chamber by squeezing it together.

Apply the constricting band above the intended IV site.

Choose the appropriate drip set and attach it to the fluid.

Continued

Skill Drill 7-2: IV Therapy—cont'd

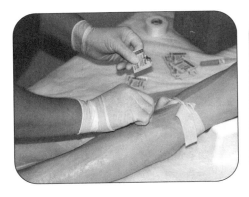

Clean the area using an aseptic technique. Use an alcohol pad to cleanse in a circular motion from the inside out. Use a second alcohol pad to wipe straight down the center.

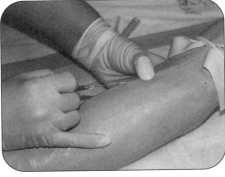

Occlude the catheter to prevent blood leaking while removing the stylet.

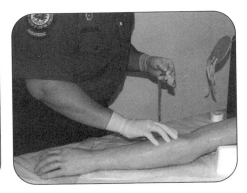

Apply gloves prior to contact with patient. Palpate a suitable vein.

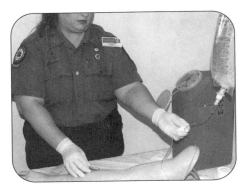

Open the IV line to ensure fluid is flowing and the IV is patent. Observe for any swelling or infiltration around the IV site.

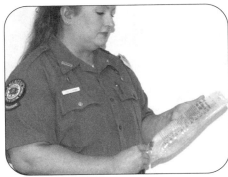

Choose the appropriate fluid and examine for clarity and check the expiration date.

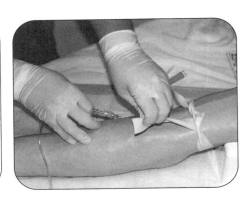

Remove the constricting band.

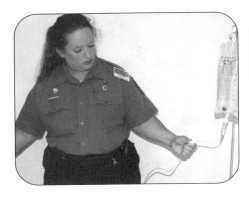

Flush or "bleed" the tubing to remove any air bubbles by opening the roller clamp.

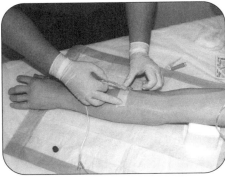

Secure the catheter with tape or a commercial device.

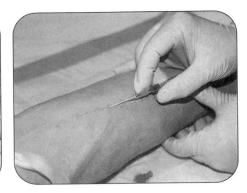

Observe for "flashback" as blood enters the catheter.

Skill Drill 7-4: Determining if an IV is Viable

Test your knowledge by placing the correct words in the photo captions.

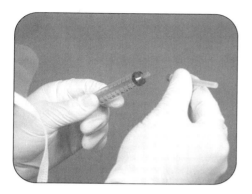

1. Select and assemble a sterile

_____

_____ and a large-

guage needle.

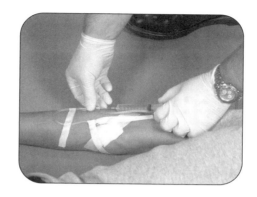

2. Select an injection port close to the

IV site and wipe it with an

_____

_____.

_____ the plunger

of the syringe and insert the syringe

into the _____.

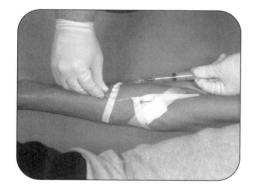

3. _____ the line be-

tween the IV site and the port and

pull back on the plunger to draw

clean _____

_____ from the bag.

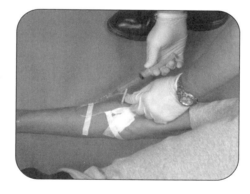

4. Once the syringe is _____, leave it in place and

switch your hand from the tubing between the port and the

_____ _____ to between the

port and the IV bag, then pinch the _____.

Gently apply _____ to the plunger to disrupt the

occlusion and reestablish _____. Ensure that the

line is free and the rate is sufficient. If the occlusion does not

_____, discontinue the IV and reestablish it in

the _____ extremity or at a proximal location on

the _____ extremity.

Workbook Activities

The following activities have been designed to help you. Your instructor may require you to complete some or all of these activities as a regular part of your EMT-I training program. You are encouraged to complete any activity that your instructor does not assign as a way to enhance your learning in the classroom.

Chapter Review

The following exercises provide an opportunity to refresh your knowledge of this chapter.

Matching

Match each of the items in the left column to the appropriate definition in the right column.

_____ **1.** Fahrenheit

_____ **2.** Liter

_____ **3.** Gram

_____ **4.** Celsius

_____ **5.** Medical asepsis

_____ **6.** Meter

_____ **7.** Enteral medication

_____ **8.** Grain

_____ **9.** Percutaneous

_____ **10.** Bolus

_____ **11.** Vial

_____ **12.** Buccal

_____ **13.** Ampule

_____ **14.** Nebulizer

A. device for producing fine spray or mist

B. basic unit of length

C. preventing contamination

D. approximate weight of a drop of water

E. sealed glass container; single dose container

F. given through the GI tract

G. in a mass

H. basic unit of volume

I. may contain single or multiple doses

J. system in which water freezes at 0°

K. relating to the cheek or mouth

L. basic unit of weight

M. administered directly through the skin

N. system in which water boils at 212°

Multiple Choice

Read each item carefully, then select the best response.

_____ **1.** Which is not a basic unit in the metric system?

    A. Liter

    B. Milliliter

    C. Meter

    D. Gram

Medication Administration

_____ **2.** All of the following are units of volume in the Apothecary system EXCEPT:

  A. minim.

  B. pint.

  C. milliliter.

  C. quart.

`1999` _____ **3.** Which of the following routes is not considered parenteral?

  A. Rectal

  B. Subcutaneous

  C. Intravenous

  D. Intraosseous

`1999` _____ **4.** Subcutaneous injections:

  A. usually are 1 mL or less.

  B. use a 24- to 26-gauge needle.

  C. are administered in the upper arm, anterior thigh, or abdomen.

  D. all of the above.

`1999` _____ **5.** Intramuscular injections:

  A. are given into the tissue above the muscle.

  B. allow for a very small volume of medication.

  C. are given at a 90° angle.

  D. carry no potential for nerve damage.

`1999` _____ **6.** The fastest route of medication delivery is:

  A. transdermal.

  B. subcutaneous.

  C. intramuscular.

  D. intravascular.

`1999` _____ **7.** Nitroglycerin is administered SL, which means:

  A. under the tongue.

  B. under the skin.

  C. swallowed.

  D. in the cheek.

1999 _____ **8.** The morphine on your ambulance is packaged as 10 mg/10 mL. Medical control ordered 5 mg. How many milliliters of the drug would you administer?

    A. 1.0

    B. 5.0

    C. 0.5

    D. 10.0

1999 _____ **9.** When medical control gives a medication order, you should:

    A. give exactly what was ordered, even if it seems inappropriate.

    B. give part of the dose to see if it will work.

    C. repeat the order back, word for word, for verification.

    D. ask if he or she is sure of the order.

1999 _____ **10.** MDI means:

    A. mega dose inhaler.

    B. monitored dose inhaler.

    C. many dose inhaler.

    D. metered-dose inhaler.

Vocabulary EMT-I vocab explorer web

Define the following terms in the space provided.

1. Bolus:

_____

_____

_____

2. Concentration:

_____

_____

_____

3. Medical asepsis:

_____

_____

_____

4. Nebulizer:

_____

_____

_____

5. Ampule:

_____

_____

_____

6. Vial:

_____

_____

_____

Fill-in

Read each item carefully, then complete the statement by filling in the missing word(s).

1. Drugs are packaged in different units of _____ and _____.

2. On the Celsius scale, water freezes at _____ and boils at _____.

1999 **3.** Most drugs used in pediatric emergency medicine are based on the child's weight in _____.

1999 **4.** The EMT-I's _____ and/or _____ govern medication administration.

1999 **5.** Many medications used to treat respiratory emergencies are administered via the _____ route.

1999 **6.** _____ medications are given through the GI tract, while _____ are given any route other than the GI tract.

1999 **7.** _____ is the most common route for administration of drugs in the prehospital setting.

1999 **8.** _____ are designed to contain a single dose of medication, but _____ may contain single or multiple doses.

1999 **9.** _____ involves injecting sterile water from one vial into a vial that contains powder, making solutions for injection.

1999 **10.** _____ are separated into a glass drug cartridge and a syringe.

True/False

If you believe the statement to be more true than false, write the letter "T" in the space provided. If you believe the statement to be more false than true, write the letter "F."

_____ **1.** To convert a larger unit of weight to a smaller one, multiply the larger unit of weight by 1000.

`1999` _____ **2.** One kilogram equals 2.6 lb.

`1999` _____ **3.** The "desired dose" is the amount of drug that you think you should give to a patient.

`1999` _____ **4.** The concentration of a drug is the total weight contained in a specific volume.

`1999` _____ **5.** The most common inhaled medication is albuterol.

`1999` _____ **6.** BSI is not needed to administer a nebulized medication.

`1999` _____ **7.** The gauge of the needle refers to the length.

`1999` _____ **8.** Subcutaneous injections are given into the loose connective tissue between the dermis and the muscle layer.

`1999` _____ **9.** Intramuscular injections allow for administration of larger volumes of medication that the subcutaneous route.

`1999` _____ **10.** A bolus is a single dose give by the IV route.

Short Answer

Complete this section with short written answers in the space provided.

1. List the "six rights" of medication administration.

_____

_____

_____

2. List the steps of administering a medication by subcutaneous injection.

_____

_____

_____

3. Where are these muscles located?

Vastus lateralis:

_____

_____

_____

Rectus femoris:

_____

_____

_____

Gluteus maximus:

_____

_____

_____

Deltoid:

_____

_____

_____

4. List the steps of giving an IV bolus.

_____

_____

_____

Word Fun EMT-I vocab explorer web

The following crossword puzzle is an activity provided to reinforce correct spelling and understanding of medical terminology associated with emergency care and the EMT-I.

Use the clues in the column to complete the puzzle.

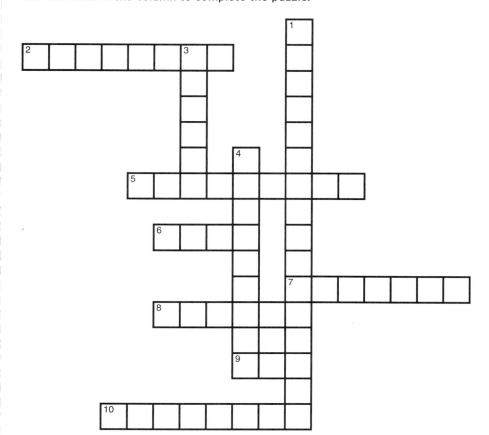

Across

2. 2.2 lb.

5. Glass cartridge and syringe

6. Single or multiple dose

7. Through the GI tract

8. Decimal system based on multiples of 10

9. Metered-dose inhaler

10. Continuous flow

Down

1. Responsible for approving and ordering medications

3. Single-dose container

4. 0.001 g

Ambulance Calls

The following real case scenario provides an opportunity to explore the concerns associated with patient management. Read each scenario, then answer each question in detail.

1. Your cardiac arrest patient has now converted back to a perfusing rhythm. Medical control has ordered 1 mg/kg of Lidocaine (packaged 100 mg/10 mL) as a bolus followed by a 2 mg/min infusion. Your patient weighs 175 lb. Calculate the doses.

2. You 11-year-old patient's mother tells you he weighs about 88 pounds. You have an order to give an IV bolus of 20 ml/kg. How much total fluid would you bolus?

1999 **3.** Your patient is experiencing chest pain. He meets all of the protocol requirements for aspirin and nitroglycerin. Medical control also orders up to 10 mg of morphine. How would you administer each of these medications?

_____

_____

_____

_____

_____

_____

_____

_____

Skill Drills

1999 **Skill Drill 8-1: Administering Medication Via Small-Volume Nebulizer**
Test your knowledge by placing the following photos in the correct order. Number the first step with a "1," the second step with a "2," etc.

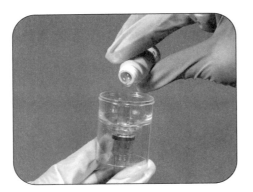

Add premixed medication to the bowl of the nebulizer.

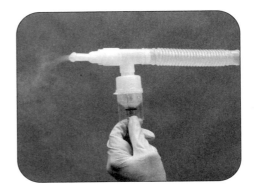

Connect the T piece with the mouthpiece to the top of the bowl, connect it to the oxygen tubing, and set the flowmeter at 6 L/min.

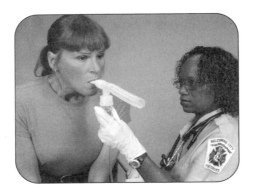

Instruct the patient to breathe as deeply as possible and hold his or her breath for 3 to 5 seconds before exhaling. Monitor the patient for effects.

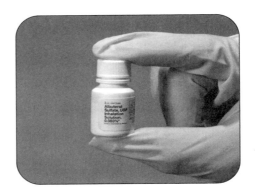

Check the medication and the expiration date.

1999 **Skill Drill 8-3: Drawing Medication From a Vial**

Test your knowledge by filling in the correct words in the photo captions.

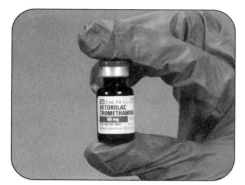

1. Check the medication and its

_____

_____.

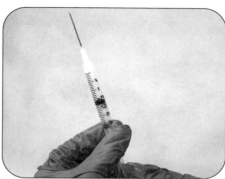

2. Determine the amount of medication needed, and draw that amount of _____ into the syringe.

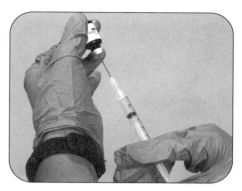

3. Invert the vial, and insert the needle through the _____

_____.

_____ the air in the syringe, and release the

_____, keeping the tip of the needle within the medication.

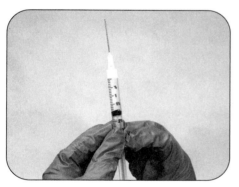

4. _____ the needle, and expel any air in the syringe.

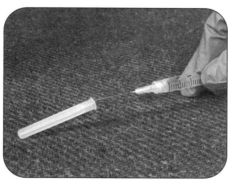

5. Recap the needle using the

_____ method.

1999 **Skill Drill 8-4: Administering Medication Via the Subcutaneous Route**

Test your knowledge by placing the following photos in the correct order. Number the first step with a "1," the second step with a "2," etc.

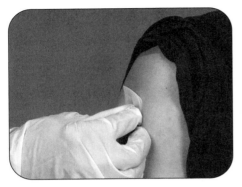

———————————

Using aseptic technique, cleanse the injection area.

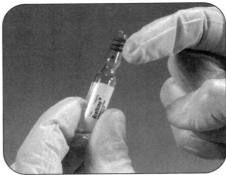

———————————

Check the medication to be sure that it is the correct one, that it is not discolored, and that the expiration date has not passed.

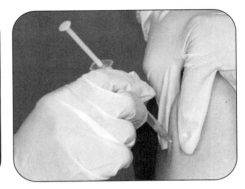

———————————

Pinch the skin surrounding the area, and insert the needle at a 45° angle. Pull back on the plunger to aspirate for blood. If there is no blood, inject the medication, remove the needle, and hold pressure over the area.

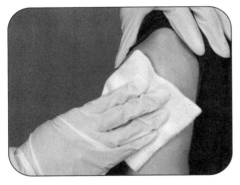

———————————

To disperse the medication, rub the area in a circular motion. Monitor the patient's condition.

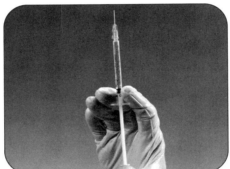

———————————

Assemble and check the equipment. Draw up the correct dose of medication.

1999 Skill Drill 8-6: Administering Medication Via the Intravenous Bolus Route
Test your knowledge by filling in the correct words in the photo captions.

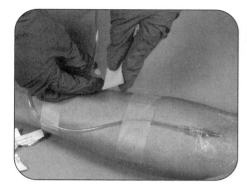
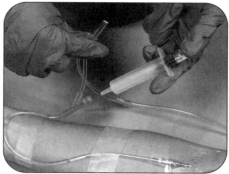
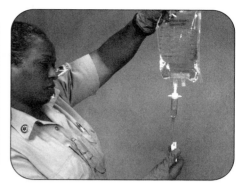
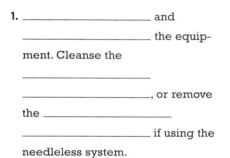

1. _____ and _____ the equipment. Cleanse the _____ _____, or remove the _____ _____ if using the needleless system.

2. Insert the needle into the port, and pinch off the _____ _____ proximal to the administration port. Administer the correct _____ at the appropriate _____.

3. _____ the IV line to flush the medication into the vein, allowing it to run briefly wide open, or flush with a _____ _____ of normal saline. Readjust the IV _____ _____ to the original setting, and monitor the patient's condition.

Workbook Activities

The following activities have been designed to help you. Your instructor may require you to complete some or all of these activities as a regular part of your EMT-I training program. You are encouraged to complete any activity that your instructor does not assign as a way to enhance your learning in the classroom.

Chapter Review

The following exercises provide an opportunity to refresh your knowledge of this chapter.

Matching

Match each of the terms in the left column to the appropriate definition in the right column.

_____ **1.** Oropharynx	**A.** measure of depth of breathing
_____ **2.** Ventilation	**B.** terminates inhalation
_____ **3.** Chemoreceptors	**C.** compression of the cricoid cartilage
_____ **4.** Tonsil tip	**D.** result of hyperventilation
_____ **5.** Surfactant	**E.** pH below 7
_____ **6.** pH	**F.** alveoli collapse
_____ **7.** Nasal cannula	**G.** holds 400 L of oxygen
_____ **8.** Tidal volume	**H.** has floating ball and calibrated tube
_____ **9.** Metabolic acidosis	**I.** amount of air moved in and out of lungs per minute
_____ **10.** Gastric distention	**J.** delivers specific concentrations of oxygen
_____ **11.** Glottic opening	**K.** related to hypoventilation
_____ **12.** D cylinder	**L.** delivers nearly 100% oxygen
_____ **13.** Respiration	**M.** excessive loss of acids
_____ **14.** Venturi mask	**N.** oral cavity
_____ **15.** Minute volume	**O.** air in lungs after maximal exhalation
_____ **16.** NRB mask	**P.** measurement of hydrogen ions
_____ **17.** Acidic	**Q.** not affected by gravity
_____ **18.** Pressure compensated flow meter	**R.** fluid that keeps alveoli expanded
_____ **19.** Sellick maneuver	**S.** delivers 24% to 44% oxygen
_____ **20.** Hering–Breuer reflex	**T.** acidosis not related to respiratory system
_____ **21.** Metabolic alkalosis	**U.** Yankauer tip
_____ **22.** Atelectasis	**V.** pH above 7
_____ **23.** Bourdon-gauge flowmeter	**W.** narrowest portion of adult trachea
_____ **24.** Basic	**X.** monitor(s) chemical composition of body fluids
_____ **25.** Residual volume	**Y.** exchange of gases
_____ **26.** M cylinder	**Z.** movement of air in and out of lungs
_____ **27.** Respiratory alkalosis	**AA.** inflation of stomach with air

Airway Management and Ventilation

_____ **28.** BVM with reservoir

_____ **29.** French catheter

_____ **30.** Respiratory acidosis

BB. holds 3,450 L oxygen

CC. delivers up to 90% oxygen

DD. whistle tip

Multiple Choice

Read each item carefully, then select the best response.

_____ **1.** The purpose of advanced airway management is to protect and improve _____ in patients by using a tube to create a direct channel to the trachea.

A. respiration

B. ventilation

C. oxygenation

D. patency

_____ **2.** The upper airway includes all of the following except the:

A. nose.

B. mouth.

C. larynx.

D. pharynx.

_____ **3.** The _____ is located at the glottic opening and prevents food and liquid from entering the lower airway during swallowing.

A. larynx

B. vocal cords

C. epiglottis

D. carina

_____ **4.** Gas exchange occurs in the:

A. alveoli.

B. nares.

C. bronchioles.

D. trachea.

_____ **5.** During inspiration:

A. the diaphragm contracts and the ribs move up and out.

B. the diaphragm relaxes and the ribs move up and out.

C. the diaphragm contracts and the ribs move down and in.

D. the diaphragm relaxes and the ribs move down and in.

_____ **6.** After _____ minutes without oxygen, cells in the brain and nervous system may die.

    A. 2 to 3

    B. 3 to 5

    C. 4 to 6

    D. 5 to 8

_____ **7.** Conditions leading to lower oxygen concentrations in the bloodstream include:

    A. excessive bleeding.

    B. decreased mechanical effort.

    C. pneumonia.

    D. all of the above.

_____ **8.** Causes of respiratory acidosis include:

    A. cardiac arrest.

    B. headache.

    C. fever.

    D. overzealous BVM ventilation.

_____ **9.** Causes of metabolic alkalosis include:

    A. excessive vomiting.

    B. eating disorders.

    C. excessive water intake.

    D. all of the above.

_____ **10.** A/An _____ is a hard plastic device used to prevent the tongue from obstructing the glottis.

    A. stylet

    B. oropharyngeal airway

    C. Yankauer tip

    D. Magill forceps

_____ **11.** Oxygen is stored in _____ cylinders.

    A. green

    B. aluminum or steel

    C. seamless

    D. all of the above

_____ **12.** All adult BVM devices should have a:

    A. 2-way valve.

    B. pop-off valve.

    C. disposable self-inflating bag.

    D. all of the above.

_____ **13.** Patients with gastric distention are prone to:

    A. gas.

    B. vomiting.

    C. sepsis.

    D. hypoxia.

_____ **14.** To perform the Sellick maneuver, apply pressure to the:

    A. thyroid cartilage.

    B. cricoid cartilage.

    C. cricothyroid membrane.

    D. trachea.

1999 _____ **15.** The curved laryngoscope blade is inserted just in front of the epiglottis, into the _____, allowing you to see the glottic opening and vocal cords.
   A. uvula
   B. vallecula
   C. larynx
   D. pharynx

1999 _____ **16.** The proper sized tube for adult male patients ranges from _____ mm.
   A. 6.5 to 8.0
   B. 7.0 to 8.0
   C. 7.5 to 8.5
   D. 8.0 to 9.0

1999 _____ **17.** The proper sized tube for adult female patients ranges from _____ mm.
   A. 6.5 to 8.0
   B. 7.0 to 8.0
   C. 7.5 to 8.5
   D. 8.0 to 9.0

1999 _____ **18.** A plastic-coated wire called a _____ may be inserted into the ET tube to add rigidity and shape to the tube.
   A. Murphy eye
   B. stylet
   C. pipe cleaner
   D. vallecula

1999 _____ **19.** Confirm placement of the ET tube by listening with a stethoscope over both lungs and over the _____ as you ventilate the patient through the tube.
   A. stomach
   B. heart
   C. diaphragm
   D. ribs

1999 _____ **20.** The best way to confirm placement of an ET tube is by:
   A. x-ray.
   B. auscultating over both lung fields and over the epigastrium.
   C. visualizing the cuff passing through the vocal cords.
   D. seeing the chest rise and fall.

Vocabulary EMT-I vocab explorer web

Define the following terms in the space provided.

1. Pin-indexing system:

_____

_____

_____

2. Combitube:

_____

_____

_____

3. Hering–Breuer reflex:

_____

_____

_____

4. Sellick maneuver:

_____

_____

_____

Fill-in
Read each item carefully, then complete the statement by filling in the missing word.

1. The backup system known as the _____ stimulates breathing when the arterial oxygen

level falls.

2. _____ is a condition in which the systolic blood pressure drops more than 10 mm Hg

with inspiration.

3. Any acidosis that is not related to the respiratory system is considered _____ in origin.

4. The _____ is the most common cause of upper airway obstruction in the patient with

an altered mental status.

5. A fixed suctioning unit should generate airflow of more than _____ and a vacuum of

more than _____ when the tubing is clamped.

6. Oxygen does not _____ or _____; however, it does support

_____.

True/False
If you believe the statement to be more true than false, write the letter "T" in the space provided. If you believe the statement to be more false than true, write the letter "F."

_____ **1.** Primary control of breathing comes from the medulla and pons.

_____ **2.** Aspirin overdose is a major cause of metabolic acidosis.

_____ **3.** The head tilt–chin lift is the preferred method for opening the airway of a trauma patient.

_____ **4.** A foreign body that completely blocks the airway of a patient is a true emergency that will result in death if not treated immediately.

_____ **5.** Any patient found unresponsive must be managed as if he or she has a compromised airway.

_____ **6.** Suctioning is the most effective method of dislodging and forcing an object out of the airway.

1999 _____ **7.** The use of an orogastric (OG) tube over a nasogastric (NG) tube is generally safer for patients with a decreased level of consciousness and/or severe facial trauma.

_____ **8.** The PtL and Combitube are inserted blindly.

_____ **9.** A sealed cuff placed below the level of the vocal cords is the only form of definitive airway management.

Short Answer

Complete this section with short written answers in the space provided.

1. List the three main components to the buffer system found in the body.

_____

_____

_____

2. What is the formula for determining duration of oxygen flow?

_____

_____

_____

3. List the methods of ventilation in order of preference.

_____

_____

_____

4. List the contraindications for multilumen airways.

_____

_____

_____

1999 **5.** List the steps of orotracheal intubation by direct laryngoscopy.

_____

_____

_____

1999 **6.** List four complications of endotracheal intubation.

_____

_____

_____

Word Fun **EMT-I** vocab explorer web

The following crossword puzzle is an activity provided to reinforce correct spelling and understanding of medical terminology associated with emergency care and the EMT-I. Use the clues in the column to complete the puzzle.

Across

2. Between base of tongue and epiglottis

4. Used to gain direct view of patient's throat

6. Pressure on cricoid cartilage

Down

1. Removes substances from stomach

3. Vocal cord spasm

5. Small metal rod inserted into an ET tube

Ambulance Calls

The following case scenarios provide an opportunity to explore the concerns associated with patient management. Read each scenario, then answer each question in detail.

1. You are dispatched to a possible cardiac arrest. You are only a block from the call and arrive to find a 72-year-old male who is still pink and warm. No one is performing CPR.

   How would you best manage this patient?

   _____

   _____

   _____

   _____

   _____

   _____

   _____

2. You are called to a residence where an unresponsive 7-year-old has possibly ingested drain cleaner by accident. He is breathing shallowly at a rate of 8 breaths/min. He has no gag reflex.

   How would you best manage this patient?

   _____

   _____

   _____

   _____

   _____

   _____

   _____

3. You are dispatched to the scene of a motor vehicle crash where your patient, the unrestrained 18-year-old driver, is breathing at a rate of 4 breaths/min and has weak radial pulses. He is also trapped in the vehicle and the fire department has not yet arrived.

How would you best manage this patient?

_____

_____

_____

_____

_____

_____

_____

_____

Skill Drills EMT-I `video clips` `web`

Skill Drill 9-2: Positioning an Unresponsive Patient

Test your knowledge of skill drills in this chapter by placing the photos below in the correct order. Number the first step with a "1," the second step with a "2," etc.

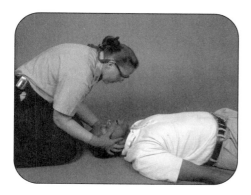

_____

Open and assess the patient's airway and breathing status.

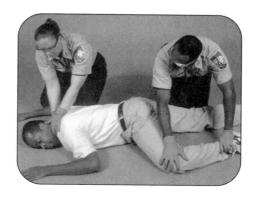

_____

Support the head while your partner straightens the patient's legs.

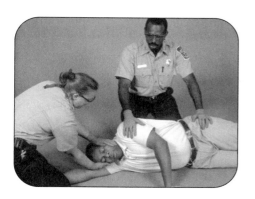

_____

Roll the patient as a unit with the person at the head calling the count to begin the move.

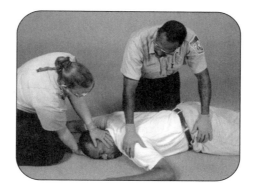

_____

Have your partner place his or her hand on the patient's far shoulder and hip.

Skill Drill 9-7: Managing Severe Airway Obstruction in an Unconscious Adult or Child
Test your knowledge of this skill drill by filling in the correct words in the photo captions.

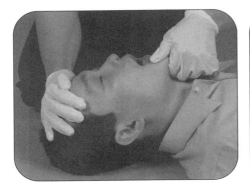

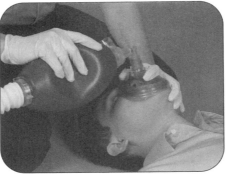

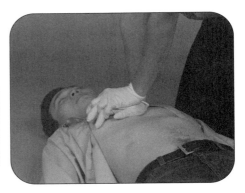

1. Open the airway and attempt
_____.

2. If unsuccessful, _____
the airway and _____
ventilation.

3. Provide _____ .

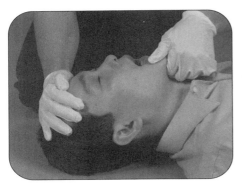

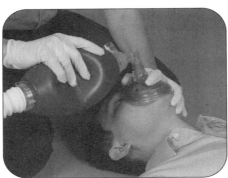

4. Open the patient's _____
and perform a _____
if the object is visible.

5. Attempt to _____.
Repeat steps _____ to
_____ until successful or help
arrives.

1999 **Skill Drill 9-23: Intubation of the Trachea with Direct Laryngoscopy**
Test your knowledge of this skill drill by filling in the correct words in the photo captions.

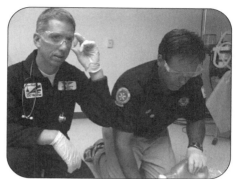

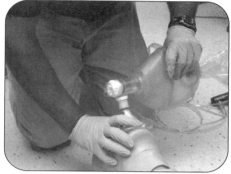

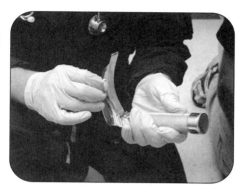

1. Use _____ precautions (_____ and face shield).

2. Preoxygenate the patient whenever possible with a _____ device and 100% oxygen.

3. _____, _____, and _____ your equipment.

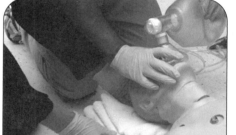

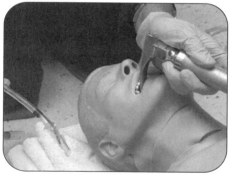

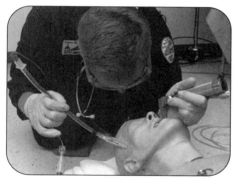

4. Place the patient's head in the _____ position.

5. Insert the blade into the _____ side of the patient's mouth and displace the tongue to the _____.

6. Gently lift the long axis of the laryngoscope handle until you can visualize the _____ and the _____.

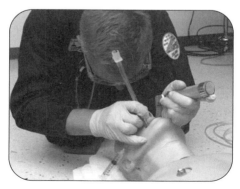

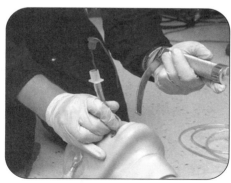

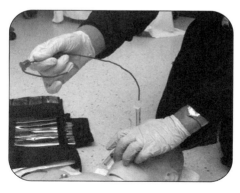

7. Insert the _____ through the right corner of the mouth and place it between the vocal cords.

8. Remove the _____ from the patient's mouth.

9. Remove the _____ from the ET tube.

Skill Drill 9-23: Intubation of the Trachea with Direct Laryngoscopy—cont'd
Test your knowledge of this skill drill by filling in the correct words in the photo captions.

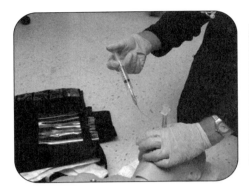

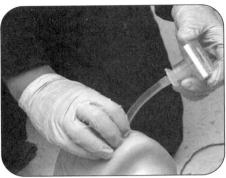

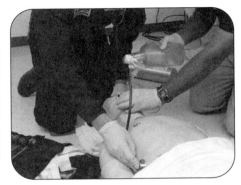

10. Inflate the distal cuff of the ET tube with _____ mL of air and detach the syringe.

11. Attach the end-tidal _____ detector to the _____.

12. Attach the _____ device, ventilate, and auscultate over the apices and bases of both _____ and over the _____.

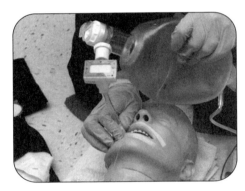

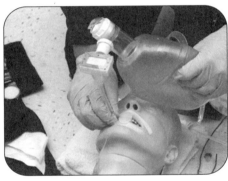

13. _____ the ET tube.

14. Place a _____ in the patient's mouth.

Skill Drill 9-29: Securing an Endotracheal Tube
Test your knowledge of this skill drill by placing the photos below in the correct order. Number the first step with a "1," the second step with a "2," etc.

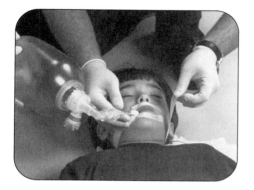

_____

Reinforce the tape around the child's neck.

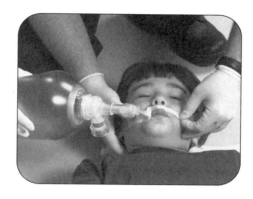

_____

With the tube positioned at the corner of the mouth, tear a strip of tape and anchor one end to the side of the face. Wrap it around the tube several times and anchor the other end over the maxilla.

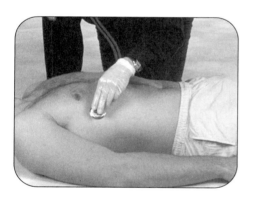

_____

Reconfirm tube placement by auscultating over the lungs and at the epigastrium.

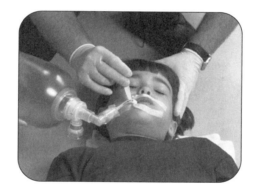

_____

Wrap another piece of tape around the tube, and anchor it over the mandible.

Workbook Activities

The following activities have been designed to help you. Your instructor may require you to complete some or all of these activities as a regular part of your EMT-I training program. You are encouraged to complete any activity that your instructor does not assign as a way to enhance your learning in the classroom.

Chapter Review

The following exercises provide an opportunity to refresh your knowledge of this chapter.

Matching

Match each of the terms in the left column to the appropriate definition in the right column.

_____ **1.** Triage

_____ **2.** Sclera

_____ **3.** Subcutaneous

_____ **4.** Paradoxical motion

_____ **5.** Conjunctiva

_____ **6.** Crepitus

_____ **7.** Accessory muscles

_____ **8.** Breath sounds

_____ **9.** Chief complaint

_____ **10.** Diffuse pain

_____ **11.** Focal pain

_____ **12.** Frostbite

_____ **13.** Jaundice

_____ **14.** Orientation

_____ **15.** OPQRST

_____ **16.** Palpate

_____ **17.** Responsiveness

_____ **18.** Retractions

A. indication of air movement in the lungs

B. lining of the eyelid

C. movements in which the skin pulls in around emphysema the ribs during inspiration

D. white part of the eyes

E. the mental status of a patient

F. the six pain questions

G. yellow skin color resulting from liver disease or dysfunction

H. a crackling sound

I. examine by touch

J. damage to tissues as the result of exposure to cold

K. the way in which a patient responds to external stimuli

L. pain not identified as being specific to a single location

M. secondary muscles of respiration

N. air under the skin

O. motion of a segment of chest wall that is opposite the normal movement during breathing

P. the reason a patient called for help

Q. pain easily identified as being specific to a location

R. a process of identifying the severity of each patient's condition; sorting

Patient Assessment

Multiple Choice

Read each item carefully, then select the best response.

_____ **1.** The scene size-up consists of all of the following EXCEPT:
   A. determining mechanism of injury.
   B. requesting additional assistance.
   C. determining level of responsiveness.
   D. PPE/BSI.

_____ **2.** Possible dangers you may observe during the scene size-up include:
   A. oncoming traffic.
   B. unstable surfaces.
   C. downed electrical lines.
   D. all of the above.

_____ **3.** With a traumatic injury, the body has been exposed to some force or energy that has resulted in:
   A. a temporary injury.
   B. permanent damage.
   C. death.
   D. all of the above.

_____ **4.** With _____, the force of the injury occurs over a broad area, and the skin is usually not broken.
   A. motor vehicle crashes
   B. blunt trauma
   C. penetrating trauma
   D. gunshot wounds

_____ **5.** With _____, the force of the injury occurs at a small point of contact between the skin and the object.
   A. motor vehicle crashes
   B. blunt trauma
   C. penetrating trauma
   D. falls

_____ **6.** You can use the mechanism of injury as a kind of guide to predict the potential for a serious injury by evaluating:

    A. the amount of force applied to the body.

    B. the length of time the force was applied.

    C. the areas of the body that are involved.

    D. all of the above.

_____ **7.** In penetrating trauma, the severity of injury depends on all of the following, EXCEPT:

    A. the geographic location.

    B. the characteristics of the penetrating object.

    C. the amount of force or energy.

    D. the part of the body affected.

_____ **8.** In motor vehicle crashes, the amount of force that is applied to the body is directly related to the _____ of the crash.

    A. distance

    B. location

    C. speed

    D. time

_____ **9.** Your evaluation should also be based, to some extent, on:

    A. the patient's position in the car.

    B. the use of seat belts.

    C. how the patient's body shifts during the crash.

    D. all of the above.

_____ **10.** Ejection from the vehicle dramatically increases the risk of:

    A. head injury.

    B. spinal cord injury.

    C. death.

    D. all of the above.

_____ **11.** In falls, the amount of force that is applied to the body is directly related to the:

    A. surface landed on.

    B. distance fallen.

    C. past medical history.

    D. how the patient landed.

_____ **12.** In order to quickly determine the nature of illness, talk with:

    A. the patient.

    B. family members.

    C. bystanders.

    D. all of the above.

_____ **13.** When considering the need for additional resources, questions to ask include all of the following, EXCEPT:

    A. How many patients are there?

    B. Is it raining?

    C. Who contacted EMS?

    D. Does the scene pose a threat to you or your patient's safety?

_____ **14.** The initial assessment includes evaluation of all of the following, EXCEPT:

    A. mental status.

    B. pupils.

    C. airway.

    D. circulation.

_____ **15.** The best indicator of brain function is the patient's:

A. pulse rate.

B. pupillary response.

C. mental status.

D. respiratory rate and depth.

_____ **16.** An altered mental status may be caused by:

A. head trauma.

B. hypoxemia.

C. hypoglycemia.

D. all of the above.

_____ **17.** All of the following are signs of inadequate breathing EXCEPT:

A. tightness in the chest.

B. two- to three-word dyspnea.

C. use of accessory muscles.

D. nasal flaring.

_____ **18.** Airway obstruction in an unconscious patient is most commonly due to:

A. vomitus.

B. the tongue.

C. dentures.

D. food.

_____ **19.** Signs of airway obstruction in an unconscious patient include:

A. obvious trauma, blood, or other obstruction.

B. noisy breathing.

C. extremely shallow or absent breathing.

D. all of the above.

_____ **20.** The _____ of the patient's pulse will give you a general idea of the overall status of the patient's cardiac function.

A. rate

B. rhythm

C. strength

D. all of the above

_____ **21.** In infants younger than 1 year old, you should palpate the _____ artery to assess pulse.

A. carotid

B. brachial

C. radial

D. femoral

_____ **22.** In almost all instances, controlling external bleeding is accomplished by:

A. direct pressure.

B. elevation.

C. pressing pressure points.

D. tourniquet.

_____ **23.** Assessing the _____ is one of the most important and readily accessible ways of evaluating circulation.

A. pulse

B. respirations

C. skin

D. capillary refill

_____ **24.** Skin color depends on:

   A. pigmentation.

   B. blood oxygen levels.

   C. the amount of blood circulating through the vessels of the skin.

   D. all of the above.

_____ **25.** In deeply pigmented skin, you should look for changes in color in areas of the skin that have less pigment, including:

   A. the sclera.

   B. the conjunctiva.

   C. the mucous membranes of the mouth.

   D. all of the above.

_____ **26.** Other conditions, not related to the body's circulation, such as _____, may slow capillary refill.

   A. local circulatory compromise

   B. hypothermia

   C. age

   D. all of the above

1999 _____ **27.** Once a medical patient has been assessed to be in cardiac arrest:

   A. attach a cardiac monitor as soon as possible.

   B. interpret the cardiac rhythm.

   C. perform immediate defibrillation if indicated.

   D. all of the above.

_____ **28.** If a patient has inadequate circulation, you must take immediate action to do all of the following, EXCEPT:

   A. restore or improve circulation.

   B. apply an AED.

   C. control severe bleeding.

   D. improve oxygen delivery to the tissues.

_____ **29.** Any patient with impaired circulation should receive high-flow oxygen via a nonrebreathing mask or assisted ventilations to improve oxygen delivery at the _____ level.

   A. alveoli

   B. capillary

   C. cellular

   D. pulmonary

_____ **30.** While initial treatment is important, it is essential to remember that immediate _____ is one of the keys to the survival of any high-priority patient.

   A. airway control

   B. bleeding control

   C. transport

   D. application of oxygen

_____ **31.** Goals of the focused history and physical exam include:

   A. identifying the patient's chief complaint.

   B. understanding the specific circumstances surrounding the chief complaint.

   C. directing further physical examination.

   D. all of the above.

_____ **32.** Understanding the _____ helps you to understand the severity of the patient's problem and provide invaluable information to hospital staff as well.

   A. chief complaint

   B. mechanism of injury

   C. physical exam

   D. focused history

_____ **33.** Seat belts that are worn improperly, across the abdomen rather than across the pelvic bones, increase the potential for:

   A. down-and-under pathway injuries.

   B. ejections.

   C. internal injuries.

   D. lumbar spine fractures.

_____ **34.** An integral part of the rapid trauma assessment is evaluation using the mnemonic:

   A. AVPU.

   B. DCAP-BTLS.

   C. OPQRST.

   D. SAMPLE.

_____ **35.** It is particularly important to evaluate the neck before:

   A. log rolling the patient.

   B. examining the chest.

   C. covering it with a cervical collar.

   D. checking for the presence of a carotid pulse.

_____ **36.** To check for motor function, you should ask the patient:

   A. to wiggle his or her fingers or toes.

   B. to identify which extremity you are touching.

   C. if he or she can feel your touch.

   D. all of the above.

_____ **37.** The "E" in SAMPLE stands for:

   A. eating habits.

   B. emergency medications.

   C. events leading up to the episode.

   D. episodes experienced previously.

_____ **38.** When assessing a complaint of dizziness, you should evaluate all of the following, EXCEPT:

   A. pulse.

   B. blood pressure.

   C. movement.

   D. skin.

_____ **39.** Patients who require a complete rapid trauma assessment, short scene time, and immediate transport to the hospital, include all of the following, EXCEPT:

   A. any patient who experienced a significant mechanism of injury.

   B. any patient hit from the rear complaining of neck pain.

   C. any patient who is unresponsive or disoriented.

   D. any patient who is extremely intoxicated from drugs or alcohol.

_____ **40.** The "S" in the mnemonic OPQRST stands for:

   A. signs.

   B. symptoms.

   C. severity.

   D. syncope.

_____ **41.** A patient who points to a single place for his or her pain has what is known as:

   A. diffuse pain.

   B. focal pain.

   C. radiating pain.

   D. referred pain.

_____ **42.** _____ is pain that exists in more than one place without a "trail" of pain in between.

    A. Focal pain

    B. Diffuse pain

    C. Referred pain

    D. Gall bladder pain

_____ **43.** When assessing a chief complaint of chest pain, you should evaluate:

    A. skin color.

    B. pulse.

    C. breath sounds.

    D. all of the above.

_____ **44.** Baseline vital signs provide useful information about the:

    A. overall function of the patient's heart.

    B. overall function of the patient's lungs.

    C. patient's stability.

    D. all of the above.

_____ **45.** If you have successfully stabilized the ABCs on any patient who is unconscious, confused, or unable to relate the chief complaint adequately, you should:

    A. try to obtain information from family members.

    B. perform a rapid assessment.

    C. look for clues from medication bottles.

    D. transport immediately.

_____ **46.** When performing a detailed physical exam, depending on what is learned, you should be prepared to:

    A. return to the initial assessment if a potentially life-threatening condition is identified.

    B. provide treatment for problems that were identified during the exam.

    C. modify any treatment that is underway on the basis of any new information.

    D. all of the above.

_____ **47.** Your report for the unresponsive medical patient should include documentation of the:

    A. cause of unresponsiveness.

    B. diagnosis.

    C. treatment and response to treatment.

    D. patients address.

_____ **48.** During the assessment of the head:

    A. palpate around the face for tenderness.

    B. monitor the airway carefully.

    C. remember that loose teeth and foreign objects may block the airway.

    D. all of the above.

_____ **49.** When listening to heart sounds, the PMI is normally found at the 5th intercostal space, just medial to the midclavicular line. This is the location of the:

    A. tricuspid valve.

    B. mitral valve.

    C. pulmonic valve.

    D. aortic valve.

_____ **50.** The Cincinnati Stroke Scale is a quick field assessment tool to look for signs of stroke. The assessment includes:

    A. facial symmetry.

    B. drooling.

    C. arm strength.

    D. balance.

_____ **51.** When performing a detailed exam, check the neck for:

    A. subcutaneous emphysema.

    B. jugular vein distention.

    C. crepitus.

    D. all of the above.

_____ **52.** The purpose of the ongoing assessment is to ask and answer the following questions, EXCEPT:

    A. Is treatment improving the patient's condition?

    B. What is the patient's diagnosis?

    C. Has an already identified problem gotten better? Worse?

    D. What is the nature of any newly identified problems?

_____ **53.** Having patients clench their teeth is a quick assessment for function of:

    A. CN II.

    B. CN V.

    C. CN IX.

    D. CN XI.

_____ **54.** When reevaluating any interventions you started, take a moment to ensure that:

    A. oxygen is still flowing.

    B. backboard straps are still tight.

    C. bleeding has been controlled.

    D. all of the above.

_____ **55.** During the ongoing assessment, you must modify treatment to address changes in the patient's condition, including:

    A. constant monitoring of the airway.

    B. security of splints.

    C. integrity of bandages.

    D. all of the above.

_____ **56.** Choosing one hospital over another depends on:

    A. specialized care the hospital offers.

    B. local protocol.

    C. patient request.

    D. any of the above.

_____ **57.** _____ provide step-by-step approaches to the care of patients with a variety of cardiac and respiratory emergencies.

    A. Protocols

    B. Standing orders

    C. Algorithms

    D. Ambiguity

_____ **58.** The greatest challenge for the EMT-I is to access and implement a treatment plan for a patient with _____ injuries.

    A. critical

    B. potentially critical

    C. non-life threatening

    D. all of the above

Vocabulary EMT-I vocab explorer web
Define the following terms in the space provided.

1. Blunt trauma:

_____

_____

_____

2. Penetrating trauma:

_____

_____

_____

3. Mechanism of injury:

_____

_____

_____

4. Capillary refill:

_____

_____

_____

5. Golden hour:

_____

_____

_____

Fill-in
Read each item carefully, then complete the statement by filling in the missing word(s).

1. _____ is the cornerstone of prehospital care.

2. The best way to reduce your risk of exposure is to follow _____ precautions.

3. You cannot help your patient if you become a _____ yourself.

4. You should park your unit in a place that will offer you and your partner the greatest

_____ but also rapid access to the patient and your equipment.

5. Risk for serious injury varies depending on whether seat belts are used and whether they are worn

_____ .

6. Any patient who has fallen more than _____ times his or her own height should be considered at risk for serious injury.

7. In gunshot wounds, the area that is involved may be predicted by creating an imaginary line between the _____ and the _____, if one exists, although this is only an approximation at best.

8. _____ is a process of identifying the severity of each patient's condition.

9. The _____ is based on your immediate assessment of the environment, the presenting signs and symptoms, mechanism of injury in a trauma patient, and the patient's chief complaint.

10. The first steps in caring for any patient focus on finding and treating the most _____ illnesses and injuries.

11. With an unresponsive patient or one with a decreased level of consciousness, you should immediately assess the _____ of the airway.

12. If a patient seems to have difficulty breathing, you should immediately _____ the airway.

13. Assess the skin temperature by touching the patient's skin with your _____ or the back of your hand.

14. Correct identification of high-priority patients is an essential aspect of the _____ and helps to improve patient outcome.

1999 **15.** Although patients with traumatic cardiac arrest will likely require intravenous fluid therapy for blood loss, certain _____ will be needed to treat the cardiac arrest itself.

16. Wheezing breath sounds suggest an _____ of the lower airways and wet breath sounds indicate _____ or _____.

17. The prehospital setting is one of controlled _____, at best; your sources of information can be overwhelming or severely limited. You must be able to _____ this information in a very short time, separate relevant from irrelevant data and provide the most appropriate care for the patient.

18. _____ patients are perhaps the most challenging to manage.

19. Patient's conditions are often _____, requiring frequent assessments and modifications in treatment.

True/False

If you believe the statement to be more true than false, write the letter "T" in the space provided. If you believe the statement to be more false than true, write the letter "F."

_____ 1. Responsiveness is evaluated with the mnemonic DCAP-BTLS.

_____ 2. The detailed physical exam is normally performed en route to the hospital.

_____ 3. The damage associated with a gunshot wound is easily evaluated by drawing an imaginary line between the entrance and exit wounds.

_____ 4. Capillary refill can be checked in children by squeezing an entire arm or leg at a distal point.

_____ 5. An ongoing assessment is not necessary for stable patients.

_____ 6. Some patients may self-treat or self-medicate before calling 9-1-1.

_____ 7. Distinguishing between medical and trauma patients is less important than identifying and treating their problems appropriately.

_____ 8. Because capillary refill is checked in different parts of the body for adults and children, add 1 to 2 seconds to the normal time frame when assessing capillary refill in children.

_____ 9. The apparent absence of a palpable pulse in a responsive patient is not caused by cardiac arrest.

_____ 10. A patient with a poor general impression is considered a priority patient.

_____ 11. A rapid trauma assessment is not necessary for a patient without a significant mechanism of injury.

_____ 12. Airbags prevent steering wheel injuries.

_____ 13. In the case of a medical problem, the detailed assessment looks at body areas, prioritizing them by systems.

_____ 14. A detailed assessment of the chest wall cannot be completed unless the entire chest wall is visualized.

`1999` _____ 15. During the ongoing assessment, treatment should be modified based on reassessment findings.

`1999` _____ 16. During the ongoing assessment, you must repeat the initial assessment, but you should not reestablish patient priorities.

`1999` _____ 17. The cardiac monitor is of no benefit in determining deterioration of the patient's condition.

_____ 18. Invasive procedures such as IV therapy were intended for the prehospital environment.

Short Answer

Complete this section with short written answers in the space provided.

1. List the three factors affecting the degree of injury resulting from penetrating trauma.

_____

_____

_____

2. What is the single goal of initial assessment?

_____

_____

_____

3. On what is the general impression based?

_____

_____

_____

4. What do the letters ABC stand for in the assessment process?

_____

_____

_____

5. Describe the difference between diffuse and focal pain.

_____

_____

_____

6. What four questions are asked when assessing orientation and what purpose do these questions serve?

_____

_____

_____

7. What are the three goals of the focused history and physical exam?

_____

_____

_____

8. List the elements of DCAP-BTLS.

_____

_____

_____

9. List at least five significant mechanisms of injury in an adult.

_____

_____

_____

10. List seven essential elements that form the foundation of critical thinking.

_____

_____

_____

11. List the "6 Rs" of clinical decision making.

_____

_____

_____

Word Fun EMT-I vocab explorer web

The following crossword puzzle is an activity provided to reinforce correct spelling and understanding of medical terminology associated with emergency care and the EMT-I. Use the clues in the column to complete the puzzle.

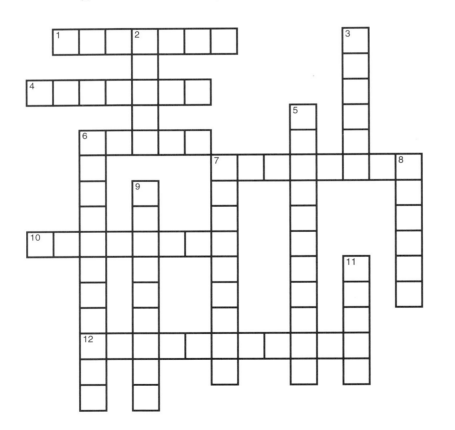

Across

1. Pain not associated with a single site
4. Coarse breath sounds
6. Rattling, moist sounds
7. Grating or grinding
10. Involuntary muscle contraction, to protect
12. Times four

Down

2. Pain in a single area
3. Pain assessment acronym
5. Below 95°F
6. Skin pulls in around ribs
7. Formation of clots
8. Acronym for history
9. Distal discomfort or pain
11. Broad area trauma without broken skin

Ambulance Calls

The following real case scenarios provide an opportunity to explore the concerns associated with patient management. Read each scenario, then answer each question in detail.

1. You are dispatched to a motor vehicle collision where you find a 32-year-old male with extensive trauma to the face and gurgling in his airway. He is responsive only to pain. You also note that the windshield is spider-webbed and there is deformity to the steering wheel. He is not wearing a seat belt.

   How would you best manage this patient? What clues tell you the transport status?

   _____

   _____

   _____

   _____

   _____

   _____

   _____

2. You are called to the scene where a 75-year-old female complains of being "weak." Family members tell you she is not acting right. She does not seem to notice as you approach. She is breathing adequately and her pulse is strong at a rate of 72. She appears to be in no obvious distress.

   How would you best manage this patient? What would you ask family members?

   _____

   _____

   _____

   _____

   _____

   _____

   _____

3. You are working a wreck involving a 24-year-old male unrestrained driver who is confused and anxious. You have him immobilized on a long backboard and have him on oxygen via nonrebreathing mask. His ABCs are within normal limits. He has a hematoma just above his left orbit but no signs of bleeding or shock.

How would you transport this patient? What would you do en route?

_____

_____

_____

_____

_____

_____

_____

_____

Skill Drills EMT-I video clips web

Skill Drill 10-1: Performing a Rapid Trauma Assessment

Test your knowledge of this skill drill by placing the photos below in the correct order. Number the first step with a "1," the second step with a "2," etc.

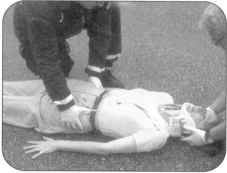

Assess the abdomen.

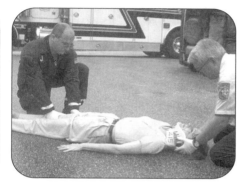

Assess the pelvis.

Assess the extremities.

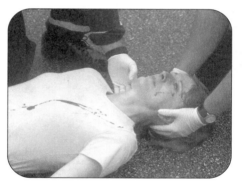

Assess the neck.

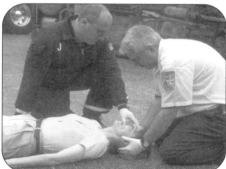

Check the ABCs, continue spinal immobilization, and assess mental status. Assess the head.

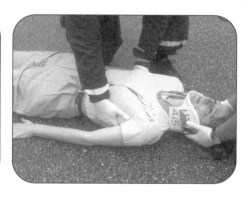

Assess the chest, including breath sounds.

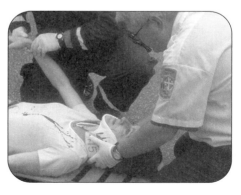

Fully immobilize the spine and assess baseline vital signs and obtain a SAMPLE history.

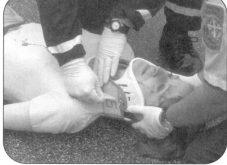

Apply a cervical collar.

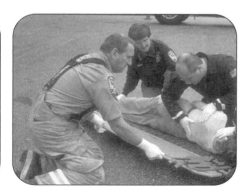

Log roll the patient, and assess the back.

Skill Drill 10-2: Performing a Rapid Medical Assessment: Unresponsive Patient
Test your knowledge of this skill drill by placing the photos below in the correct order. Number the first step with a "1," the second step with a "2," etc.

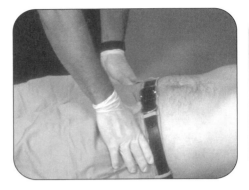

_____

Assess the pelvis.

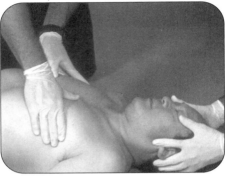

_____

Assess the chest.

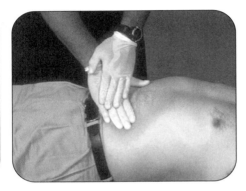

_____

Assess the abdomen.

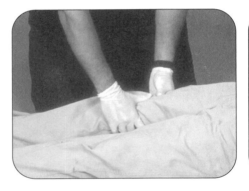

_____

Assess the extremities.

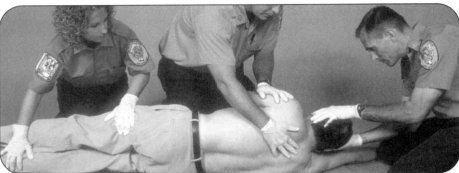

_____

Assess the back.

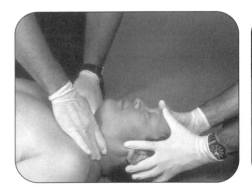

_____

Assess the neck.

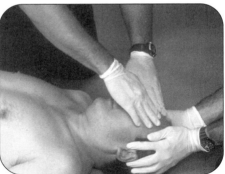

_____

Assess the head.

Skill Drill 10-3: Performing the Detailed Physical Exam

Test your knowledge of this skill drill by placing the photos below in the correct order. Number the first step with a "1," the second step with a "2," etc.

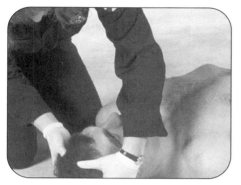
_____

Observe and palpate the head.

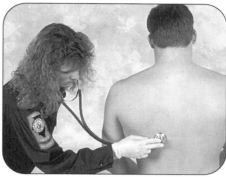
_____

In a medical patient, listen for posterior breath sounds.

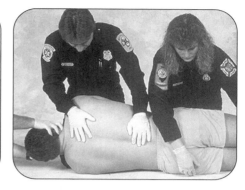
_____

Assess the back, unless the patient is immobilized. Complete assessment of the respiratory system. Complete assessment of the cardiovascular system.

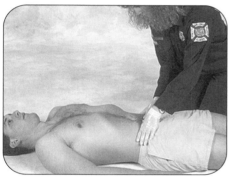
_____

Observe the abdomen and pelvis.

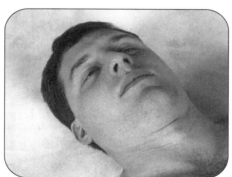
_____

Observe the face.

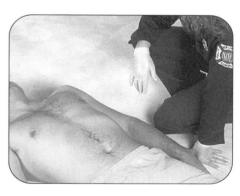
_____

Inspect the chest.

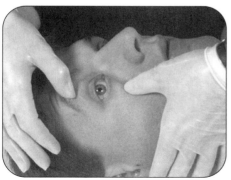
_____

Inspect the area around the eyes and eyelids.

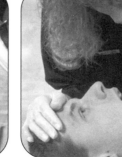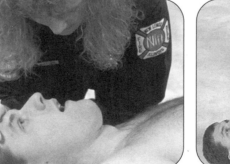
_____

Check for unusual breath odors.

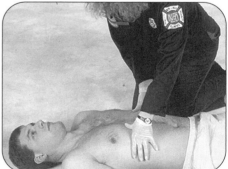
_____

Gently palpate the ribs.

Continued

Skill Drill 10-3: Performing the Detailed Physical Exam—continued

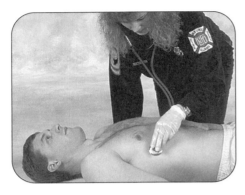

Listen to breath sounds.

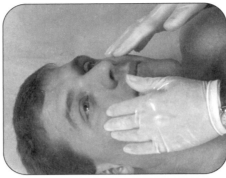

Palpate the maxillae.

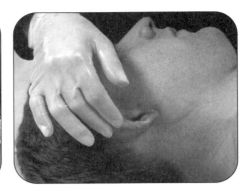

Look behind the ears for Battle's sign.

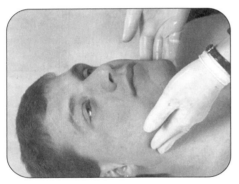

Palpate the mandible.

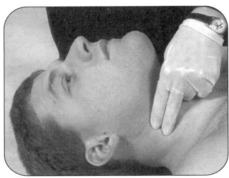

Observe for distended or pulsating jugular veins.

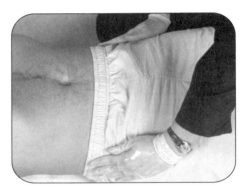

Gently compress the pelvis.

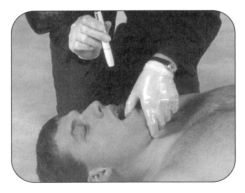

Assess the mouth.

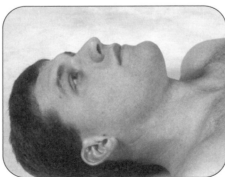

Inspect the neck.

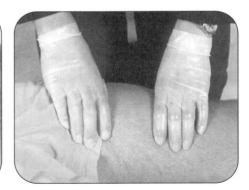

Inspect all four extremities; assess distal circulation and motor and sensory function. Assess for the presence of edema and pitting edema.

Skill Drill 10-3: Performing the Detailed Physical Exam—continued

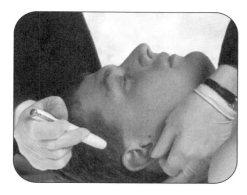

Check the ears.

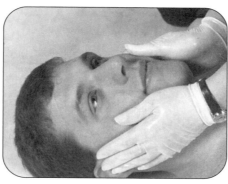

Palpate the zygomas.

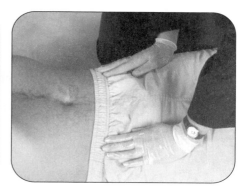

Gently press the iliac crest.

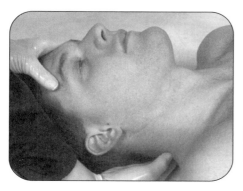

Palpate the neck, front and back.

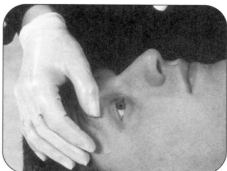

Examine the sclera and conjunctiva of the eyes.

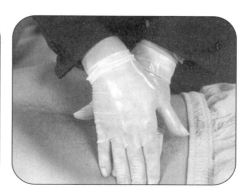

Gently palpate the abdomen.

Workbook Activities

The following activities have been designed to help you. Your instructor may require you to complete some or all of these activities as a regular part of your EMT-I training program. You are encouraged to complete any activity that your instructor does not assign as a way to enhance your learning in the classroom.

Chapter Review

The following exercises provide an opportunity to refresh your knowledge of this chapter.

Matching

Match each of the terms in the left column to the appropriate definition in the right column.

_____ 1. Base station

_____ 2. Mobile radio

_____ 3. Portable radio

_____ 4. Repeater

_____ 5. Telemetry

_____ 6. UHF range

_____ 7. VHF range

_____ 8. Cellular telephone

_____ 9. Dedicated line

_____ 10. MED channels

_____ 11. Scanner

_____ 12. Channel

_____ 13. Rapport

A. "hot line"

B. a trusting relationship built with your patient

C. communication through an interconnected series of repeater stations

D. assigned frequency used to carry voice and/or data communications

E. radio receiver that searches across several frequencies until the message is completed

F. VHF and UHF channels designated exclusively for EMS use

G. vehicle-mounted device that operates at a lower frequency than a base station

H. a process in which electronic signals are converted into coded, audible signals

I. radio frequencies between 30 and 300 MHz

J. hand-carried or hand-held devices that operate at 1 to 5 watts

K. special base station radio that receives messages and signals on one frequency and then automatically retransmits them on a second frequency

L. radio frequencies between 300 and 3,000 MHz

M. radio hardware containing a transmitter and receiver that is located in a fixed location

Multiple Choice

Read each item carefully, then select the best response.

_____ 1. The base station may be used:

A. in a single place by an operator speaking into a microphone that is connected directly to the equipment.

B. remotely through telephone lines.

C. by radio from a communications center.

D. all of the above.

CHAPTER 11

Communications and Documentation

_____ **2.** The transmission range of a(n) _____ is more limited than that of mobile or base station radios.

    A. portable radio

    B. 800 MHz radio

    C. cellular phone

    D. UHF radio

_____ **3.** Base stations:

    A. usually have more power than mobile or portable radios.

    B. have higher, more efficient antenna systems.

    C. allow for communication with field units at much greater distances.

    D. all of the above.

_____ **4.** _____ are helpful when you are away from the ambulance and need to communicate with dispatch, another unit, or medical control.

    A. Base stations

    B. Portable radios

    C. Mobile radios

    D. Cellular phones

_____ **5.** Digital signals are also used in some kinds of paging and tone-alerting systems because they transmit _____ and allow more choices and flexibility.

    A. numerically

    B. faster

    C. alphanumerically

    D. encoded messages

_____ **6.** Once connected to a cellular network, you can call any other telephone in the world and can send _____ signals.

    A. voice

    B. data

    C. telemetry

    D. all of the above

_____ **7.** As with all repeater-based systems, a cellular telephone is useless if the equipment:

    A. fails.

    B. loses power.

    C. is damaged by severe weather or other circumstances.

    D. all of the above.

_____ **8.** In the simplex mode, all of the following are true EXCEPT:

  A. when one party transmits, the other must wait to reply.

  B. you must push a button to talk.

  C. it is called a "pair of frequencies."

  D. radio transmissions can occur in either direction but not simultaneously in both.

_____ **9.** _____ communications can simultaneously transmit two or more different types of information such as voice and telemetry.

  A. Simplex

  B. Duplex

  C. Multiplex

  D. Med channel

_____ **10.** Principal EMS-related responsibilities of the FCC include:

  A. monitoring radio operations.

  B. establishing limitations for transmitter power output.

  C. allocating specific radio frequencies for use by EMS providers.

  D. all of the above.

_____ **11.** Responsibilities of the dispatcher include all of the following EXCEPT:

  A. properly screening and assigning priority to each call.

  B. selecting and alerting the appropriate EMS response units.

  C. maintaining a record of the incident.

  D. providing emergency medical care to the telephone caller.

_____ **12.** In order to dispatch the appropriate unit to the necessary location, the dispatcher must find out:

  A. the exact location of the patient.

  B. the nature of the problem.

  C. the severity of the problem.

  D. all of the above.

_____ **13.** Determination of the level and type of response necessary is based on:

  A. the dispatcher's perception of the nature and severity of the problem.

  B. the anticipated response time to the scene.

  C. the level of training.

  D. all of the above.

_____ **14.** Information given to the responding unit(s) should include all of the following, EXCEPT:

  A. the number of patients.

  B. the time the unit will arrive.

  C. the exact location of the incident.

  D. responses by other public safety agencies.

_____ **15.** You must consult with medical control to:

  A. notify the hospital of an incoming patient.

  B. request advice or orders from medical control.

  C. advise the hospital of special situations.

  D. all of the above.

_____ **16.** The patient report commonly includes all of the following EXCEPT:

  A. a list of the patient's medications.

  B. the patient's age and gender.

  C. a brief history of the patient's current problem.

  D. your estimated time of arrival.

_____ **17.** In most areas, medical control is provided by the _____ who work at the receiving hospital.
A. nurses
B. physicians
C. interns
D. staff

_____ **18.** For _____ reasons, the delivery of sophisticated care, such as assisting patients in taking medications, must be done in association with physicians.
A. logical
B. ethical
C. legal
D. all of the above

_____ **19.** Standard radio operating procedures are designed to:
A. reduce the number of misunderstood messages.
B. keep transmissions brief.
C. develop effective radio discipline.
D. all of the above.

_____ **20.** All of the following should be contained in the patient report EXCEPT:
A. patient's name.
B. patient's age.
C. chief complaint.
D. description of the scene.

_____ **21.** Be sure that you report all patient information in a(n) _____ manner.
A. objective
B. accurate
C. professional
D. all of the above

_____ **22.** Medical control guides the treatment of patients in the system through all of the following EXCEPT:
A. hands-on care.
B. protocols.
C. direct orders.
D. post-call review.

_____ **23.** Depending on how the protocols are written, you may need to call medical control for direct orders to:
A. administer certain treatments.
B. transport a patient.
C. request assistance from other agencies.
D. immobilize a patient.

_____ **24.** The delivery of EMS involves an impressive array of:
A. assessments.
B. stabilization.
C. treatments.
D. all of the above.

_____ **25.** During transport:
A. you must periodically reassess the patient's overall condition.
B. it is not necessary to report changes in the patient's condition.
C. you are required to check vital signs once.
D. it is safe to finish your paperwork once treatment is provided because the patient's condition will remain stable.

_____ **26.** While en route to and from the scene, you should report all of the following to the dispatcher EXCEPT:

A. any special hazards.

B. traffic delays.

C. abandoned vehicles in the median.

D. road construction.

_____ **27.** Situations that might require special preparation on the part of the hospital include:

A. HazMat situations.

B. mass-casualty incidents.

C. rescues in progress.

D. all of the above.

_____ **28.** The _____ officially occurs during your oral report at the hospital, not as a result of your radio report en route.

A. patient report

B. transfer of care

C. termination of services

D. all of the above

_____ **29.** Effective communication between the EMT-I and health care professionals in the receiving facility is an essential cornerstone of _____ patient care.

A. efficient

B. effective

C. appropriate

D. all of the above

_____ **30.** Components that must be included in the oral report during transfer of care include:

A. the patient's name.

B. any important history.

C. vital signs assessed.

D. all of the above.

_____ **31.** Your _____ are critically important in gaining the trust of both the patient and family.

A. gestures

B. body movements

C. attitude toward the patient

D. all of the above

_____ **32.** If the patient is hearing impaired, you should:

A. stand on the patient's left side.

B. shout.

C. speak clearly and distinctly.

D. use baby talk.

_____ **33.** When caring for visually impaired patients, you should:

A. use sign language.

B. touch the patient only when necessary to render care.

C. try to avoid sudden movements.

D. never walk them to the ambulance.

_____ **34.** When attempting to communicate with non-English-speaking patients, you should:

A. use short, simple questions and simple words whenever possible.

B. always use medical terms.

C. shout.

D. position yourself so the patient can read your lips.

_____ **35.** The patient information that is included in the minimum data set includes all of the following EXCEPT:

   A. the chief complaint.

   B. the time that the EMS unit arrived at the scene.

   C. respirations and effort.

   D. skin color and temperature.

_____ **36.** The administrative information that is included in the minimum data set includes:

   A. the time that patient care was transferred.

   B. the chief complaint.

   C. skin color and temperature.

   D. systolic blood pressure for patients older than 3 years.

_____ **37.** Functions of the prehospital care report include:

   A. continuity of care.

   B. education.

   C. research.

   D. all of the above.

_____ **38.** A good prehospital care report documents:

   A. the care that was provided.

   B. the patient's condition on arrival.

   C. any changes.

   D. all of the above.

_____ **39.** When completing the narrative section, be sure to:

   A. describe what you see and what you do.

   B. only include positive findings.

   C. record your conclusions about the incident.

   D. use appropriate radio codes.

_____ **40.** Instances in which you may be required to file special reports with appropriate authorities include:

   A. gunshot wounds.

   B. dog bites.

   C. suspected physical, sexual, or substance abuse.

   D. all of the above.

Vocabulary EMT-I vocab explorer web

Define the following terms in the space provided.

1. Simplex:

_____

_____

_____

2. Standing orders:

_____

_____

_____

3. Federal Communications Commission (FCC):

_____

_____

_____

4. Duplex:

_____

_____

_____

5. Prehospital care report:

_____

_____

_____

Fill-in

Read each item carefully, then complete the statement by filling in the missing word(s).

1. Written communications, in the form of a written _____, provide you with an opportunity to communicate the patient's story to others who may participate in the patient's care in the future.

2. A two-way radio consists of two units: a _____ and a _____.

3. A _____, also known as a hot line, is always open or under the control of the individuals at each end.

4. The 800 MHz radio frequency offers excellent penetration of buildings and has minimal interference and reduced channel noise. It also allows for _____ multiple agencies or systems that can share frequencies.

5. With _____, electronic signals are converted into coded audible signals.

6. Low-power portable radios that communicate through a series of interconnected repeater stations called "cells" are known as _____.

7. _____ are commonly used in EMS operations to alert on- and off-duty personnel.

8. When the first call to 9-1-1 comes in, the dispatcher must try to judge its relative _____ in order to begin the appropriate EMS response using emergency medical dispatch protocols.

9. The principal reason for radio communication is to facilitate communication between you and

_____.

10. You could be successfully sued for _____ if you describe a patient in a way that injures his or her reputation.

11. Regardless of your system's design, your link to _____ is vital in maintaining the high quality of care that your patient requires and deserves.

12. To ensure complete understanding, once you receive an order from medical control, you must _____ the order back, word for word, and then receive confirmation.

13. By their very nature, _____ do not require direct communication with medical control.

14. Maintaining _____ with your patient builds trust and lets the patient know that he or she is your first priority.

15. Children can easily see through lies or deception, so you must always be _____ with them.

16. If the patient does not speak any English, find a family member or friend to act as a(n)

_____.

17. The national EMS community has identified a _____ that should enable communication and comparison of EMS runs between agencies, regions, and states.

18. A properly written report is _____, _____, _____, _____, and free of any nonprofessional or extraneous information.

19. Your best protection, and the patient's best opportunity for proper treatment, depend on a PCR that is

_____, _____, and completed in a _____ manner.

20. _____ adult patients have the right to refuse treatment.

True/False

If you believe the statement to be more true than false, write the letter "T" in the space provided. If you believe the statement to be more false than true, write the letter "F."

_____ **1.** The two-way radio is actually at least two units: a transmitter and a receiver.

_____ **2.** Base stations typically have more power and much higher and more efficient antenna systems than mobile or portable radios.

_____ **3.** A cellular telephone is just another kind of portable radio that is available for EMS use.

_____ **4.** The transmission range of a mobile radio is more limited than that of a portable radio.

_____ **5.** A dedicated line, a special telephone line used for specific point-to-point communications, is always open or under the control of the individuals at each end.

        6. The written report is a vital part of providing emergency medical care and ensuring the continuity of patient care.

        7. EMS systems that use repeaters are unable to get good signals from portable radios.

        8. Small changes in your location will not significantly affect the quality of your transmission.

        9. When used improperly or not understood, codes create confusion rather than clear it up.

        10. Radio equipment that is operating properly should be serviced at least every 2 years.

        11. Your reporting responsibilities end when you arrive at the hospital.

        12. Special cleansing solvents should be used on the exterior surface of radio equipment.

        13. In report writing, the format chosen is not as important as knowing how to differentiate subjective from objective information.

        14. Patients deserve to know that you can provide medical care and that you are concerned about their well-being.

Short Answer

Complete this section with short written answers in the space provided.

1. List the five principal FCC responsibilities related to EMS.

2. List five guidelines for effective radio communications.

3. List the six functions of a prehospital care report.

4. Describe the two types of written report forms generally in use in EMS systems.

5. You have documented that the patient fell 3 feet. You meant to state that he fell 30 feet. How would you correct your documentation?

6. List four items of supportive information that should be recorded on the PCR.

_____

_____

_____

Word Fun EMT-I vocab explorer web

The following crossword puzzle is an activity provided to reinforce correct spelling and understanding of medical terminology associated with emergency care and the EMT-I. Use the clues in the column to complete the puzzle.

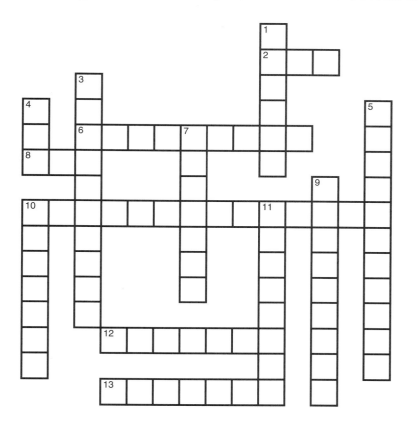

Across

  2. Frequencies between 300 and 3,000 MHz

  6. Point-to-point

  8. Agency with jurisdiction over radios

  10. Outline specific directions, protocols

  12. Trusting relationship

  13. Radio receiver that searches

Down

  1. Transmit and receive simultaneously

  3. Frequencies for exclusive EMS usage

  4. Frequencies between 30 and 300 MHz

  5. Hardware in a fixed location

  7. Assigned frequency

  9. Electronic signals converted into coded audible signals

  10. Transmit in both ways, but not at the same time

  11. Receives on one, transmits on another

Ambulance Calls

The following real case scenarios provide an opportunity to explore the concerns associated with patient management. Read each scenario, then answer each question in detail.

1. You are in the dispatch office filling in for the EMS dispatcher who needed to use the restroom. The phone rings and you answer it to find a hysterical female screaming about a child falling in an old well. All you can get out of her is that he is 5 years old and is not making any noise. The address is on the computer display.

   How would you best manage this situation and what additional help would you need?

   _____

   _____

   _____

   _____

   _____

   _____

   _____

   _____

2. You are called to a special school for deaf children where a 6-year-old female fell on the playground and twisted her ankle. Her mother has been notified, and will meet you at the emergency room. The patient is sitting beside the monkey bars when you arrive.

   How would you best manage this patient?

   _____

   _____

   _____

   _____

   _____

   _____

   _____

   _____

3. You are dispatched to the local park where a collision occurred between a bicycle and a pedestrian. Your patient, a 25-year-old male, was walking his dog when the cyclist swerved to miss a squirrel and collided with him, knocking him to the ground. You notice he has deformity to his right forearm and the dog is a seeing-eye dog.

How would you best manage this patient? The dog?

_____

_____

_____

_____

_____

_____

_____

Workbook Activities

The following activities have been designed to help you. Your instructor may require you to complete some or all of these activities as a regular part of your EMT-I training program. You are encouraged to complete any activity that your instructor does not assign as a way to enhance your learning in the classroom.

Chapter Review

The following exercises provide an opportunity to refresh your knowledge of this chapter.

Matching

Match each of the terms in the left column to the appropriate definition in the right column.

_____ **1.** Cavitation

_____ **2.** Deceleration

_____ **3.** Kinetic energy

_____ **4.** Mechanism of injury

_____ **5.** Potential energy

_____ **6.** Blunt trauma

_____ **7.** Penetrating trauma

_____ **8.** Work

A. impact on the body by objects that cause injury without penetrating soft tissue or internal organs and cavities

B. force acting over a distance

C. product of mass, gravity, and height

D. injury caused by objects that pierce the surface of the body

E. how trauma occurs

F. energy of moving objects

G. slowing

H. emanation of pressure waves that can damage nearby structures

Multiple Choice

Read each item carefully, then select the best response.

_____ **1.** Trauma centers that have 24-hour in-house availability of qualified attending surgeons would be designated as:

    A. Level 1.

    B. Level 2.

    C. Level 3.

    D. Level 4.

_____ **2.** The following are concepts of energy typically associated with injury EXCEPT:

    A. potential energy.

    B. thermal energy.

    C. kinetic energy.

    D. work.

CHAPTER 12

Trauma Systems and Mechanism of Injury

_____ **3.** The energy of a moving object is called:
   A. potential energy.
   B. thermal energy.
   C. kinetic energy.
   D. work.

_____ **4.** Energy can be:
   A. created.
   B. destroyed.
   C. converted.
   D. all of the above.

_____ **5.** In an energy exchange, _____ are more likely to splinter or fragment.
   A. air density particles
   B. water density particles
   C. solid density particles
   D. high density particles

_____ **6.** The amount of kinetic energy that is converted to do work on the body dictates the _____ of the injury.
   A. location
   B. severity
   C. cause
   D. speed

_____ **7.** Potential energy is mostly associated with the energy of:
   A. falling objects.
   B. motor vehicle crashes.
   C. pedestrian vs. bicycle crashes.
   D. gunshot wounds.

_____ **8.** Motor vehicle crashes are classified traditionally as:
   A. frontal.
   B. rollover.
   C. lateral.
   D. all of the above.

_____ 9. The three collisions in a frontal impact include all of the following EXCEPT:

    A. car vs. object.

    B. passenger vs. vehicle.

    C. flying objects vs. passengers.

    D. internal organs vs. solid structures of the body.

_____ 10. The mechanism of injury provides information about the severity of the collision and therefore has a(n) _____ effect on patient care.

    A. direct

    B. positive

    C. indirect

    D. negative

_____ 11. Your index of suspicion for the presence of life-threatening injuries should automatically increase if you see:

    A. seats torn from their mountings.

    B. collapsed steering wheels.

    C. intrusion into the passenger compartment.

    D. all of the above.

_____ 12. Trauma to the brain that results from striking the front and back of the skull is known as:

    A. frontal-occipital injury.

    B. front to back injury.

    C. coup–contrecoup injury

    D. none of the above.

_____ 13. In a motor vehicle crash, as the passenger's head hits the windshield the brain continues to move forward until it strikes the inside of the skull, resulting in a _____ injury.

    A. compression

    B. laceration

    C. lateral

    D. motion

_____ 14. Your quick initial assessment of the patient and the evaluation of the _____ can help to direct lifesaving care and provide critical information to the hospital staff.

    A. scene

    B. index of suspicion

    C. mechanism of injury

    D. abdominal area

_____ 15. A contusion to a patient's forehead along with a spider-webbed windshield suggests possible injury to the:

    A. nose.

    B. brain.

    C. face.

    D. heart.

_____ 16. Significant mechanisms of injury include:

    A. moderate intrusions from a lateral impact.

    B. severe damage from the rear.

    C. collisions in which rotation is involved.

    D. all of the above.

_____ 17. Significant clues to the possibility of severe injuries include:

    A. death of a passenger.

    B. a blown-out tire.

    C. broken glass.

    D. a deployed air bag.

_____ **18.** When properly applied, seat belts are successful in:

    A. restraining the passengers in a vehicle.

    B. preventing a second collision inside the motor vehicle.

    C. decreasing the severity of the third collision.

    D. all of the above.

_____ **19.** Airbags decrease injury to all of the following EXCEPT:

    A. chest.

    B. heart.

    C. face.

    D. head.

_____ **20.** Signs of most injuries sustained in a motor vehicle crash can be found by simply inspecting the _____ during extrication of the patient.

    A. head and neck

    B. chest

    C. interior of the vehicle

    D. torso

_____ **21.** Passengers in the back seat wearing only a lap belt might have a higher incidence of injuries to the thoracic and lumbar spine in a _____ impact.

    A. frontal

    B. lateral

    C. rear-end

    D. rollover

_____ **22.** _____ impacts are probably the number one cause of death associated with motor vehicle crashes.

    A. Frontal

    B. Lateral

    C. Rear-end

    D. Rollover

_____ **23.** In a frontal collision, organ collision may cause:

    A. severe bleeding.

    B. stretching of the brain stem.

    C. a pneumothorax.

    D. all of the above.

_____ **24.** In lateral impacts, the _____ move(s) the upper torso with the vehicle, restricting multiple collisions.

    A. lap belt

    B. shoulder restraint

    C. air bag

    D. child safety seats

_____ **25.** The most common life-threatening element in a rollover is _____ or partial ejection of the passenger from the vehicle.

    A. "sandwiching"

    B. centrifugal force

    C. ejection

    D. spinal cord injury

_____ **26.** There is a _____ increase in brain injury in those motorcycle riders who do not wear helmets.

   A. 30%

   B. 100%

   C. 300%

   D. 1000%

_____ **27.** A fall from more than _____ times the patient's height is considered to be significant.

   A. two

   B. three

   C. four

   D. five

_____ **28.** Factors that should be taken into account when evaluating the fall patient include:

   A. the height of the fall.

   B. the surface struck.

   C. the part of the body that hit first.

   D. all of the above.

_____ **29.** Low-energy penetrating trauma may be caused accidentally by impalement or intentionally by:

   A. a knife.

   B. a pair of scissors.

   C. an ice pick.

   D. all of the above.

_____ **30.** The area that is damaged by medium- and high-velocity projectiles can be _____ than the diameter of the projectile itself.

   A. slightly larger

   B. many times larger

   C. slightly smaller

   D. many times smaller

_____ **31.** Exit wounds are larger than entrance wounds because of all of the following EXCEPT:

   A. the speed of the bullet.

   B. the size of the bullet.

   C. tumbling of the bullet.

   D. pressure waves.

_____ **32.** When you notice a collapsed steering wheel during scene size-up, you should suspect serious _____ injuries even if the driver shows no visible signs of injury.

   A. head

   B. chest

   C. abdominal

   D. pelvic

_____ **33.** Rupture of gas-containing organs occurs in the _____ phase of a blast injury.

   A. primary

   B. secondary

   C. tertiary

   D. all of the above

_____ **34.** Injuries sustained during the _____ phase of a blast injury are similar to those sustained in a fall or vehicle ejection.

   A. primary

   B. secondary

   C. tertiary

   D. all of the above

Vocabulary

Define the following terms in the space provided.

1. Newton's First Law:

_____

_____

_____

2. Newton's Second Law:

_____

_____

_____

3. Newton's Third Law:

_____

_____

_____

4. Mesentery:

_____

_____

_____

Fill-in

Read each item carefully, then complete the statement by filling in the missing word(s).

1. _____ are the leading cause of death and disability in the United States among children and young adults.

2. Certain injury _____ occur with certain types of injury _____.

3. The _____ is the EMT-I's concern for potentially serious underlying and unseen injuries.

4. _____ occurs to the body when the body's tissues are exposed to energy levels beyond their tolerance.

5. The formula for calculating kinetic energy is _____.

6. _____ of the crash scene may provide valuable information to the staff and treating physicians of the trauma center.

7. Air bags provide the final capture point of the passengers and decrease the severity of _____ injuries.

8. Seat belts that buckle automatically at the shoulder but require the passengers to buckle the lap portion can result in the body _____ forward underneath the shoulder restraint when the lap portion is not attached.

9. Because rear-facing car seats rest in close proximity to the dashboard, rapid inflation of the air bag could cause _____ or _____ to the infant.

10. _____ are known to cause whiplash-type injuries.

11. _____ hold the lower torso close to the seat and away from the dash or steering column.

12. Air bags alone are _____ effective.

13. With falls, head-first impact may result in _____ from compression, along with _____ or _____ of the brain.

True/False

If you believe the statement to be more true than false, write the letter "T" in the space provided. If you believe the statement to be more false than true, write the letter "F."

_____ 1. Work is defined as force acting over distance.

_____ 2. Energy can be both created and destroyed.

_____ 3. The energy of a moving object is called potential energy.

_____ 4. If only one body system is involved in trauma, the EMT-I should maintain a high index of suspicion for serious unseen injuries.

_____ 5. When passengers are riding in a vehicle equipped with airbags but are not restrained by seat belts, they are often thrown forward in an act of emergency braking.

_____ 6. Rear-end collisions often cause whiplash injuries.

_____ 7. The cervical spine has little tolerance for lateral bending.

_____ 8. Never place a child or infant in the front seat of a vehicle with air bags.

_____ 9. The injury potential of a fall is related to the height from which the patient fell.

_____ 10. Injuries are the leading cause of death and injuries among 1- to 34-year-olds in the United States.

Short Answer

Complete this section with short written answers in the space provided.

1. Describe potential energy.

_____

_____

_____

2. List the three series of collisions typical with motor vehicles.

_____

_____

_____

3. List the three factors to consider when evaluating a fall.

_____

_____

_____

4. Describe the phenomenon of cavitation as it relates to an injury from a bullet.

_____

_____

_____

5. Why is it important to try to determine the type of gun and ammunition used when you are caring for a gunshot victim?

_____

_____

_____

6. List three components of EMS trauma systems.

_____

_____

_____

7. List three situations when air transport is a viable option.

_____

_____

_____

8. List the injury patterns.
Front-end collision:

_____

_____

_____

Rear-end collision:

_____

_____

_____

Lateral impact:

_____

_____

_____

9. What are the three phases of impact in pedestrian vs. motor vehicle accidents?

_____

_____

_____

Word Fun

The following crossword puzzle is an activity provided to reinforce correct spelling and understanding of medical terminology associated with emergency care and the EMT-I. Use the clues in the column to complete the puzzle.

Across

1. Pressure waves from speed
4. Slowing down
5. Force acting over distance
7. Cause or reason for injury
8. Impact on the body without penetrating soft tissue

Down

2. The result of body tissues being exposed to energy levels beyond their tolerance
3. Product of mass × gravity × height
6. Energy from a moving object

Ambulance Calls

The following real case scenarios provide an opportunity to explore the concerns associated with patient management. Read each scenario, then answer each question in detail.

1. You are called to the scene of a rollover motor vehicle crash. Your patient is a 25-year-old male, restrained driver, complaining of chest pain. He is alert and oriented and his vital signs are within normal limits.

   How would you best manage this patient?

   _____

   _____

   _____

   _____

   _____

   _____

   _____

2. You are dispatched to the scene of a fall from the roof of a two-story house. Your patient, a 32-year-old male, was found lying on the ground with obvious deformity to his right lower leg. He is alert and oriented and tells you he slipped on a hammer. Bleeding is controlled and his airway is intact.

   How would you best manage this patient?

   _____

   _____

   _____

   _____

   _____

   _____

   _____

3. You are dispatched to a domestic dispute with shots fired. Police have secured the scene and located a patient in the bedroom who has a single small caliber gunshot wound to the RUQ of his abdomen. He is responsive to verbal stimuli and is notably pale and diaphoretic.

How would you best manage this patient?

_____

_____

_____

_____

_____

_____

_____

_____

4. You are called to the residence of a 19-year-old male who was stabbed in the abdomen with an ice pick. The scene is safe, and the patient is lying on the floor with the ice pick impaled in his LLQ. Bystanders tell you he did not fall. He is alert and complaining of severe pain.

How would you best manage this patient?

_____

_____

_____

_____

_____

_____

_____

Workbook Activities

The following activities have been designed to help you. Your instructor may require you to complete some or all of these activities as a regular part of your EMT-I training program. You are encouraged to complete any activity that your instructor does not assign as a way to enhance your learning in the classroom.

Chapter Review

The following exercises provide an opportunity to refresh your knowledge of this chapter.

Matching

Match each of the terms in the left column to the appropriate definition in the right column.

_____ **1.** Shock

_____ **2.** Perfusion

_____ **3.** Chronotropic

_____ **4.** Pulse pressure

_____ **5.** Hemophilia

_____ **6.** Cardiogenic shock

_____ **7.** Hematuria

_____ **8.** Sphincter

_____ **9.** Cardiac output

_____ **10.** Neurogenic shock

_____ **11.** Hemorrhage

_____ **12.** Inotropic

_____ **13.** PASG

_____ **14.** Hematochezia

_____ **15.** Anaphylaxis

_____ **16.** Hypovolemic shock

_____ **17.** Dromotropic

_____ **18.** Melena

A. blood in the urine

B. bleeding

C. influences contractibility

D. dark, tarry stools

E. used to stabilize a fractured pelvis

F. regulates blood flow in capillaries

G. hypoperfusion

H. distributive shock caused by allergic reaction

I. influences heart rate

J. sufficient circulation to meet cell needs

K. difference in systolic and diastolic blood pressure

L. condition of low blood volume

M. influences conductivity

N. congenital condition in which a patient lacks one or more normal clotting factors

O. spinal vascular shock

P. HR x SV

Q. pump failure

R. bright red blood in the stool

Multiple Choice

Read each item carefully, then select the best response.

_____ **1.** Shock:

    A. refers to a state of collapse and failure of the cardiovascular system.

    B. results in the inadequate flow of blood to the body's cells.

    C. results in failure to rid cells of metabolic wastes.

    D. all of the above.

Hemorrhage and Shock

_____ **2.** _____ is the circulation of blood within an organ or tissue in adequate amounts to meet the cells' current needs for oxygen, nutrients, and waste removal.

A. Anatomy

B. Perfusion

C. Physiology

D. Conduction

_____ **3.** The _____ only require(s) a minimal blood supply when at rest.

A. lungs

B. kidneys

C. muscles

D. heart

_____ **4.** The brain and spinal cord cannot go for more than _____ minutes without perfusion or the nerve cells will be permanently damaged.

A. 30 to 45

B. 12 to 20

C. 8 to 10

D. 4 to 6

_____ **5.** An organ or tissue that is considerably _____ is much better able to resist damage from hypoperfusion.

A. warmer

B. colder

C. younger

D. older

_____ **6.** The body will not tolerate an acute blood loss of greater than _____ of blood volume.

A. 10%

B. 20%

C. 30%

D. 40%

_____ **7.** If the typical adult loses more than 1 liter of blood, significant changes in vital signs such as _____ will occur.

A. increased heart rate

B. increased respiratory rate

C. decreased blood pressure

D. all of the above

_____ **8.** Significant blood loss demands your immediate attention as soon as the _____ has/have been managed.

    A. fractures

    B. extrication

    C. airway

    D. none of the above

_____ **9.** Even though the body is very efficient at controlling bleeding on its own, it may fail in situations such as:

    A. when medications interfere with normal clotting.

    B. when damage to the vessel is so large that a clot cannot completely block the hole.

    C. when only part of the vessel wall is cut, preventing it from constricting.

    D. all of the above.

_____ **10.** Coffee-ground emesis is a sign of:

    A. upper GI bleeding.

    B. lower GI bleeding.

    C. liver injury.

    D. spleen injury.

_____ **11.** A lack of one or more of the blood's clotting factors is called:

    A. deficiency.

    B. hemophilia.

    C. platelet anomaly.

    D. anemia.

_____ **12.** The first step in controlling bleeding is:

    A. direct pressure.

    B. maintaining the airway.

    C. taking BSI precautions.

    D. elevation.

_____ **13.** When applying a bandage to hold a dressing in place, stretch the bandage tight enough to control bleeding but not so tight as to decrease _____ to the extremity.

    A. blood flow

    B. pulses

    C. oxygen

    D. CRTs

_____ **14.** If bleeding continues after applying a pressure dressing, you should do all of the following EXCEPT:

    A. remove the dressing and apply another sterile dressing.

    B. apply manual pressure through the dressing.

    C. add more gauze over the first dressing.

    D. secure both dressings tighter with a roller bandage.

_____ **15.** Bleeding from hemorrhoids causes _____.

    A. melena.

    B. hematochezia.

    C. hematuria.

    D. all of the above.

_____ **16.** Contraindications to the use of the PASG include:

    A. pulmonary edema.

    B. pregnancy.

    C. penetrating chest trauma.

    D. all of the above.

_____ **17.** A tourniquet is rarely needed to control bleeding and often _____ problems.

   A. resolves

   B. decreases

   C. creates

   D. all of the above

_____ **18.** When applying a tourniquet, make sure you:

   A. use the narrowest bandage possible to minimize the area restricted.

   B. cover the tourniquet with a bandage.

   C. never pad underneath the tourniquet.

   D. do not loosen the tourniquet after you have applied it.

_____ **19.** You should not attempt to stop the blood flow from the nose or ears following a head injury because:

   A. it should be collected to reinfuse at the hospital.

   B. it could collect within the head and increase the pressure in the brain.

   C. it is contaminated.

   D. you could fracture the skull with the pressure needed to staunch the flow of blood.

_____ **20.** _____ develops when the heart muscle can no longer generate enough pressure to circulate the blood to all organs.

   A. Pump failure

   B. Cardiogenic shock

   C. A myocardial infarction

   D. Congestive heart failure

_____ **21.** Hypovolemic shock is caused by:

   A. blood loss.

   B. thermal burns.

   C. dehydration.

   D. all of the above.

_____ **22.** In anaphylactic shock:

   A. there is blood loss.

   B. there is a strong possibility of direct cardiac muscle injury.

   C. there is widespread vascular dilation resulting in relative hypovolemia.

   D. there is vascular damage.

_____ **23.** Damage to the _____ may cause significant injury to the part of the nervous system that controls the size and muscular tone of the blood vessels.

   A. cervical vertebrae

   B. skull

   C. spinal cord

   D. peripheral nerves

_____ **24.** Neurogenic shock usually results from damage to the spinal cord at the:

   A. cervical level.

   B. thoracic level.

   C. lumbar level.

   D. sacral level.

Labeling
Label the following diagrams with the correct terms.

Perfusion

A. _____

B. _____

C. _____

D. _____

E. _____

F. _____

G. _____

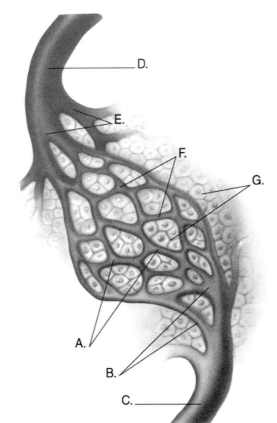

Arterial Pressure Points

A. _____

B. _____

C. _____

D. _____

E. _____

F. _____

G. _____

H. _____

I. _____

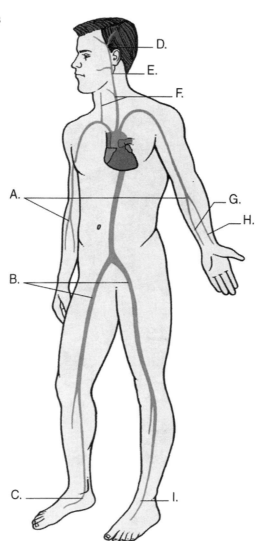

Cardiovascular System

A. _____

B. _____

C. _____

D. _____

E. _____

F. _____

G. _____

H. _____

I. _____

J. _____

Vocabulary EMT-I

Define the following terms in the space provided.

1. Perfusion:

_____

_____

_____

2. Shock:

_____

_____

_____

3. Autonomic nervous system:

_____

_____

_____

4. Pressure point:

_____

_____

_____

5. Pulse pressure:

_____

_____

_____

Fill-in

Read each item carefully, then complete the statement by filling in the missing word(s).

1. The circulation of blood in adequate amounts to meet cellular needs is called _____.

2. The _____ monitors the body's needs from moment to moment and adjusts the blood flow as required.

3. The brain and spinal cord generally cannot go longer than _____ minutes without adequate perfusion, or permanent nerve cell damage may occur.

4. The body will not tolerate an acute blood loss of greater than _____.

5. Because internal bleeding is not visible, you must rely on _____ to determine the extent and severity of the hemorrhage.

6. _____ may be helpful when a vessel has been severed, especially if it has retracted into the surrounding tissue.

7. Bleeding from the nose or ears following a head injury may indicate a _____, and you should not attempt to stop the blood flow.

8. As perfusion decreases, the body attempts to compensate by redirecting blood flow from _____ organs to _____ organs.

9. A decrease in systolic blood pressure to less than _____ stimulates the vasomotor center to increase arterial pressure by constricting vessels.

10. _____ _____ occurs as perfusion decreases.

1999 **11.** Positive cardiac _____ drugs may be administered to some patients in shock to increase the strength of contraction of the heart.

12. Maintenance of _____ is always an important element of the treatment for a patient in shock.

13. The presence of radial pulses equates to a systolic blood pressure of _____, which is sufficient to

perfuse the brain and other vital organs.

True/False

If you believe the statement to be more true than false, write the letter "T" in the space provided. If you believe the statement to be more false than true, write the letter "F."

_____ **1.** Venous blood tends to spurt and is difficult to control.

_____ **2.** The human body is tolerant of blood losses greater than 20% of blood volume.

_____ **3.** The first step in controlling external bleeding is application of the PASG.

_____ **4.** The first step in preparing to treat a bleeding patient is BSI.

_____ **5.** A properly applied tourniquet should be loosened by the EMT-I every 10 minutes.

_____ **6.** If a wound continues to bleed after it is bandaged, you should remove the bandage and start over again.

_____ **7.** Before inflation of any compartment of the PASG, you must auscultate breath sounds for pulmonary edema.

_____ **8.** Shock is considered to be hypothermia until proven otherwise.

1999 _____ **9.** The cardiac monitor should be placed on all patients in shock to detect possible dysrhythmias.

Short Answer

Complete this section with short written answers in the space provided.

1. List, in the proper sequence, the methods by which an EMT-I should attempt to control external bleeding.

_____

_____

_____

2. Discuss compensated shock.

_____

_____

_____

3. Discuss decompensated shock.

_____

_____

_____

4. Discuss irreversible shock.

_____

_____

_____

Word Fun EMT-I vocab explorer web

The following crossword puzzle is an activity provided to reinforce correct spelling and understanding of medical terminology associated with emergency care and the EMT-I. Use the clues in the column to complete the puzzle.

Across

3. Discoloration of skin from closed wound

5. Mass of blood in soft tissues

6. Lack of normal clotting factors

7. Circulatory system failure

8. Low blood volume; inadequate perfusion

9. Circulation of blood within the body

Down

1. Nosebleed

2. Bleeding

4. Formation of clots to stop bleeding

Ambulance Calls

The following real case scenarios provide an opportunity to explore the concerns associated with patient management. Read each scenario, then answer each question in detail.

1. You are dispatched to a school playground for an 8-year-old male complaining of a minor laceration to his left wrist with uncontrollable hemorrhaging. The teacher tells you that he has a history of hemophilia. The blood is steady but not spurting and is dark in color.

How would you best manage this patient?

_____

_____

_____

_____

_____

_____

_____

_____

2. You are called to the scene of a motor vehicle crash with major damage to the front of the vehicle where your patient was the restrained driver. She is a 23-year-old female with no pertinent medical history, according to a passenger in the vehicle. She is responsive to pain and showing signs of hypovolemic shock. Her only visible injury is a bruise to her right upper quadrant.

How would you best manage this patient?

_____

_____

_____

_____

_____

_____

_____

3. You are dispatched to aid a 22-year-old male with a history of depression. Upon arrival, police on scene tell you he tried to commit suicide by cutting his wrist. He has a laceration to the right radial artery with bright red, spurting blood. He has lost what looks to be possibly 2 pints of blood.

How would you best manage this patient?

_____

_____

_____

_____

_____

_____

_____

4. You are working a standby at a local high school football game when a player "goes down" on the field. The coach signals you. Your patient is a 17-year-old who has an altered LOC and difficulty breathing. He is not moving.

How would you best manage this patient?

_____

_____

_____

_____

_____

_____

_____

_____

Skill Drills EMT-I video clips web

Skill Drill 13-1: Controlling External Bleeding
Test your knowledge of this skill drill by filling in the correct words in the photo captions.

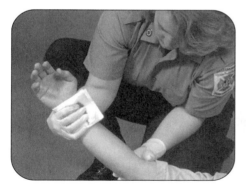
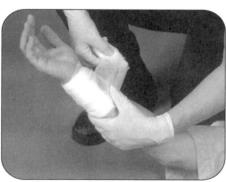
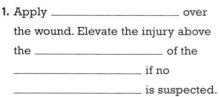

1. Apply _____ over the wound. Elevate the injury above the _____ of the _____ if no _____ is suspected.

2. Apply a _____.

3. Apply pressure at the appropriate _____ while continuing to hold _____.

Skill Drill 13-2: Applying a Pneumatic Antishock Garment (PASG)

Test your knowledge of this skill drill by placing the photos below in the correct order. Number the first step with a "1," the second step with a "2," etc.

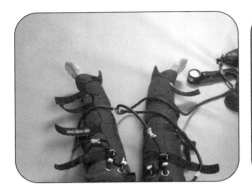

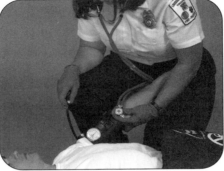

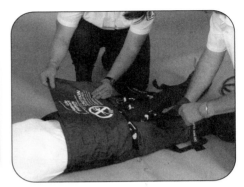

Inflate with the foot pump until the patient's blood pressure reaches 90 to 100 mm Hg or the Velcro crackles. Monitor radial pulses.

Check the patient's blood pressure again. Monitor vital signs.

Rapidly expose and examine the areas to be covered by the PASG. Pad any exposed bone ends.

Apply the garment so that the top is below the lowest rib.

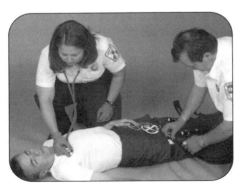

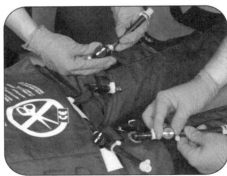

Open the stopcocks.

Auscultate breath sounds for pulmonary edema before inflation of any compartment.

Close and fasten both leg compartments and the abdominal compartment.

Skill Drill 13-4: Treating Shock

Test your knowledge of this skill drill by placing the photos below in the correct order. Number the first step with a "1," the second step with a "2," etc.

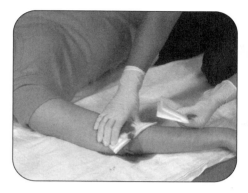

_____

Control obvious external bleeding.

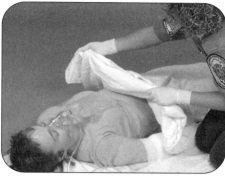

_____

Place blankets under and over the patient.

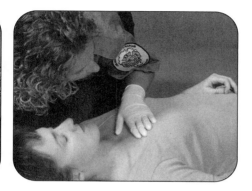

_____

Keep the patient supine, open the airway, and check breathing and pulse.

Give high-flow oxygen and assist ventilations if needed.

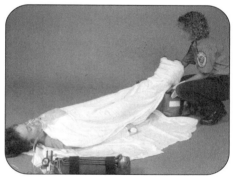

_____

If no fractures are suspected, elevate the legs 6" to 12".

Start an IV and administer fluid.

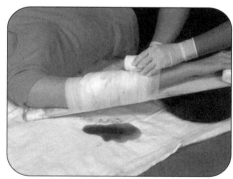

_____

Splint any broken bones or joint injuries.

Workbook Activities

The following activities have been designed to help you. Your instructor may require you to complete some or all of these activities as a regular part of your EMT-I training program. You are encouraged to complete any activity that your instructor does not assign as a way to enhance your learning in the classroom.

Chapter Review

The following exercises provide an opportunity to refresh your knowledge of this chapter.

Matching

Match each of the terms in the left column to the appropriate definition in the right column.

_____ 1. Dermis

_____ 2. Sweat glands

_____ 3. Epidermis

_____ 4. Mucous membranes

_____ 5. Sebaceous glands

_____ 6. Abrasion

_____ 7. Laceration

_____ 8. Hemothorax

_____ 9. Penetrating wound

_____ 10. Avulsion

_____ 11. Evisceration

_____ 12. Pneumothorax

A. gunshot wound

B. cool the body by discharging a substance through the pores

C. tissue hanging as a flap from wound

D. tough external layer forming a watertight covering for the body

E. razor cut

F. secrete a watery substance that lubricates the openings of the mouth and nose

G. inner layer of skin that contains the structures that give skin its characteristic appearance

H. air around the lungs

I. produce oil, which waterproofs the skin and keeps it supple

J. blood collecting inside chest

K. exposed intestines

L. skinned knee

Multiple Choice

Read each item carefully, then select the best response.

_____ 1. The _____ is (are) our first line of defense against external forces.

A. extremities

B. hair

C. skin

D. lips

_____ 2. The skin covering the _____ is quite thick.

A. lips

B. scalp

C. ears

D. eyelids

Burns and Soft-Tissue Injuries

_____ **3.** As the cells on the surface of the skin are worn away, new cells form in the _____ layer.

    A. dermal

    B. germinal

    C. epidermal

    D. subcutaneous

_____ **4.** The hair follicles, sweat glands, and sebaceous glands are found in the:

    A. dermis.

    B. germinal layer.

    C. epidermis.

    D. subcutaneous layer.

_____ **5.** The skin regulates temperature in a cold environment by:

    A. secreting sweat through sweat glands.

    B. constricting the blood vessels.

    C. dilating the blood vessels.

    D. increasing the amount of heat that is radiated from the body's surface.

_____ **6.** Closed soft-tissue injuries are characterized by all of the following EXCEPT:

    A. pain at the site of injury.

    B. swelling beneath the skin.

    C. damage to the protective layer of skin.

    D. a history of blunt trauma.

_____ **7.** A(n) _____ occurs whenever a large blood vessel is damaged and bleeds.

    A. contusion

    B. hematoma

    C. crushing injury

    D. avulsion

_____ **8.** A(n) _____ is usually associated with extensive tissue damage.

    A. contusion

    B. hematoma

    C. crushing injury

    D. avulsion

_____ **9.** A hematoma can result from:

    A. a soft-tissue injury.

    B. a fracture.

    C. any injury to a large blood vessel.

    D. all of the above

_____ **10.** A(n) _____ occurs when a great amount of force is applied to the body for a long period of time.

    A. contusion

    B. hematoma

    C. crushing injury

    D. avulsion

_____ **11.** More extensive closed injuries may involve significant swelling and bleeding beneath the skin, which could lead to:

    A. compartment syndrome.

    B. contamination.

    C. hypovolemic shock.

    D. hemothorax.

_____ **12.** The "S" in ICES stands for:

    A. swelling.

    B. soft tissue.

    C. splinting.

    D. shock.

_____ **13.** Open soft-tissue wounds include all of the following EXCEPT:

    A. abrasions.

    B. contusions.

    C. lacerations.

    D. avulsions.

_____ **14.** An abrasion is:

    A. superficial.

    B. deep.

    C. full thickness.

    D. none of the above.

_____ **15.** A laceration may be:

    A. superficial.

    B. deep.

    C. jagged.

    D. all of the above.

_____ **16.** Bleeding from avulsions can usually be controlled by:

    A. elevation.

    B. pressure dressings.

    C. tourniquets.

    D. pressure points.

_____ **17.** The amount of damage from a gunshot wound is directly related to the:

    A. size of the entrance wound.

    B. size of the bullet.

    C. size of the exit wound.

    D. speed of the bullet.

_____ **18.** Because shootings usually end up in court, it is important to factually and completely document:

    A. the circumstances surrounding any gunshot injury.

    B. the patient's condition.

    C. the treatment given.

    D. all of the above.

_____ **19.** All open wounds are assumed to be _____ and present a risk of infection.

    A. contaminated

    B. life threatening

    C. minimal

    D. extensive

_____ **20.** Before you begin caring for a patient with an open wound, you should:

    A. survey the scene.

    B. follow BSI precautions.

    C. be sure the patient has an open airway.

    D. all of the above.

_____ **21.** Splinting an extremity, even when there is no fracture, can help by:

    A. reducing pain.

    B. minimizing damage to an already injured extremity.

    C. making it easier to move the patient.

    D. all of the above.

_____ **22.** On inhalation, pressure inside the chest cavity _____, allowing air to enter.

    A. increases

    B. decreases

    C. equalizes

    D. stabilizes

_____ **23.** Treatment for evisceration includes:

    A. pushing the exposed organs back into the abdominal cavity.

    B. covering the organs with dry dressings.

    C. flexing the knees and legs to relieve pressure on the abdomen.

    D. applying moist adherent dressings.

_____ **24.** An open neck injury may result in (an) _____ if enough air is sucked into a blood vessel.

    A. hypovolemic shock

    B. tracheal deviation

    C. air embolism

    D. subcutaneous emphysema

_____ **25.** Burns may result from:

    A. heat.

    B. toxic chemicals.

    C. electricity.

    D. all of the above.

_____ **26.** Mechanisms of burn injury include:

    A. scalding.

    B. steam.

    C. flames.

    D. all of the above.

_____ **27.** Burns cause local and systemic responses such as:

   A. release of catecholamines.

   B. vasoconstriction.

   C. fluid shift.

   D. all of the above.

_____ **28.** The burn process releases _____ from dead or dying cells into the bloodstream that may plug tubules in the kidneys, leading to renal failure.

   A. catecholamines

   B. hemoglobin

   C. myoglobin

   D. sodium

_____ **29.** Factors that help determine the severity of a burn include:

   A. the depth of the burn.

   B. the extent of the burn.

   C. whether or not there are critical areas involved.

   D. all of the above.

_____ **30.** _____ burns involve only the epidermis.

   A. Full-thickness

   B. Second-degree

   C. Superficial

   D. Third-degree

_____ **31.** _____ burns cause intense pain.

   A. First-degree

   B. Second-degree

   C. Superficial

   D. Third-degree

_____ **32.** _____ burns may involve subcutaneous layers, muscle, bone, or internal organs.

   A. Superficial

   B. Partial-thickness

   C. Full-thickness

   D. Second-degree

_____ **33.** With _____ burns, the area is dry and leathery and may appear white, dark brown, or even charred.

   A. first-degree

   B. second-degree

   C. partial-thickness

   D. third-degree

_____ **34.** Significant airway burns may be associated with:

   A. singeing of the hair in the nostrils.

   B. hoarseness.

   C. hypoxia.

   D. all of the above.

_____ **35.** The size of the patient's palm is roughly equal to _____ of the patient's total body surface area.

   A. 1%

   B. 3%

   C. 5%

   D. 10%

1999 _____ **36.** Treatment for chemical burns includes:
   A. ECG monitoring.
   B. pain medication.
   C. steroids for inflammation.
   D. all of the above.

_____ **37.** If an acid or strong alkali has burned the eye, flush for:
   A. 5 minutes.
   B. 10 minutes.
   C. 20 minutes.
   D. 30 minutes.

_____ **38.** The most important consideration when dealing with electrical burns is:
   A. BSI precautions.
   B. scene safety.
   C. level of responsiveness.
   D. airway.

_____ **39.** Electrical injuries may cause:
   A. cardiac dysrhythmias.
   B. thermal injuries.
   C. vascular injuries.
   D. all of the above.

_____ **40.** Treatment of electrical burns includes:
   A. maintaining the airway.
   B. monitoring the patient closely for respiratory or cardiac arrest.
   C. splinting any suspected injuries.
   D. all of the above.

_____ **41.** Radiation particles that can be stopped by paper are _____ particles.
   A. alpha
   B. beta
   C. gamma
   D. all of the above

_____ **42.** _____ rays have enough energy to pass entirely through a body.
   A. Alpha
   B. Beta
   C. Gamma
   D. All of the above

_____ **43.** The amount of radiation exposure depends on:
   A. time.
   B. distance.
   C. shielding.
   D. all of the above.

1999 _____ **44.** Treatment for radiation burns includes:
   A. IV access.
   B. ECG monitoring.
   C. early intubation for unresponsive patients.
   D. all of the above.

_____ **45.** All of the following, EXCEPT _____, may be used as an occlusive dressing.

    A. gauze pads

    B. Vaseline gauze

    C. aluminum foil

    D. plastic

_____ **46.** Using elastic bandages to secure dressings may result in _____ if the injury swells or if improperly applied.

    A. additional tissue damage

    B. loss of a limb

    C. impaired circulation

    D. all of the above

1999 _____ **47.** Treatment for the burn injury patient includes:

    A. ECG monitoring.

    B. early intubation with inhalation injury.

    C. analgesics.

    D. all of the above.

Labeling EMT-I anatomy review web

Label the following diagrams with the correct terms.

Skin

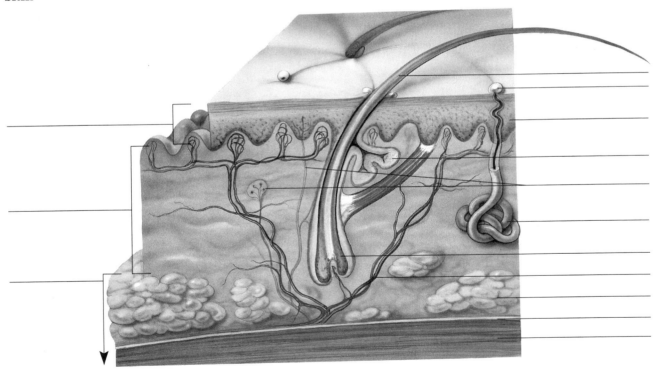

Classifications of Burns

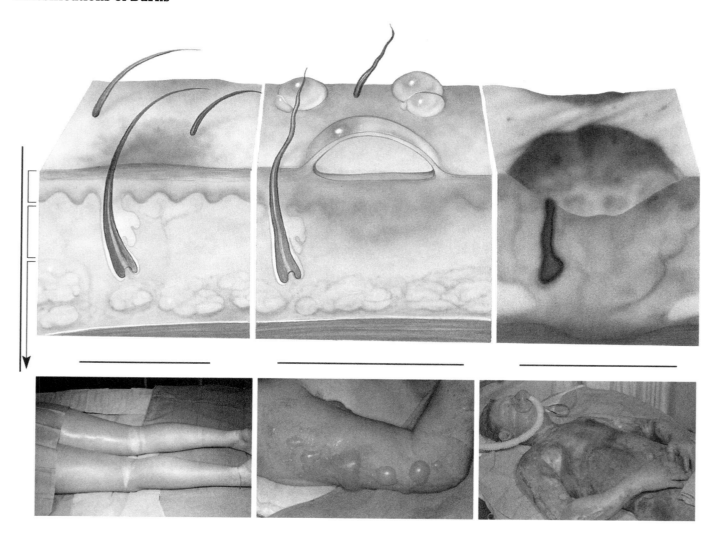

Rule of Nines

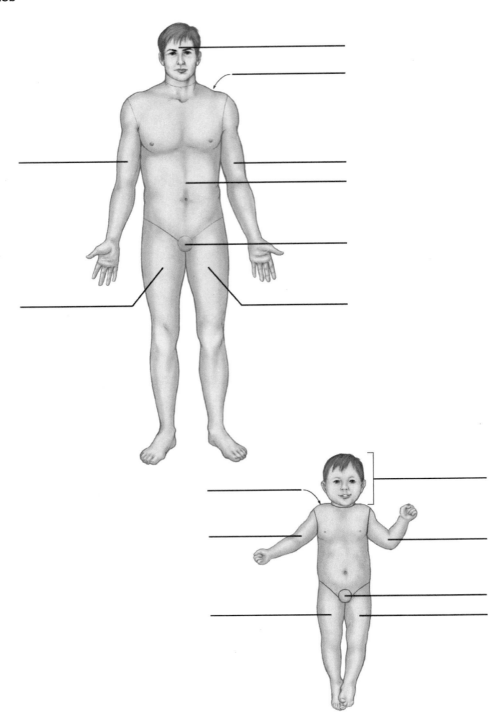

Vocabulary

Define the following terms in the space provided.

1. Partial-thickness burn:

_____

_____

_____

2. Closed injury:

_____

_____

_____

3. Evisceration:

_____

_____

_____

4. Compartment syndrome:

_____

_____

_____

5. Contamination:

_____

_____

_____

6. Tetany:

_____

_____

_____

7. Eschar:

_____

_____

_____

Fill-in

Read each item carefully, then complete the statement by filling in the missing word(s).

1. Mucous membranes are _____.

2. A person will sweat in an effort to _____ the body.

3. Nerve endings are located in the _____.

4. Below the dermis lies the _____ tissue.

5. In cold weather, skin blood vessels will _____.

6. The skin protects the body by keeping _____ out and _____ in.

7. Because nerve endings are present, injury to the _____ may be painful.

8. A major function of the skin is regulating body _____.

9. The external layer of skin is the _____ and the inner layer is the _____.

10. When the vessels of the skin dilate, heat is _____ from the body.

11. Exercise great care when _____ an impaled object because a small amount of movement

on the proximal end will cause a significant amount of movement on the distal end.

1999 **12.** Consider _____ if signs of rapid airway swelling are present.

13. Burns around the face or exposure to superheated air tend to result in _____ and

_____ compromise.

14. Always brush _____ off the skin and clothing before flushing the patient with water.

15. With electrical burns, _____ and _____ are common entrance sites and

_____ are common exit sites.

True/False

If you believe the statement to be more true than false, write the letter "T" in the space provided. If you believe the statement to be more false than true, write the letter "F."

_____ **1.** Partial-thickness burns involve the epidermis and some portion of the dermis.
_____ **2.** Blisters are commonly seen with superficial burns.
_____ **3.** Severe burns are usually a combination of superficial, partial-thickness, and full-thickness burns.
_____ **4.** The rule of nines allows you to estimate the percentage of body surface area that has been burned.
_____ **5.** Two factors, depth and extent, are critical in assessing the severity of a burn.
_____ **6.** Your first responsibility with a burn patient is to stop the burning process.
_____ **7.** Burned areas should be immersed in cool water for up to 30 minutes.
_____ **8.** Upper airway edema is a late consequence of inhalation injury.
_____ **9.** Thermal injury to the lower airway is rare.
_____ **10.** Caustic injuries to the eyes will produce burns similar to thermal burns.
_____ **11.** Touching a patient who is still in contact with a live power line can be fatal to you.

_____ **12.** Any living tissue in the human body can be damaged by ionizing radiation.

_____ **13.** Electrical burns are always more severe than the external signs indicate.

_____ **14.** The universal dressing is ideal for covering large open wounds.

_____ **15.** Occlusive dressings are usually made of Vaseline gauze, aluminum foil, or plastic.

_____ **16.** Gauze pads prevent air and liquids from entering or exiting the wound.

_____ **17.** Elastic bandages can be used to secure dressings.

_____ **18.** Soft roller bandages are slightly elastic and the layers adhere somewhat to one another.

_____ **19.** Ecchymosis is associated with open wounds.

_____ **20.** A laceration is considered a closed wound.

Short Answer

Complete this section with short written answers in the space provided.

1. List the three major classifications of burn depth.

2. List the three general classifications of soft-tissue injuries.

3. Define the mnemonic ICES.

I: _____

C: _____

E: _____

S: _____

4. Describe the classifications of a critical burn for an infant or child.

5. What treatment should be used with a patient burned by a dry chemical?

6. Why are electrical burns particularly dangerous to a patient?

_____

_____

_____

7. Describe a sucking chest wound.

_____

_____

_____

8. List the three primary functions of dressings and bandages.

_____

_____

_____

9. List the four types of open soft-tissue injuries.

_____

_____

_____

10. List the five factors used to determine the severity of a burn.

_____

_____

_____

11. List the Parkland formula

_____

_____

_____

12. List the common signs and symptoms of a burn injury.

_____

_____

_____

13. List three types of inhalation injuries.

_____

_____

_____

14. List three types of ionizing radiation.

_____

_____

_____

Word Fun EMT-I

The following crossword puzzle is an activity provided to reinforce correct spelling and understanding of medical terminology associated with emergency care and the EMT-I.

Use the clues in the column to complete the puzzle.

Across

2. Presence of infective organisms

3. Blood collected in soft tissues

6. Bruise

7. Torn completely loose or hanging as a flap

8. Displacement of organs outside the body

9. Inner layer of skin

10. Injury from sharp, pointed objects

Down

1. Discoloration associated with closed injury

4. Lining of body cavities and passages with contact to outside

5. Assigns percentages to burns

7. Scraping injury

Ambulance Calls

The following real case scenarios provide an opportunity to explore the concerns associated with patient management. Read each scenario, then answer each question in detail.

1. You are dispatched to a residence where a 10-year-old female fell onto a jagged piece of metal and has a gaping laceration to the right upper arm that is spurting bright red blood. The mother tried to control bleeding with a towel, but it kept soaking through.

   How would you best manage this patient?

   _____

   _____

   _____

   _____

   _____

   _____

   _____

   _____

2. You are called to an industrial plant for a 26-year-old male complaining of a crush injury of his left foot. Bleeding is moderate, and a portion of the dorsal aspect is partially avulsed. He is alert and oriented.

   How would you best manage this patient?

   _____

   _____

   _____

   _____

   _____

   _____

   _____

   _____

3. You are dispatched to stand by at a structure fire. Suddenly, fire fighters emerge from the residence with a 40-year-old female who is coughing violently. She has second-degree burns to both hands and forearms and on her abdomen. She is alert and having mild difficulty breathing.

How would you best manage this patient?

_____

_____

_____

_____

_____

_____

_____

4. You are called to a residence where you find a 2-year-old female with "sock-like" burns to both feet. The skin on her feet is blistered and sloughing.

How would you best manage this patient?

_____

_____

_____

_____

_____

_____

_____

Skill Drills EMT-I video clips web

Skill Drill 14-1: Controlling Bleeding from a Soft-Tissue Injury

Test your knowledge of this skill drill by filling in the correct words in the photo captions.

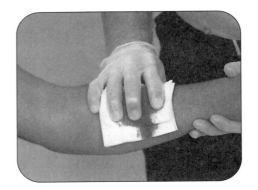

1. Apply _____ with a
   _____.

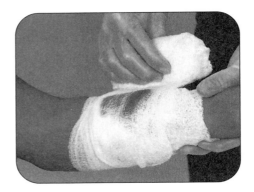

2. Maintain pressure with a
   _____ bandage.

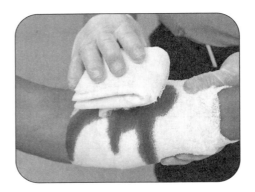

3. If bleeding continues, apply a second
   _____ and
   _____ bandage
   over the first.

4. _____ the extremity.

Skill Drill 14-2: Sealing a Sucking Chest Wound
Test your knowledge of this skill drill by filling in the correct words in the photo captions.

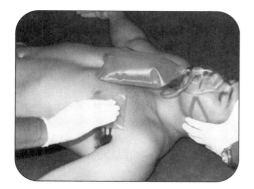

1. Keep the patient

_____ and give

_____.

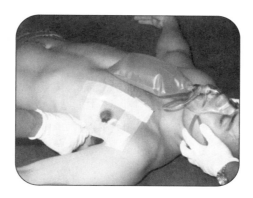

2. Seal the wound with a(n)

_____ dressing.

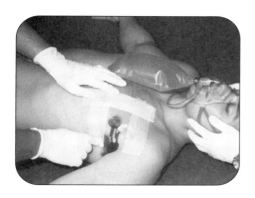

3. Follow _____ re-

garding sealing or

_____ the dressing's

fourth side.

Skill Drill 14-3: Stabilizing an Impaled Object

Test your knowledge of this skill drill by filling in the correct words in the photo captions.

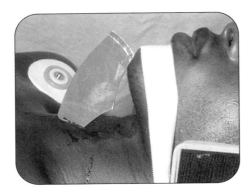

1. Do not attempt to _____ or _____ the object.

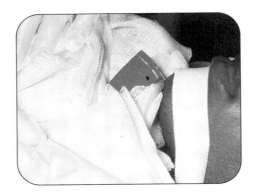

2. Control _____ and _____ the object in place using _____, _____, and/or _____.

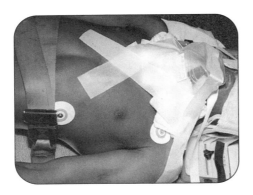

3. Tape a _____ item over the stabilized object to protect it from _____ during transport.

Chapter 14 Burns and Soft-Tissue Injuries **193**

Skill Drill 14-4: Caring for Burns
Test your knowledge of this skill drill by placing the photos below in the correct order. Number the first step with a "1," the second step with a "2," etc.

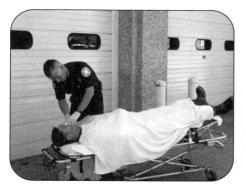

_____

Estimate the severity of the burn, then cover the area with a dry, sterile dressing or clean sheet.

Assess and treat the patient for any other injuries.

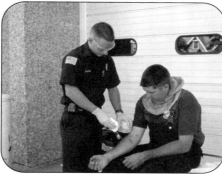

_____

Follow BSI precautions and use sterile technique to help prevent infection.

Remove the patient from the burning area; extinguish or remove hot clothing and jewelry as needed.

If the wound(s) is still burning or hot, immerse the hot area in cool, sterile water, or cover with a wet, cool dressing.

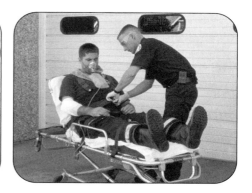

_____

Cover the patient with blankets to prevent loss of body heat.

Transport promptly.

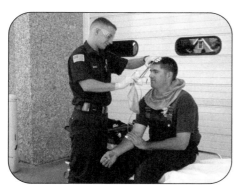

_____

Provide high-flow oxygen and continue to assess the airway.

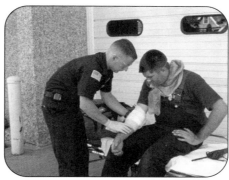

_____

Prepare for transport.

Treat for shock if needed.

Workbook Activities

The following activities have been designed to help you. Your instructor may require you to complete some or all of these activities as a regular part of your EMT-I training program. You are encouraged to complete any activity that your instructor does not assign as a way to enhance your learning in the classroom.

Chapter Review

The following exercises provide an opportunity to refresh your knowledge of this chapter.

Matching

Match each of the terms in the left column to the appropriate definition in the right column.

_____ **1.** Thoracic cage   **A.** chest rises

_____ **2.** Diaphragm   **B.** chest

_____ **3.** Exhalation   **C.** chest falls

_____ **4.** Inhalation   **D.** separates chest from abdomen

_____ **5.** Aorta   **E.** major artery in the chest

_____ **6.** Closed chest injury   **F.** penetrating wound

_____ **7.** Hemoptysis   **G.** rapid respirations

_____ **8.** Pericardium   **H.** unusually blunt trauma

_____ **9.** Open chest injury   **I.** coughing up blood

_____ **10.** Tachypnea   **J.** sac around the heart

Multiple Choice

Read each item carefully, then select the best response.

_____ **1.** Air is supplied to the lungs via the:

    A. esophagus.

    B. trachea.

    C. nares.

    D. oropharynx.

_____ **2.** The _____ separates the thoracic cavity from the abdominal cavity.

    A. diaphragm

    B. mediastinum

    C. xyphoid process

    D. inferior border of the ribs

Thoracic Trauma

_____ **3.** On inhalation, all of the following occur EXCEPT:

   A. the intercostal muscles contract, elevating the rib cage.

   B. the diaphragm contracts.

   C. the pressure inside the chest increases.

   D. air enters through the nose and mouth.

_____ **4.** Blunt trauma to the chest may:

   A. bruise the lungs and heart.

   B. fracture whole areas of the chest wall.

   C. damage the aorta.

   D. all of the above.

_____ **5.** Symptoms of chest injury include:

   A. cyanosis around the lips or fingertips.

   B. rapid, weak pulse.

   C. hemoptysis.

   D. pain at the site of injury.

_____ **6.** Common causes of dyspnea include:

   A. airway obstruction.

   B. lung compression.

   C. damage to the chest wall.

   D. all of the above.

_____ **7.** _____ occurs when the chest wall does not expand on each side when the patient inhales.

   A. Flail segment

   B. Paradoxical motion

   C. Pneumothorax

   D. Hemoptysis

_____ **8.** Irritation of or damage to the pleural surfaces causes sharp or stabbing pain with each breath. This is known as:

   A. dyspnea.

   B. pneumonia.

   C. pleurisy.

   D. tachypnea.

_____ **9.** Bowel sounds heard in the lower hemithorax could indicate:

   A. pneumothorax.

   B. diaphragmatic rupture.

   C. evisceration.

   D. hemothorax.

1999 _____ **10.** When assessing the ECG of a patient with thoracic trauma, note any:

   A. ST-segment elevation.

   B. ST-segment depression.

   C. dysrhythmias.

   D. all of the above.

1999 _____ **11.** Management for patients with thoracic trauma includes:

   A. early intubation.

   B. antiarrhythmics.

   C. analgesics.

   D. all of the above.

_____ **12.** Rib fractures are most often caused by:

   A. pneumothorax.

   B. blunt trauma.

   C. penetrating trauma.

   D. subcutaneous emphysema.

_____ **13.** _____, or collapse of the alveoli, decreases the surface area for gas exchange.

   A. Atelectesis

   B. Subcutaneous emphysema

   C. Hemoptysis

   D. Hemothorax

_____ **14.** Assessment findings in the patient with fractured ribs would include all of the following EXCEPT:

   A. pain on palpation.

   B. deep breathing.

   C. crepitus.

   D. guarding or splinting.

_____ **15.** The mortality rate in patients with a sternal fracture is:

   A. 10 to 25%.

   B. 15 to 35%.

   C. 25 to 45%.

   D. 50 to 100%.

_____ **16.** The principle reason for concern about a patient who has a chest injury is:

   A. hemoptysis.

   B. cyanosis.

   C. that the body has no means of storing oxygen.

   D. a rapid, weak pulse and low blood pressure.

_____ **17.** A _____ results when an injury allows air to enter through a hole in the chest wall or the surface of the lung as the patient attempts to breathe, causing the lung on that side to collapse.

   A. tension pneumothorax

   B. hemothorax

   C. hemopneumothorax

   D. pneumothorax

_____ **18.** Management of thoracic trauma includes:

   A. a 20-mL/kg bolus of isotonic crystalloid solution.

   B. a possible need for early endotrachael intubation.

   C. analgesics for pain per protocol.

   D. all of the above.

_____ **19.** A spontaneous pneumothorax:

    A. presents with a sudden sharp chest pain.

    B. presents with increasing difficulty breathing.

    C. should be treated the same as a traumatic pneumothorax.

    D. all of the above.

_____ **20.** As a pneumothorax develops tension:

    A. air gradually increases the pressure in the chest.

    B. it causes the complete collapse of the affected lung.

    C. it prevents blood from returning through the venae cavae to the heart.

    D. all of the above.

_____ **21.** Common signs and symptoms of tension pneumothorax include:

    A. increasing respiratory distress.

    B. distended neck veins.

    C. tracheal deviation away from the injured site.

    D. all of the above.

_____ **22.** A hemothorax results from blood collecting in the pleural space from:

    A. a bleeding rib cage.

    B. a bleeding lung.

    C. a bleeding great vessel.

    D. all of the above.

_____ **23.** All of the following are signs or symptoms of a tension pneumothorax EXCEPT:

    A. tachycardia.

    B. anxiety.

    C. hypertension.

    D. cyanosis.

_____ **24.** Assessment findings of narrowing pulse pressure, neck vein distension, and muffled heart tones are classic signs of cardiac tamponade and are known as:

    A. Grey Turner's sign.

    B. Beck triad.

    C. Cushing triad.

    D. Cullen's sign.

1999 _____ **25.** ECG changes seen in patients with myocardial contusions include all EXCEPT:

    A. persistant bradycardia.

    B. atrial fibrillation.

    C. PVCs.

    D. ST-segment elevation.

_____ **26.** A fractured rib that penetrates into the pleural space may lacerate the surface of the lung, causing a:

    A. tension pneumothorax.

    B. hemothorax.

    C. hemopneumothorax.

    D. all of the above.

_____ **27.** In what is called paradoxical movement, the detached portion of the chest wall:

    A. moves opposite of normal.

    B. moves out instead of in during inhalation.

    C. moves in instead of out during expiration.

    D. all of the above.

_____ **28.** Traumatic asphyxia:

    A. is bruising of the lung.

    B. occurs when three or more adjacent ribs are fractured in two or more places.

    C. is a sudden, severe compression of the chest.

    D. all of the above.

_____ **29.** Traumatic asphyxia results in a very characteristic appearance, including:

    A. distended neck veins.

    B. cyanosis.

    C. hemorrhage into the sclera of the eye.

    D. all of the above.

_____ **30.** Signs and symptoms of a pericardial tamponade include:

    A. low blood pressure.

    B. a weak pulse.

    C. muffled heart tones.

    D. all of the above.

_____ **31.** Large blood vessels in the chest thatm when injured, can result in massive hemorrhaging include all of the following EXCEPT:

    A. the pulmonary arteries.

    B. the femoral arteries.

    C. the aorta.

    D. four main pulmonary veins.

Labeling

Label the following diagrams with the correct terms.

Anterior Aspect of the Chest

A. _____

B. _____

C. _____

D. _____

E. _____

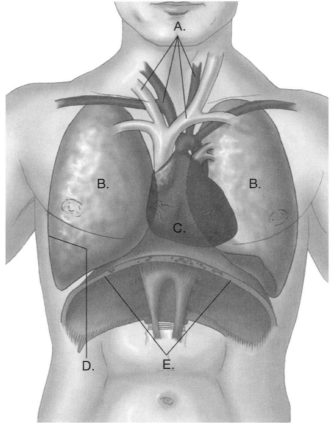

Ribs

A. _____

B. _____

C. _____

D. _____

E. _____

F. _____

G. _____

H. _____

I. _____

J. _____

K. _____

L. _____

M. _____

N. _____

O. _____

P. _____

Q. _____

R. _____

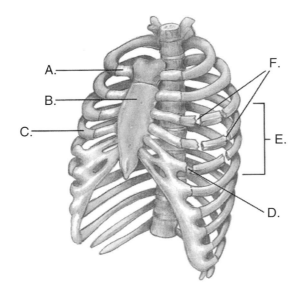

Flail Chest

A. _____

B. _____

C. _____

D. _____

E. _____

F. _____

Hemothorax and Hemopneumothorax

A. _____

B. _____

C. _____

D. _____

E. _____

F. _____

G. _____

H. _____

I. _____

J. _____

K. _____

L. _____

Vocabulary EMT-I

Define the following terms in the space provided.

1. Flail chest:

_____

_____

_____

2. Paradoxical motion:

_____

_____

_____

3. Pericardial tamponade:

_____

_____

_____

4. Spontaneous pneumothorax:

_____

_____

_____

5. Sucking chest wound:

_____

_____

_____

6. Tension pneumothorax:

_____

_____

_____

7. Paper bag syndrome:

_____

_____

_____

8. Chemoreceptors:

_____

_____

_____

9. Bradypnea:

_____

_____

_____

Fill-in

Read each item carefully, then complete the statement by filling in the missing word.

1. The esophagus is located in the _____ portion of the chest.

2. During inhalation, the pressure in the chest _____.

3. In the anterior chest, ribs connect to the _____.

4. The trachea divides into the right and left main stem _____.

5. The _____ nerves supply the diaphragm.

6. Contents of the chest are protected by the _____.

7. The chest extends from the lower end of the neck to the _____.

8. _____ line the area between the lungs and chest wall.

9. The great vessel located in the chest is the _____.

10. During inhalation, the diaphragm _____.

11. _____ _____ are among the most important factors that influence the

rate and depth of breathing. These include changing levels of _____

_____, _____, and _____ _____.

12. Any injury that compromises the chest _____ _____ decreases air

exchange and subsequent oxygenation.

13. Nerves supplying the diaphragm exit the spinal cord at _____, _____,

and _____.

14. Thoracic trauma may impair _____ _____, decreasing blood pressure

and perfusion to vital organs.

15. Loss of peripheral pulse during inspiration suggests _____ _____.

16. A blow significant enough to fracture the sternum causes severe _____ of the thoracic

cage.

17. An open or penetrating wound to the chest is often called a _____

_____ _____.

18. With pulmonary contusions, the degree of respiratory compromise is directly related to the

_____ of the contused area.

19. The most common site of aortic rupture is the _____ _____.

20. The majority of tracheobronchial injuries occur within 3 cm of the _____.

True/False

If you believe the statement to be more true than false, write the letter "T" in the space provided. If you believe
the statement to be more false than true, write the letter "F."

_____ **1.** Dyspnea is difficulty with breathing.

_____ **2.** Tachypnea is slow respirations.

_____ **3.** Distended neck veins may be a sign of a tension pneumothorax.

_____ **4.** Rib fractures are common in children.

_____ **5.** Narrowing pulse pressure is related to spontaneous pneumothorax.

_____ **6.** Laceration of the large blood vessels in the chest can cause minimal hemorrhage.

_____ **7.** The thoracic cage extends from the lower end of the neck to the umbilicus.

_____ **8.** Patients with spinal cord injuries at C3 or above can lose their ability to breathe entirely.

_____ **9.** Almost one third of people who are killed immediately in car crashes die as a result of traumatic rupture of the myocardium.

_____ **10.** Pulmonary contusion is the most common injury from blunt thoracic trauma.

_____ **11.** You should tape a flail segment circumferentially around the chest.

_____ **12.** A fracture to the upper four ribs is a sign of a very severe mechanism of injury.

_____ **13.** The most common cause of a flail segment is a fall.

_____ **14.** Assessment findings of a flail chest would include paradoxical motion, pleuritic pain, crepitus, and tachypnea.

1999 _____ **15.** Monitor the ECG and be alert for cardiac dysrhythmias in patients with a flail chest.

1999 _____ **16.** Tracheal deviation away from the affected side is a finding that is always present in patients with a tension pneumothorax.

_____ **17.** Hypovolemia and respiratory compromise produce signs and symptoms of massive hemothorax.

_____ **18.** Conduction defects do not occur in patients with a myocardial contusion.

Short Answer

Complete this section with short written answers in the space provided.

1. List the signs and symptoms associated with a chest injury.

_____

_____

_____

1999 **2.** List the steps of needle decompression.

_____

_____

_____

3. Describe the method(s) for immobilizing a flail chest wall segment.

_____

_____

_____

4. Define traumatic asphyxia and describe its signs.

_____

_____

_____

Word Fun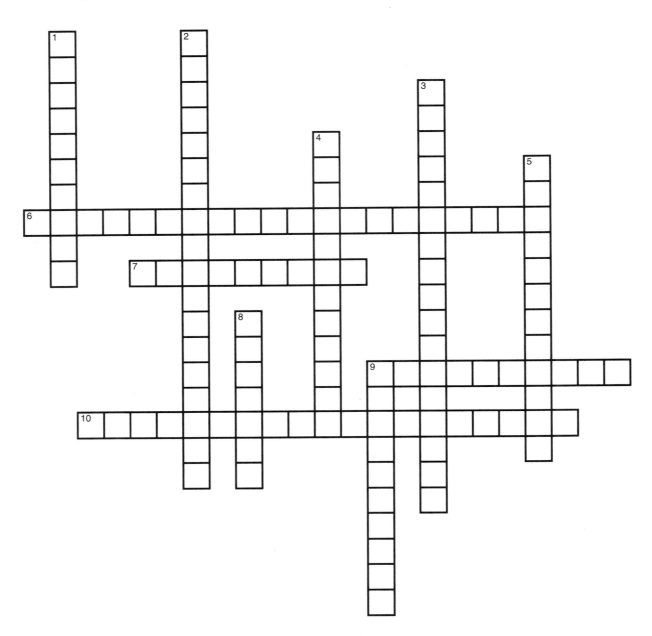

The following crossword puzzle is an activity provided to reinforce correct spelling and understanding of medical terminology associated with emergency care and the EMT-I. Use the clues in the column to complete the puzzle.

Across

6. Buildup of blood in sac around heart

7. Rapid breathing

9. Blood in pleural cavity

10. Accumulation of air in pleural cavity, causing pressure in cavity to rise

Down

1. Results from at least three fractured ribs in two or more places

2. Bruise of the lung

3. Opposite movement from normal

4. One-way valve allowing air to leave

5. Air in the pleural cavity

8. Difficulty breathing

9. Spitting or coughing up blood

Ambulance Calls

The following real case scenarios provide an opportunity to explore the concerns associated with patient management. Read each scenario, then answer each question in detail.

1. You are dispatched to a head-on motor vehicle crash. Your patient, a 67-year-old male unrestrained driver, is unresponsive and has a very weak pulse and decreasing respirations as you pull him from the vehicle. Once you have him immobilized on the long backboard, he becomes apneic and pulseless. How would you best manage this patient?

_____

_____

_____

_____

_____

_____

_____

2. Your patient, a 22-year-old male, is complaining of a sudden onset of right-sided chest pain with a sudden onset of difficulty breathing. He tells you he was out running when it started. How would you best manage this patient?

_____

_____

_____

_____

_____

_____

_____

_____

3. You are dispatched to a lumberyard where a 27-year-old male was crushed by a piece of heavy equipment. Coworkers pulled the equipment off the patient. He presents with distended neck veins, cyanosis, and bloodshot eyes.

How would you best manage this patient?

_____

_____

_____

_____

_____

_____

_____

4. You are called to a motor vehicle crash where a single vehicle left the roadway and struck a tree. The driver was unrestrained and is now complaining of severe pain to the left upper chest on inspiration. There is deformity to the ribs.

How would you best manage this patient?

_____

_____

_____

_____

_____

_____

_____

Skill Drills

1999 Skill Drill 15-1: Decompression of a Tension Pneumothorax

Test your knowledge by filling in the correct words in the photo captions.

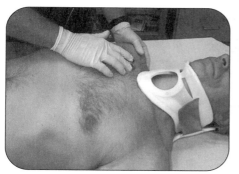

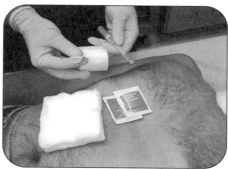

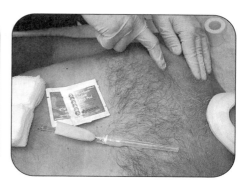

1. _____ the patient.

2. _____ and _____ necessary equipment. Obtain orders from _____ _____.

3. _____ the appropriate site.

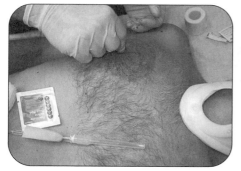

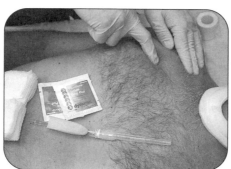

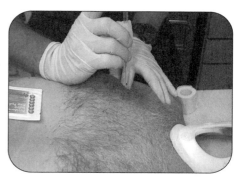

4. _____ the appropriate area using an _____ technique.

5. Make a _____ valve, or _____ valve.

6. Insert the needle at a _____ angle.

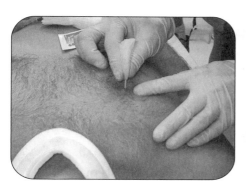

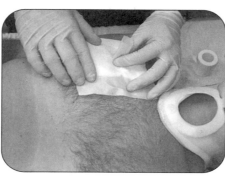

7. Remove the needle and listen for the _____ of _____. Properly _____ of the needle in the _____ _____.

8. Secure the _____ in place. _____ the patient closely for recurrence of the _____ _____.

Workbook Activities

The following activities have been designed to help you. Your instructor may require you to complete some or all of these activities as a regular part of your EMT-I training program. You are encouraged to complete any activity that your instructor does not assign as a way to enhance your learning in the classroom.

Chapter Review

The following exercises provide an opportunity to refresh your knowledge of this chapter.

Matching

Match each of the terms in the left column to the appropriate definition in the right column.

_____ **1.** Hollow organs

_____ **2.** Solid organs

_____ **3.** Peritonitis

_____ **4.** Genitourinary system

_____ **5.** Filtering system

_____ **6.** Evisceration

_____ **7.** Hematuria

_____ **8.** Peritoneal cavity

A. blood in urine

B. organs outside of the body

C. abdominal lining inflammation

D. kidneys, liver, spleen

E. kidneys

F. abdomen

G. stomach, bladder, ureters

H. controls reproductive functions and the waste discharge system

Multiple Choice

Read each item carefully, then select the best response.

_____ **1.** The abdomen contains several organs that make up the:

  A. digestive system.

  B. urinary system.

  C. genitourinary system.

  D. all of the above.

_____ **2.** Hollow organs of the abdomen include the:

  A. stomach.

  B. ureters.

  C. bladder.

  D. all of the above.

_____ **3.** Solid organs of the abdomen include all of the following EXCEPT:

  A. the liver.

  B. the spleen.

  C. the gallbladder.

  D. the pancreas.

CHAPTER 16

Abdomen and Genitalia Injuries

_____ **4.** The first signs of peritonitis include:

   A. severe abdominal pain.

   B. tenderness.

   C. muscular spasm.

   D. all of the above.

_____ **5.** Late signs of peritonitis may include:

   A. a soft abdomen.

   B. nausea.

   C. normal bowel sounds.

   D. all of the above.

_____ **6.** _____ takes place in the solid organs.

   A. Digestion

   B. Excretion

   C. Energy production

   D. All of the above

_____ **7.** Because solid organs have a rich supply of blood, any injury can result in major:

   A. hemorrhaging.

   B. damage.

   C. pain.

   D. guarding.

_____ **8.** A patient who has abdominal bleeding may experience all of the following EXCEPT:

   A. pain or tenderness.

   B. rigidity.

   C. urticaria.

   D. distention.

_____ **9.** The major soft-tissue landmarks is/are the _____, which overlie(s) the fourth lumbar vertebra.

   A. iliac crests

   B. umbilicus

   C. pubic symphysis

   D. anterior iliac spines

_____ **10.** The abdomen is divided into four:
  A. quadrants.
  B. planes.
  C. sections.
  D. angles.

_____ **11.** Injuries to the abdomen may involve:
  A. hollow organs.
  B. open injuries.
  C. solid organs.
  D. all of the above.

_____ **12.** Open abdominal injuries are also known as:
  A. blunt injuries.
  B. eviscerations.
  C. penetrating injuries.
  D. peritoneal injuries.

_____ **13.** Closed abdominal injuries may result from:
  A. a stab wound.
  B. seat belts.
  C. a gunshot wound.
  D. all of the above.

_____ **14.** The major complaint of patients with abdominal injury is:
  A. pain.
  B. tachycardia.
  C. rigidity.
  D. swelling.

_____ **15.** The most common sign of significant abdominal injury is:
  A. pain.
  B. tachycardia.
  C. rigidity.
  D. distention.

_____ **16.** Late signs of abdominal injury include all of the following EXCEPT:
  A. distention.
  B. increased blood pressure.
  C. rigidity.
  D. shallow respirations.

_____ **17.** Your primary concern when dealing with an unresponsive patient with an open abdominal injury is:
  A. covering the wound with a moist dressing.
  B. maintaining the airway.
  C. controlling the bleeding.
  D. monitoring vital signs.

_____ **18.** A patient with blunt abdominal trauma may present with:
  A. severe bruises on the abdominal wall.
  B. laceration of the liver or spleen.
  C. rupture of the intestine.
  D. all of the above.

_____ **19.** It is imperative that a patient who has received severe blunt abdominal trauma be:
  A. log rolled onto a backboard.
  B. transported rapidly.
  C. given oxygen.
  D. all of the above.

_____ **20.** When used alone, diagonal shoulder safety belts can cause:

    A. a bruised chest.

    B. a lacerated liver.

    C. decapitation.

    D. all of the above.

_____ **21.** When evaluating a patient involved in a motor vehicle crash where airbags have deployed, it is important to look for:

    A. debris inside the vehicle.

    B. condition of the tires.

    C. damage to the steering column underneath the airbag.

    D. all of the above.

_____ **22.** Patients with penetrating abdominal injuries often complain of:

    A. pain.

    B. nausea.

    C. vomiting.

    D. all of the above.

_____ **23.** When caring for a patient with a penetrating abdominal injury, you should assume that the object:

    A. has penetrated the peritoneum.

    B. entered the abdominal cavity.

    C. possibly injured one or more organs.

    D. all of the above.

_____ **24.** When treating a patient with an evisceration, you should:

    A. attempt to replace the abdominal contents.

    B. cover the protruding organs with a dry sterile dressing.

    C. cover the protruding organs with moist adherent dressings.

    D. cover the protruding contents with moist sterile gauze compresses.

_____ **25.** The solid organs of the urinary system include the:

    A. kidneys.

    B. ureters.

    C. bladder.

    D. urethra.

_____ **26.** All of the male genitalia lie outside the pelvic cavity, with the exception of the:

    A. urethra.

    B. penis.

    C. seminal vesicles.

    D. testes.

_____ **27.** Suspect kidney damage if the patient has a history or physical evidence of:

    A. an abrasion, laceration, or contusion in the flank.

    B. a penetrating wound in the region of the lower rib cage or the upper abdomen.

    C. fractures on either side of the lower rib cage.

    D. all of the above.

_____ **28.** Signs of injury to the kidney may include:

    A. bruises or lacerations on the overlying skin.

    B. shock.

    C. hematuria.

    D. all of the above.

_____ **29.** Suspect a possible injury of the urinary bladder with all of the following findings EXCEPT:

  A. bruising to the left upper quadrant.

  B. blood at the urethral opening.

  C. blood at the tip of the penis or a stain on the patient's underwear.

  D. physical signs of trauma on the lower abdomen, pelvis, or perineum.

_____ **30.** When treating a patient with an amputation of the penile shaft, your top priority is:

  A. locating the amputated part.

  B. controlling bleeding.

  C. keeping the remaining tissue dry.

  D. delaying transport until bleeding is controlled.

_____ **31.** Treatment of injuries involving the external male genitalia includes:

  A. making the patient as comfortable as possible.

  B. using sterile moist compresses to cover areas that have been stripped of skin.

  C. applying direct pressure with dry sterile gauze dressings to control bleeding.

  D. all of the above.

_____ **32.** In cases of sexual assault, you must treat the medical injuries but also provide:

  A. privacy.

  B. support.

  C. reassurance.

  D. all of the above.

1999 _____ **33.** Treatment for patients with abdominal injury includes:

  A. analgesics

  B. a fluid bolus to maintain radial pulses.

  C. ECG monitoring.

  D. all of the above.

Labeling EMT-I anatomy review web

Label the following diagrams with the correct terms.

Hollow Organs

A. _____

B. _____

C. _____

D. _____

E. _____

F. _____

G. _____

H. _____

I. _____

J. _____

K. _____

Solid Organs

A. _____

B. _____

C. _____

D. _____

E. _____

F. _____

G. _____

H. _____

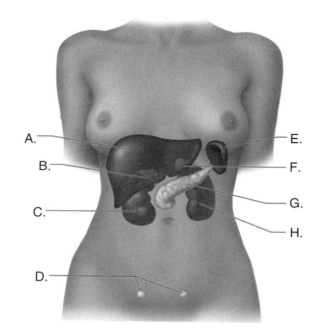

Male Reproductive System

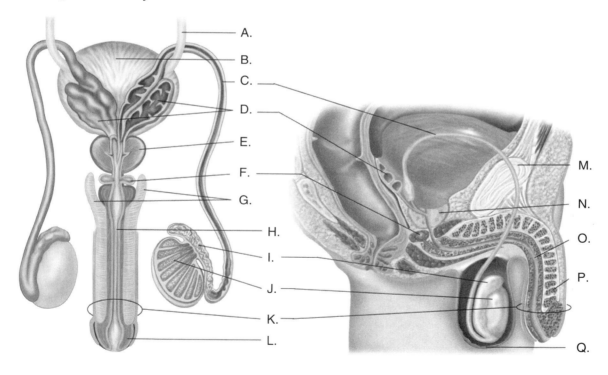

A. _____   F. _____   J. _____   N. _____

B. _____   G. _____   K. _____   O. _____

C. _____   H. _____   L. _____   P. _____

D. _____   I. _____   M. _____   Q. _____

E. _____

Female Reproductive System

A. _____   E. _____   I. _____

B. _____   F. _____   J. _____

C. _____   G. _____   K. _____

D. _____   H. _____   L. _____

Vocabulary EMT-I vocab explorer web

Define the following terms in the space provided.

1. Closed abdominal injury:

_____

_____

_____

2. Open abdominal injury:

_____

_____

_____

3. Guarding:

_____

_____

_____

Fill-in

Read each item carefully, then complete the statement by filling in the missing word(s).

1. Severe bleeding may occur with injury to _____ organs.

2. The _____ system is responsible for filtering waste.

3. Kidneys are located in the _____ space.

4. Injuries to the kidneys or bladder will not have obvious _____ _____,

but there are usually more subtle clues such as lower rib pain or a possible pelvic fracture.

5. When ruptured, the organs of the abdominal cavity can spill their contents into the peritoneal cavity,

causing an intense inflammatory reaction called _____.

6. Blood within the peritoneal cavity does not provoke a(n) _____ _____

and may not cause pain or tenderness.

7. Closed abdominal injuries are also known as _____ injuries.

1999 **8.** Consider _____ for patients with injuries to the external genitalia.

True/False

If you believe the statement to be more true than false, write the letter "T" in the space provided. If you believe the statement to be more false than true, write the letter "F."

_____ **1.** Hollow organs will bleed profusely if injured.

_____ **2.** The most common sign of an abdominal injury is an elevated heart rate.

_____ **3.** Patients with abdominal injuries should be kept supine with head elevated.

_____ **4.** Peritoneal irritation is a response to hollow organ injury.

_____ **5.** Eviscerated organs should be covered with a dry dressing.

_____ **6.** Injuries to the kidneys usually occur in isolation.

_____ **7.** All patients presenting with trauma-related injuries should be completely immobilized.

Short Answer

Complete this section with short written answers in the space provided.

1. List the hollow organs of the abdomen and urinary systems.

_____

_____

_____

2. List the solid organs of the abdomen and urinary systems.

_____

_____

_____

3. List the signs and symptoms of an abdominal injury.

_____

_____

_____

4. List the steps to care for a penetrating abdominal injury.

_____

_____

_____

5. List the steps to care for an open abdominal wound with exposed organs.

_____

_____

_____

6. List the major history or physical findings associated with possible kidney damage.

_____

_____

_____

Word Fun EMT-I vocab explorer web

The following crossword puzzle is an activity provided to reinforce correct spelling and understanding of medical terminology associated with emergency care and the EMT-I. Use the clues in the column to complete the puzzle.

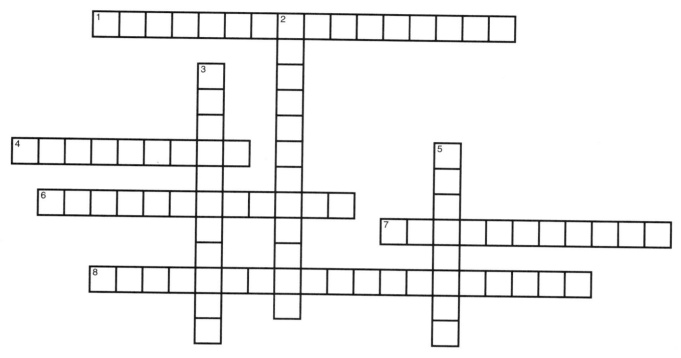

Across

1. Abdominal cavity
4. Blood in urine
6. Stomach, small intestine, bladder
7. Inflammation of the abdominal lining
8. Penetrating wound of belly

Down

2. Displacement of organs outside of abdomen
3. Liver, spleen, pancreas
5. Contraction of muscles to protect

Ambulance Calls

The following real case scenarios provide an opportunity to explore the concerns associated with patient management. Read each scenario, then answer each question in detail.

1. You are dispatched to a local bar where your patient, a 26-year-old male, was involved in an altercation. He has several superficial lacerations to his arms, and a knife is impaled in his right upper quadrant. He is lying supine on the floor. He is alert, and bar patrons tell you that he did not fall; they helped him to the floor.

   How would you best manage this patient?

   _____

   _____

   _____

   _____

   _____

   _____

   _____

   _____

2. You are called to a significant motor vehicle crash where a 21-year-old female restrained driver is complaining of pain to the abdomen but no other injury. She believes that the pain is just from the seat belt. She is alert and oriented and vital signs are all within normal limits. You explain that because of the mechanism of injury and her complaint of abdominal pain, she should be seen at the emergency room for evaluation. She agrees to go with you.

   How would you best manage this patient?

   _____

   _____

   _____

   _____

   _____

   _____

   _____

   _____

3. You are dispatched to a fall at a residence where you find a 35-year-old male who tripped and fell onto a barbed wire fence. He has a bowel evisceration and is in extreme pain. His neighbor tells you that there was no trauma involved; he slipped and fell from a standing position onto the wire, tearing open his abdomen in the process. He lowered himself to the ground before passing out. He is voice responsive and tachycardic. His breathing is 24 and deep.

How would you best manage this patient?

_____

_____

_____

_____

_____

_____

_____

4. You are called to the scene of a fistfight at the junior high school. The principal has separated the two boys involved. While one has only abrasions to his cheek and knuckles and a bloody lip, the other is in a fetal position on the floor.

How would you best manage both of these patients?

_____

_____

_____

_____

_____

_____

_____

Workbook Activities

The following activities have been designed to help you. Your instructor may require you to complete some or all of these activities as a regular part of your EMT-I training program. You are encouraged to complete any activity that your instructor does not assign as a way to enhance your learning in the classroom.

Chapter Review

The following exercises provide an opportunity to refresh your knowledge of this chapter.

Matching

Match each of the terms in the left column to the appropriate definition in the right column.

_____ 1. Cerebellum

_____ 2. Brain stem

_____ 3. Somatic nervous system

_____ 4. Autonomic nervous system

_____ 5. Spinal column

_____ 6. Central nervous system

_____ 7. Cerebral edema

_____ 8. Connecting nerves

_____ 9. Intervertebral disk

_____ 10. Meninges

A. consists of 33 bones

B. swelling of the brain

C. the brain and spinal cord

D. controls movement

E. the part of the central nervous system that controls virtually all the functions that are absolutely necessary for life

F. three distinct layers of tissue that surround and protect the brain and spinal cord within the skull and spinal cord

G. the part of the nervous system that regulates involuntary functions

H. the part of the nervous system that regulates voluntary activities

I. located in the brain and spinal cord, these connect the motor and sensory nerves

J. cushion that lies between the vertebrae

Multiple Choice

Read each item carefully, then select the best response.

_____ 1. The nervous system includes:

A. the brain.

B. the spinal cord.

C. billions of nerve fibers.

D. all of the above.

_____ 2. The nervous system is divided into two parts: the central nervous system and the:

A. autonomic nervous system.

B. peripheral nervous system.

C. sympathetic nervous system.

D. somatic nervous system.

C H A P T E R 17

Head and Spine Injuries

_____ **3.** The brain is divided into three major areas: the cerebrum, the cerebellum, and the:
  A. foramen magnum.
  B. meninges.
  C. brain stem.
  D. spinal column.

_____ **4.** Injury to the head and neck may indicate injury to the:
  A. thoracic spine.
  B. lumbar spine.
  C. cervical spine.
  D. sacral spine.

_____ **5.** The _____ is composed of three layers of tissue that surround the brain and spinal cord within the skull and spinal canal.
  A. meninges
  B. dura mater
  C. pia mater
  D. arachnoid space

_____ **6.** The skull is divided into two large structures: the cranium and the:
  A. occipital condyles.
  B. face.
  C. parietal lobe.
  D. foramen magnum.

_____ **7.** Peripheral nerves include:
  A. connecting nerves.
  B. sensory nerves.
  C. motor nerves.
  D. all of the above.

_____ **8.** The brain and spinal cord float in cerebrospinal fluid (CSF), which:
  A. acts as a shock absorber.
  B. bathes the brain and spinal cord.
  C. buffers them from injury.
  D. all of the above.

_____ **9.** The autonomic nervous system is composed of two parts: the sympathetic nervous system and the:

    A. peripheral nervous system.

    B. central nervous system.

    C. parasympathetic nervous system.

    D. somatic nervous system.

_____ **10.** The most prominent and the most easily palpable spinous process is at the _____ cervical vertebra at the base of the neck.

    A. 7th

    B. 6th

    C. 5th

    D. 4th

_____ **11.** When identifying the mechanism of injury of an unresponsive patient, _____ may have helpful information.

    A. first responders

    B. family members

    C. bystanders

    D. all of the above

_____ **12.** Emergency medical care of a patient with a possible spinal injury begins with:

    A. opening the airway.

    B. assessing the level of consciousness.

    C. scene of safety.

    D. BSI precautions.

_____ **13.** The _____ is a tunnel running the length of the spine, which encloses and protects the spinal cord.

    A. foramen magnum

    B. spinal canal

    C. foramen foranina

    D. meninges

_____ **14.** Once the head and neck are manually stabilized, you should assess:

    A. pulse.

    B. motor function.

    C. sensation.

    D. all of the above.

_____ **15.** You must maintain manual stabilization of the head until:

    A. the patient's head and torso are in line.

    B. the patient is secured to a backboard with the head immobilized.

    C. the rigid cervical collar is in place.

    D. the patient arrives at the hospital.

_____ **16.** The ideal procedure for moving a patient from the ground to the backboard is the:

    A. four-person log roll.

    B. lateral slide.

    C. four-person lift.

    D. push and pull maneuver.

_____ **17.** You can almost always control bleeding from a scalp laceration with:

    A. direct pressure.

    B. elevation.

    C. pressure point.

    D. tourniquet.

_____ **18.** You should not use a short spinal extrication device in any of the following circumstances EXCEPT when:

    A. you or the patient is in danger.

    B. the patient is conscious and complaining of lumbar pain.

    C. you need to gain immediate access to other patients.

    D. the patient's injuries justify immediate removal.

_____ **19.** Applying excessive pressure to an open wound with a skull fracture could:

    A. increase intracranial pressure.

    B. push bone fragments into the brain.

    C. increase the size of the soft-tissue injury.

    D. all of the above.

_____ **20.** When immobilizing the sitting patient, you should place the patient on the LSB and then:

    A. release the leg straps and loosen the chest strap.

    B. secure the short device and the LSB together.

    C. reassess the pulse.

    D. all of the above.

_____ **21.** Posturing is an ominous sign and indicates:

    A. increased blood pressure.

    B. increased intracranial pressure.

    C. seizure activity.

    D. decreased LOC.

1999 _____ **22.** Consider endotracheal intubation in any brain-injured patient with a GCS score of less than:

    A. 7.

    B. 8.

    C. 9.

    D. 10.

_____ **23.** A _____ is a temporary loss or alteration of a part or all of the brain's abilities to function but without actual physical damage to the brain:

    A. contusion

    B. concussion

    C. hematoma

    D. subdural hematoma

_____ **24.** Symptoms of a concussion include:

    A. dizziness.

    B. weakness.

    C. vision changes.

    D. all of the above.

_____ **25.** Intracranial bleeding outside of the dura and under the skull is known as a(n):

    A. concussion.

    B. intracerebral hemorrhage.

    C. subdural hematoma.

    D. epidural hematoma.

_____ **26.** The difference in signs and symptoms of traumatic vs. nontraumatic brain injuries is the:

    A. lack of altered mental status.

    B. lack of mechanism of injury.

    C. lack of swelling.

    D. increase in blood pressure.

_____ **27.** _____ is the most reliable sign of a closed head injury.

    A. Vomiting

    B. Decreased LOC

    C. Seizures

    D. Numbness and tingling in the extremities

_____ **28.** _____ is one of the most common, and one of the most serious, complications of a head injury.

    A. Cyanosis

    B. Hypoxia

    C. Vomiting

    D. Cerebral edema

_____ **29.** Common causes of head injuries include all of the following EXCEPT:

    A. direct blows.

    B. motor vehicle crashes.

    C. seizure activity.

    D. sports injuries.

_____ **30.** Assessment of mental status is accomplished through the use of the mnemonic:

    A. SAMPLE.

    B. OPQRST.

    C. AVPU.

    D. AEIOU-TIPS.

_____ **31.** Unequal pupil size may indicate:

    A. increased intracranial pressure.

    B. developing blood clots on the occulomotor nerve.

    C. damage to the nerves that control dilation and constriction.

    D. all of the above.

_____ **32.** Patients with head injuries often have injuries to the _____ as well.

    A. face

    B. torso

    C. cervical spine

    D. extremities

_____ **33.** The proper order of treatment for traumatic head injuries includes:

    A. scene safety, airway, LOC with c-spine control, breathing, circulation.

    B. LOC with c-spine control, airway, breathing, circulation.

    C. LOC, airway, breathing, circulation, c-spine.

    D. BSI, ABCs, LOC, c-spine control.

_____ **34.** A cervical collar should be applied to a patient with a possible spinal injury based on:

    A. the mechanism of injury.

    B. the history.

    C. signs and symptoms.

    D. all of the above.

_____ **35.** Hypotension in the brain-injured patient could indicate:

    A. decreased cerebral perfusion pressure.

    B. hypovolemia.

    C. hypoxia.

    D. herniation.

_____ **36.** Helmets must be removed in all of the following cases EXCEPT:

    A. cardiac arrest.

    B. when the helmet allows for excessive movement.

    C. when there are no impending airway or breathing problems.

    D. when a shield cannot be removed.

_____ **37.** Your best choice of action for a child involved in a motor vehicle crash and found in their car seat is to:

A. immobilize the child in the car seat.

B. rule out spinal injury and place the child with a parent.

C. pad the sides of the car seat but leave space to allow for lateral movement.

D. move the child to a pediatric immobilization device.

Labeling EMT-I anatomy review web

Label the following diagrams with the correct terms.

Brain

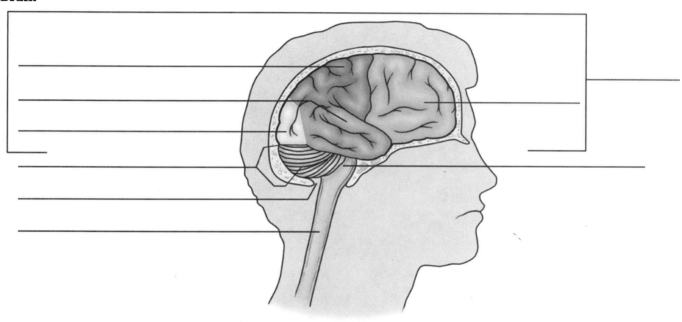

Connecting Nerves in the Spinal Cord

A. _____

B. _____

C. _____

D. _____

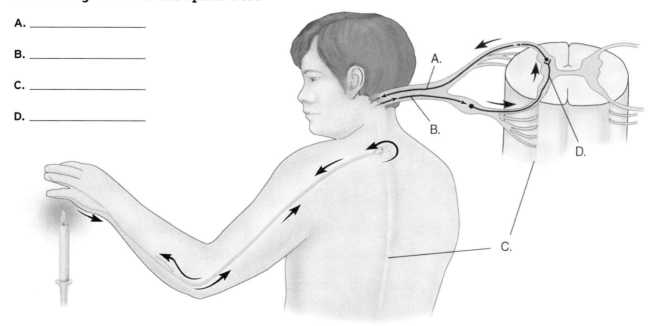

Skull

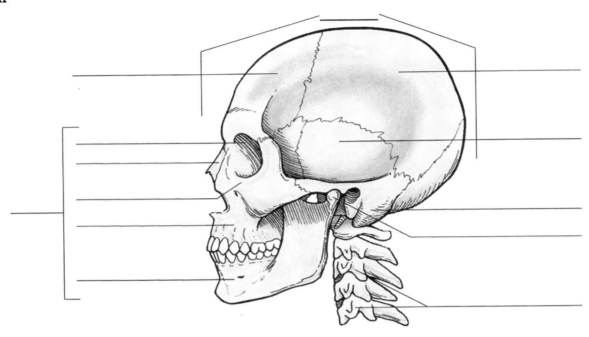

Spinal Canal

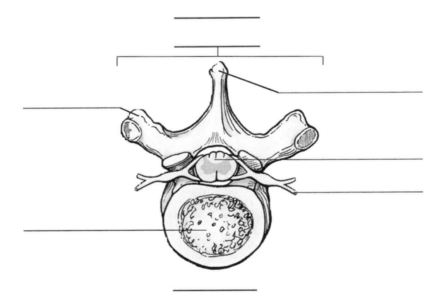

Vocabulary EMT-I vocab explorer web

Define the following terms in the space provided.

1. Retrograde amnesia:

_____

_____

_____

2. Anterograde (posttraumatic) amnesia:

_____

_____

_____

3. Closed head injury

_____

_____

_____

4. Eyes-forward position:

_____

_____

_____

5. Open head injury:

_____

_____

_____

6. Distracted:

_____

_____

_____

Fill-in

Read each item carefully, then complete the statement by filling in the missing word(s).

1. The _____ nerves carry information to the muscles.

2. The dura mater, arachnoid, and pia mater are layers of _____ within the skull and

spinal canal.

3. The brain and spinal cord are part of the _____ nervous system.

4. Within the peripheral nervous system, there are _____ pairs of spinal nerves.

5. The _____ nerves pass through holes in the skull and transmit sensations directly to the brain.

6. Vertebrae are separated by cushions called _____.

7. The skull has two large structures of bone, the _____ and the _____.

8. The _____ and _____ produce cerebrospinal fluid (CSF).

9. The _____ nervous system reacts to stress.

10. The _____ nervous system causes the body to relax.

11. _____ _____ is characterized by flexion of the arms and extension of

    the legs, and _____ _____ is characterized by extension of the arms

    and legs.

12. When treating a patient with a head injury, start a _____ IV of a(n)

    _____ crystalloid solution.

13. A single drop in the patient's SaO_2 to less than 90% _____ the brain-injured patient's

    chance of death.

True/False

If you believe the statement to be more true than false, write the letter "T" in the space provided. If you believe the statement to be more false than true, write the letter "F."

_____ 1. A distracted spine has been moved laterally.

_____ 2. If a sensory nerve in the reflex arc detects an irritating stimulus, it will bypass the motor nerve and send a message directly to the brain.

_____ 3. Voluntary activities are those actions we perform unconsciously.

_____ 4. The autonomic nervous system is composed of the sympathetic nervous system and the parasympathetic nervous system.

_____ 5. The parasympathetic nervous system reacts to stress with the fight-or-flight response whenever it is confronted with a threatening situation.

_____ 6. All patients with suspected head and/or spine injuries should have their heads realigned to an in-line neutral position.

_____ 7. When assessing a patient for possible spinal injury, you should begin with a focused history and physical exam.

1999 _____ 8. If dysrhythmias occur, treat according to standard ACLS or local protocols.

Short Answer

Complete this section with short written answers in the space provided.

1. List the five basic questions to ask a conscious patient when conducting an assessment of a head or head and spine injury.

_____

_____

_____

2. List the reasons for NOT placing the head/spine injury patient's head into a neutral in-line position.

_____

_____

_____

3. List the three major types of brain injuries.

_____

_____

_____

4. List at least five signs and symptoms of a head injury.

_____

_____

_____

5. List the three general principles for treating a head injury.

_____

_____

_____

6. List the six questions to ask yourself when deciding whether or not to remove a helmet.

_____

_____

_____

Word Fun EMT-I vocab explorer web

The following crossword puzzle is an activity provided to reinforce correct spelling and understanding of medical terminology associated with emergency care and the EMT-I. Use the clues in the column to complete the puzzle.

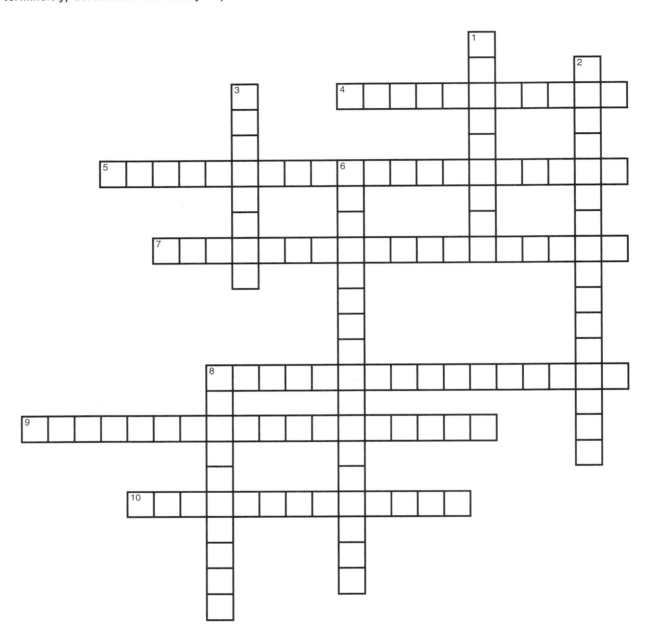

Across

4. Pulling the spine along its length
5. Voluntary part of CNS
7. Inability to remember after the event
8. Cerebral trauma without broken skin
9. Cushion between vertebrae
10. Swelling of the brain

Down

1. Controls primary life functions
2. Join motor and sensory nerves
3. Layers of tissue surrounding the brain
6. Inability to remember the event
8. Coordinates body movement

Ambulance Calls

The following real case scenarios provide an opportunity to explore the concerns associated with patient management. Read each scenario, then answer each question in detail.

1. You are dispatched to a moderate damage motor vehicle crash. Your patient is a 52-year-old female, restrained driver, hit from the rear, complaining of neck and back pain. She is alert and oriented, and her vital signs are within the normal limits. Pulse, motor, and sensory functions are intact in all extremities. How would you best manage this patient?

_____

_____

_____

_____

_____

_____

_____

2. You are called to the scene of a baseball game where a 10-year-old boy was accidentally hit with a baseball bat on the left side of his head. He has a depression in the left temporal region and severe vomiting. He is pain responsive, and bleeding is minimal. How would you best manage this patient?

_____

_____

_____

_____

_____

_____

_____

3. You are dispatched to a motor vehicle crash with major damage to the patient compartment. Your patient, an 18-month-old male, is still in his car seat in the center of the back seat. He responds appropriately, and there is no damage to his seat. He has no visible injuries, but a front seat passenger was killed.

How would you best manage this patient?

_____

_____

_____

_____

_____

_____

_____

_____

Skill Drills

Skill Drill 17-1: Performing Manual In-Line Stabilization

Test your knowledge by filling in the correct words in the photo captions.

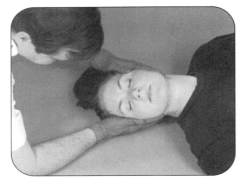

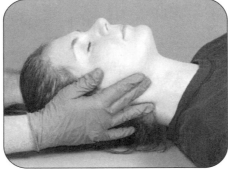

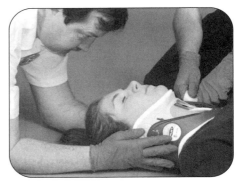

1. Kneel behind the patient and place your hands firmly around the _____ of the _____ on either _____.

2. Support the lower jaw with your _____ and _____ fingers and the head with your _____. Gently _____ the head into a _____ position, aligned with the torso. Do not _____ the head or neck excessively.

3. Continue to _____ the head manually while your partner places a rigid _____ around the neck. Maintain _____ _____ until you have the patient secured to a backboard.

Skill Drill 17-2: Immobilizing a Patient to a Long Backboard

Test your knowledge by placing the photos below in the correct order. Number the first step with a "1," the second step with a "2," etc. Also, fill in the correct words in the photo captions.

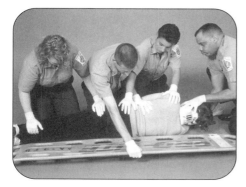

_____

On command, rescuers roll the patient _____ themselves, quickly examine the _____, slide the backboard _____ the patient, and _____ the patient onto the board.

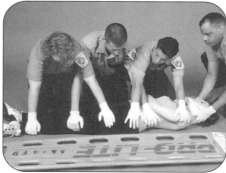

_____

Rescuers kneel on one side of the patient and place hands on the _____ _____ of the patient.

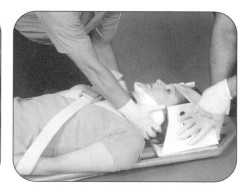

_____

Place tape across the patient's _____.

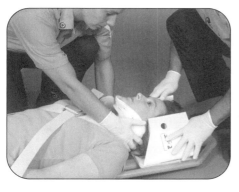

_____

Begin to secure the patient's _____ by using a _____ _____ device or _____ _____.

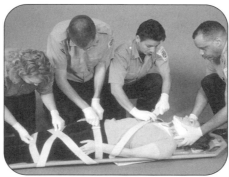

_____

Secure the _____, _____, and upper _____.

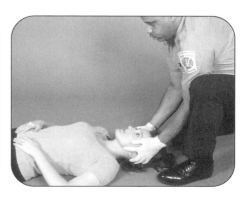

_____

Apply and maintain _____ stabilization. Assess _____ _____ in all extremities.

Continued

Skill Drill 17-2: Immobilizing a Patient to a Long Backboard—cont'd

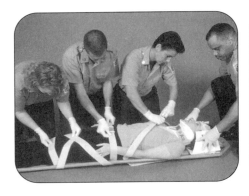

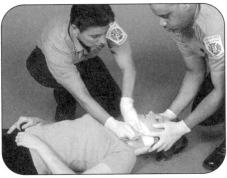

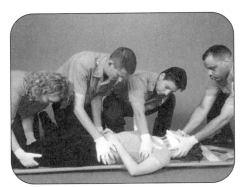

_____

Check all _____, and readjust as needed. Reassess _____ functions in all _____.

_____

Apply a _____ _____.

_____

_____ the patient on the board.

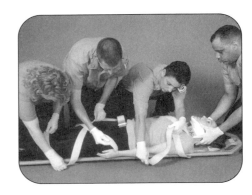

_____

Secure the _____ _____ first.

Skill Drill 17-5: Application of a Cervical Collar

Test your knowledge by placing the photos below in the correct order. Number the first step with a "1," the second step with a "2," etc.

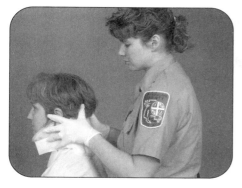

Assure proper fit, and maintain neutral, in-line stabilization.

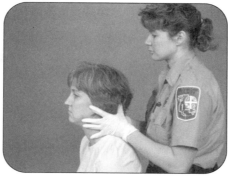

Apply in-line stabilization.

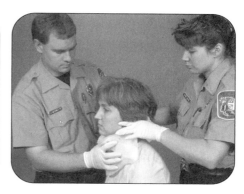

Place the chin support first.

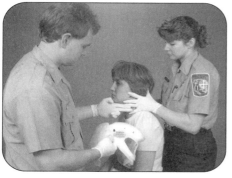

Measure the proper collar size.

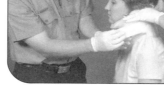

Wrap the collar around the neck, and secure the collar.

SECTION 5

TRAUMA

Workbook Activities

The following activities have been designed to help you. Your instructor may require you to complete some or all of these activities as a regular part of your EMT-I training program. You are encouraged to complete any activity that your instructor does not assign as a way to enhance your learning in the classroom.

Chapter Review

The following exercises provide an opportunity to refresh your knowledge of this chapter.

Matching

Match each of the terms in the left column to the appropriate definition in the right column.

_____ 1. Striated muscle

_____ 2. Tendons

_____ 3. Smooth muscle

_____ 4. Joint

_____ 5. Ligaments

_____ 6. Closed fracture

_____ 7. Point tenderness

_____ 8. Displaced fracture

_____ 9. Articular cartilage

_____ 10. Open fracture

_____ 11. Traction

A. Any injury that makes the limb appear in an unnatural position

B. Any fracture in which the skin has not been broken

C. A thin layer of cartilage covering the articular surface of bones in synovial joints

D. Involuntary muscle

E. Any break in the bone in which the overlying skin has been damaged as well

F. Hold joints together

G. Skeletal muscle

H. Act of exerting a pulling force on a structure

I. Contact point between two bones

J. Attach muscle to bone

K. Tenderness sharply located at the site of an injury

Multiple Choice

Read each item carefully, then select the best response.

_____ 1. Blood in the urine is known as (a):

  A. hematuria.

  B. hemotysis.

  C. hematocrit.

  D. hemoglobin.

_____ 2. Smooth muscle is found in the:

  A. back.

  B. blood vessels.

  C. heart.

  D. all of the above.

Musculoskeletal Care

_____ **3.** The bones in the skeleton produce _____ in the bone marrow.

    A. red blood cells

    B. minerals

    C. electrolytes

    D. white blood cells

_____ **4.** _____ are held together in a tough fibrous structure known as a capsule.

    A. Tendons

    B. Joints

    C. Ligaments

    D. Bones

_____ **5.** Joints are bathed and lubricated by _____ fluid.

    A. cartilaginous

    B. articular

    C. synovial

    D. cerebrospinal

_____ **6.** A _____ is a disruption of a joint in which the bone ends are no longer in contact.

    A. torn ligament

    B. dislocation

    C. fracture dislocation

    D. sprain

_____ **7.** A _____ is a joint injury in which there is both some partial or temporary dislocation of the bone ends and partial stretching or tearing of the supporting ligaments.

    A. dislocation

    B. strain

    C. sprain

    D. torn ligament

_____ **8.** A _____ is a stretching or tearing of the muscle.

    A. strain

    B. sprain

    C. torn ligament

    D. split

_____ **9.** The zone of injury includes the:

    A. adjacent nerves.

    B. adjacent blood vessels.

    C. surrounding soft tissue.

    D. all of the above.

_____ **10.** A(n) _____ fractures the bone at the point of impact.

    A. direct blow

    B. indirect force

    C. twisting force

    D. high-energy injury

_____ **11.** A(n) _____ may cause a fracture or dislocation at a distant point.

    A. direct blow

    B. indirect force

    C. twisting force

    D. high-energy injury

_____ **12.** When caring for patients who have fallen, you must identify the _____ and the mechanism of injury so that you will not overlook associated injuries.

    A. site of injury

    B. height of fall

    C. point of contact

    D. twisting forces

_____ **13.** _____ produce severe damage to the skeleton, surrounding soft tissues, and vital internal organs.

    A. Direct blows

    B. Indirect forces

    C. Twisting forces

    D. High-energy injuries

_____ **14.** Regardless of the extent and severity of the damage to the skin, you should treat any injury that breaks the skin as a possible:

    A. closed fracture.

    B. open fracture.

    C. nondisplaced fracture.

    D. displaced fracture.

_____ **15.** A(n) _____ is also known as a hairline fracture.

    A. closed fracture

    B. open fracture

    C. nondisplaced fracture

    D. displaced fracture

_____ **16.** A(n) _____ produces actual deformity, or distortion, of the limb by shortening, rotating, or angulating it.

    A. closed fracture

    B. open fracture

    C. nondisplaced fracture

    D. displaced fracture

_____ **17.** When examining an injured extremity, you should compare the injured limb to:

    A. the opposite uninjured limb.

    B. one of your limbs or one of your partner's limbs.

    C. an injury chart.

    D. none of the above.

_____ **18.** _____ is the most reliable indicator of an underlying fracture.

   A. Crepitus

   B. Deformity

   C. Point tenderness

   D. Absence of distal pulse

_____ **19.** A(n) _____ is a fracture that occurs in a growth section of a child's bone, which may prematurely stop growth if not properly treated.

   A. greenstick fracture

   B. comminuted fracture

   C. pathologic fracture

   D. epiphyseal fracture

_____ **20.** A(n) _____ is an incomplete fracture that passes only partway through the shaft of a bone but may still cause severe angulation.

   A. greenstick fracture

   B. comminuted fracture

   C. pathologic fracture

   D. epiphyseal fracture

_____ **21.** A(n) _____ is a fracture of a weakened or diseased bone, seen in patients with osteoporosis or cancer.

   A. greenstick fracture

   B. comminuted fracture

   C. pathologic fracture

   D. epiphyseal fracture

_____ **22.** A(n) _____ is a fracture in which the bone is broken into two or more fragments.

   A. greenstick fracture

   B. comminuted fracture

   C. pathologic fracture

   D. epiphyseal fracture

_____ **23.** Rapid swelling usually indicates _____ a fracture site and is typically followed by severe pain.

   A. bleeding from

   B. a laceration near

   C. compartment syndrome at

   D. all of the above

_____ **24.** Fractures are almost always associated with _____ of the surrounding soft tissue.

   A. laceration

   B. crepitus

   C. ecchymosis

   D. swelling

_____ **25.** Signs and symptoms of a dislocated joint include:

   A. marked deformity.

   B. tenderness or palpation.

   C. locked joint.

   D. all of the above.

_____ **26.** Signs and symptoms of sprains include all of the following EXCEPT:

   A. point tenderness.

   B. pain prevents the patient from moving or using the limb normally.

   C. marked deformity.

   D. instability of the joint is indicated by increased motion.

_____ **27.** Assessment of patients with musculoskeletal injuries must include:

    A. initial assessment followed by a focused physical exam.

    B. evaluation of neurovascular function.

    C. applying oxygen as needed.

    D. all of the above.

_____ **28.** Compartment syndrome:

    A. occurs within 6 to 12 hours after injury.

    B. usually is a result of excessive bleeding, a severely crushed extremity, or the rapid return of blood to an ischemic limb.

    C. is characterized by pain that is out of proportion to the injury.

    D. all of the above.

_____ **29.** Always check neurovascular function:

    A. after any manipulation of the limb.

    B. before applying a splint.

    C. after applying a splint.

    D. all of the above.

_____ **30.** Splinting will help to prevent:

    A. excessive bleeding of the tissues at the injury site caused by broken bone ends.

    B. laceration of the skin by broken bone ends.

    C. increased pain from movement of bone ends.

    D. all of the above.

_____ **31.** In-line _____ is the act of exerting a pulling force on a body structure in the direction of its normal alignment.

    A. stabilization

    B. immobilization

    C. traction

    D. direction

_____ **32.** Basic types of splints include:

    A. rigid.

    B. formable.

    C. traction.

    D. all of the above.

_____ **33.** Before applying a zippered or unzippered air splint:

    A. assess pulse and motor and sensory function.

    B. cover wounds with dry dressings.

    C. use BSI precautions.

    D. all of the above.

_____ **34.** Do not use traction splints for any of the following conditions EXCEPT:

    A. injuries of the pelvis.

    B. an isolated femur fracture.

    C. partial amputation or avulsions with bone separation.

    D. lower leg or ankle injury.

_____ **35.** Hazards associated with improper application of splints include:

    A. compression of nerves, tissues, and blood vessels.

    B. delay in transport of a patient with a life-threatening injury.

    C. reduction of distal circulation if the splint is too tight.

    D. all of the above.

_____ **36.** The _____ is one of the most commonly fractured bones in the body.

   A. scapula

   B. clavicle

   C. humerus

   D. radius

1999 _____ **37.** For patients who are at risk of hypovolemia from fractures:

   A. apply high-flow oxygen.

   B. administer an IV of crystalloid solution.

   C. consider analgesics.

   D. all of the above.

_____ **38.** Indications that blood vessels have likely been injured include:

   A. a cold, pale hand.

   B. weak or absent pulse.

   C. poor capillary refill.

   D. all of the above.

_____ **39.** Signs and symptoms associated with hip dislocation include:

   A. severe pain in the hip.

   B. lateral and posterior aspects of the hip region will be tender on palpation.

   C. you may be able to palpate the femoral head deep within the muscles of the buttock.

   D. all of the above.

_____ **40.** There is always a significant amount of blood loss, as much as _____ mL, after a fracture of the shaft of the femur.

   A. 100 to 250

   B. 250 to 500

   C. 500 to 1,000

   D. 100 to 1,500

_____ **41.** The knee is especially susceptible to _____ injuries, which occur when abnormal bending or twisting forces are applied to the joint.

   A. tendon

   B. ligament

   C. dislocation

   D. fracture-dislocation

_____ **42.** Signs and symptoms of knee ligament injury include:

   A. swelling.

   B. point tenderness.

   C. joint effusion.

   D. all of the above.

_____ **43.** Although substantial ligament damage always occurs with a knee dislocation, the more urgent injury is to the _____ artery, which is often lacerated or compressed by the displaced tibia.

   A. tibial

   B. femoral

   C. popliteal

   D. dorsalis pedis

_____ **44.** Because of local tenderness and swelling, it is easy to confuse a nondisplaced or minimally displaced fracture about the knee with a:

   A. tendon injury.

   B. ligament injury.

   C. dislocation.

   D. fracture-dislocation.

_____ **45.** Fracture of the tibia and fibula are often associated with _____ as a result of the distorted positions of the limb following injury.

    A. vascular injury

    B. muscular injury

    C. tendon injury

    D. ligament injury

_____ **46.** The _____ is the most commonly injured joint.

    A. knee

    B. elbow

    C. ankle

    D. hip

Labeling EMT-I anatomy review web

Label the following diagram with the correct terms.

Human Skeleton

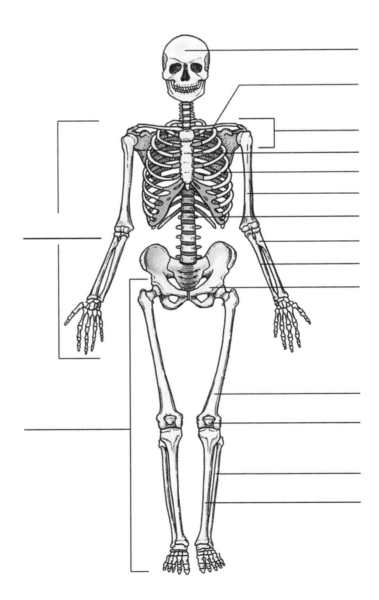

Vocabulary EMT-I vocab explorer web

Define the following terms in the space provided.

1. Acromioclavicular (A/C) joint:

_____

_____

_____

2. Compartment syndrome:

_____

_____

_____

3. Dislocation:

_____

_____

_____

4. Nondisplaced fracture:

_____

_____

_____

5. Position of function:

_____

_____

_____

6. Sling:

_____

_____

_____

7. Swathe:

_____

_____

_____

Fill-in

Read each item carefully, then complete the statement by filling in the missing word(s).

1. Atrophy is the _____ of muscle tissue.

2. Bone marrow produces _____ blood cells.

3. The knee and elbow are _____ and socket joints.

4. The _____ is one of the most commonly fractured bones in the body.

5. Always carefully assess the _____ to try to determine the amount of kinetic energy that an injured limb has absorbed.

6. Penetrating injury should alert you to the possibility of a(n) _____

   _____.

7. The _____ _____ is the most important nerve in the lower extremity; it

   controls the activity of muscles in the thigh and below the knee.

8. The _____ is the longest and largest bone in the body.

9. A grating or grinding sensation known as _____ can be felt and sometimes even heard

   when fractured bone ends rub together.

10. A dislocated joint sometimes will spontaneously _____ or return to its normal position.

11. If you suspect that a patient has compartment syndrome, splint the affected limb, keeping it at the level

    of the heart, and provide immediate transport, checking _____ _____

    frequently during transport.

12. Before applying a vacuum splint, assess _____ and _____ and

    _____ function.

True/False

If you believe the statement to be more true than false, write the letter "T" in the space provided. If you believe the statement to be more false than true, write the letter "F."

_____ 1. All extremity injuries should be splinted before moving a patient unless the patient's life is in immediate danger.

_____ 2. Splinting reduces pain and prevents the motion of bone fragments.

_____ 3. You should use traction to reduce a fracture and force all bone fragments back into alignment.

_____ 4. When applying traction, the direction of pull is always in the direction of normal alignment.

_____ 5. Cover wounds with a dry sterile dressing before applying a splint.

_____ 6. When splinting a fracture, you should be careful to immobilize only the joint above the injury site.

_____ **7.** One of the steps of the neurologic examination is to palpate the pulse distal to the point of injury.

_____ **8.** Assessment of neurovascular function should be repeated every 5 to 10 minutes until the patient arrives at the hospital.

_____ **9.** A patient's ability to sense light touch in the fingers and toes distal to the injury site is a good indication that the nerve supply is intact.

Short Answer

Complete this section with short written answers in the space provided.

1. List the four types of forces that may cause injury to a limb.

2. List five of the signs associated with a possible fracture.

3. List the four items to check when assessing neurovascular function.

4. List the general principles of splinting.

5. What are the three goals of in-line traction?

Word Fun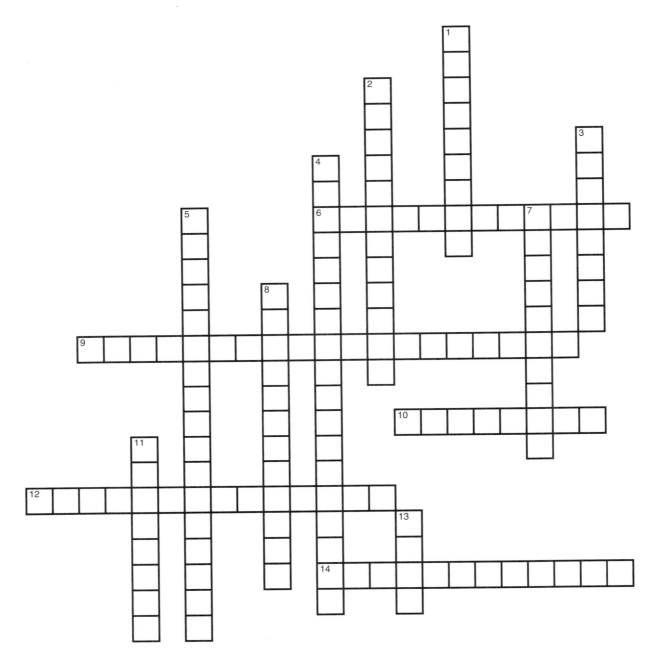

The following crossword puzzle is an activity provided to reinforce correct spelling and understanding of medical terminology associated with emergency care and the EMT-I. Use the clues in the column to complete the puzzle.

Across

6. Major lower extremity nerve
9. Elevation of pressure in fibrous tissues
10. Exerting a pulling force
12. Striated; attached to bones
14. Broken bone with overlying skin injured

Down

1. Blood in urine
2. Part of scapula that joins with humerus
3. Collarbone
4. Hand position for splinting
5. Bone fragments are separated
7. Discoloration from bleeding under skin
8. Joint between the two pubic bones
11. Grating sound of bone ends
13. Forearm bone on small finger side

Ambulance Calls

The following real case scenarios provide an opportunity to explore the concerns associated with patient management. Read each scenario, then answer each question in detail.

1. You are dispatched to a construction site for a 27-year-old male complaining of severe thoracic pain posteriorly. Coworkers tell you he was hit in the upper back by the bucket of a backhoe. He is alert and oriented, and closer inspection reveals bruising and deformity over the left scapula with pain and crepitus on palpation.

   How would you best manage this patient?

   _____

   _____

   _____

   _____

   _____

   _____

   _____

2. You are called to a local park where an 11-year-old girl fell off the parallel bars onto her right elbow. She is cradling the arm to her chest. She has obvious swelling and deformity in the area. She has good pulse, motor, and sensation at the wrist. ABCs are normal.

   How would you best manage this patient?

   _____

   _____

   _____

   _____

   _____

   _____

   _____

3. You are dispatched to a rollover motor vehicle crash. Your patient is a 29-year-old female unrestrained driver complaining of severe lower back pain. She is slightly tachycardic, but the ABCs are all normal. While performing a rapid trauma assessment, you find crepitus and an unstable pelvis. She is becoming less responsive.

How would you best manage this patient?

_____

_____

_____

_____

_____

_____

_____

4. Your 40-year-old female patient fell while shopping. She is alert and oriented and tells you that she had recent knee surgery and that weakness to the knee caused the fall. There is no deformity to her knee but there is obvious deformity to the left wrist.

How would you best manage this patient?

_____

_____

_____

_____

_____

_____

_____

Skill Drills

Skill Drill 18-1: Assessing Neurovascular Pulse

Test your knowledge of this chapter by filling in the correct words in the photo captions.

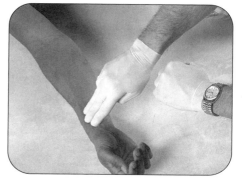

1. Palpate the _____ pulse in the upper extremity.

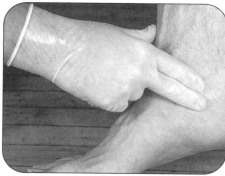

2. Palpate the _____ _____ pulse in the lower extremity.

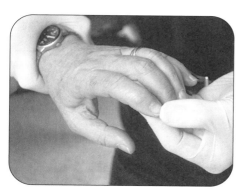

3. Assess capillary refill by blanching a fingernail or _____.

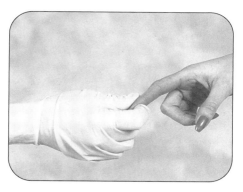

4. Assess sensation on the flesh near the _____ of the _____ finger.

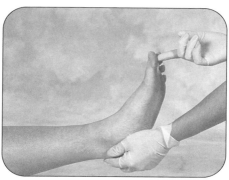

5. On the foot, first check sensation on the flesh near the _____ of the _____ _____.

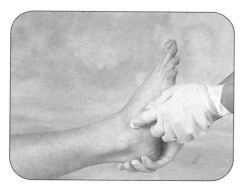

6. Also check foot sensation on the _____ of the _____.

Continued

Skill Drill 18-1: Assessing Neurovascular Pulse—cont'd

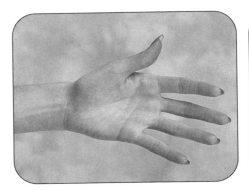

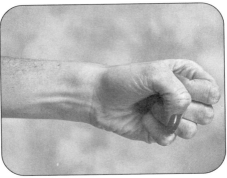

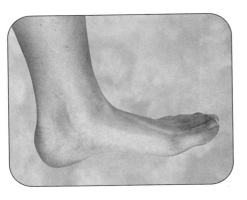

7. Evaluate motor function by asking the patient to _____ the hand. (Perform motor tests only if the hand or foot is not _____. _____ a test if it causes pain.)

8. Also ask the patient to _____ a _____.

9. To evaluate motor function in the foot, ask the patient to _____ the foot.

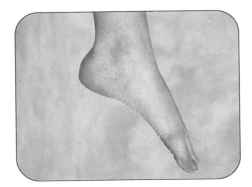

10. Also have the patient _____ the foot and _____ the toes.

Skill Drill 18-2: Caring for Musculoskeletal Injuries

Test your knowledge by placing the photos below in the correct order. Number the first step with a "1," the second step with a "2," etc.

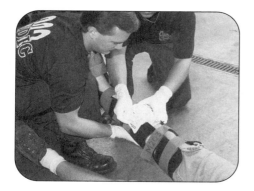

Apply cold packs if there is swelling, but do not place them directly on the skin.

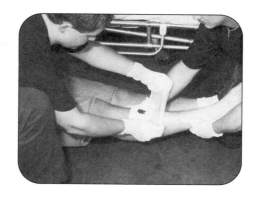

Cover open wounds with a dry, sterile dressing, and apply pressure to control bleeding.

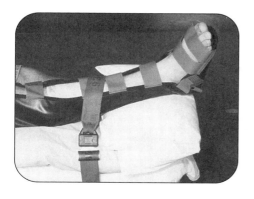

Position the patient for transport, and secure the injured area.

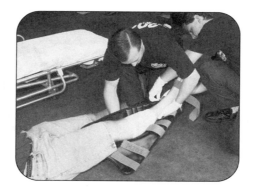

Assess pulse, motor, and sensory functions. Apply a splint, and elevate the extremity about 6" (slightly above the level of the heart).

Skill Drill 18-3: Applying a Rigid Splint

Test your knowledge by filling in the correct words in the photo captions.

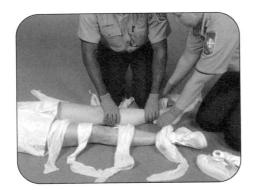

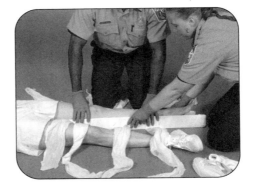

1. Assess pulse, motor, and sensory functions. Provide gentle _____ and _____ _____ of the limb.

2. Second EMT-I places the splint _____ or _____ the limb. _____ between the limb and the splint as needed to ensure even pressure and contact.

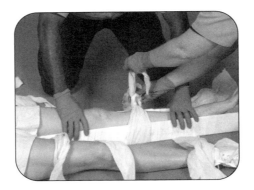

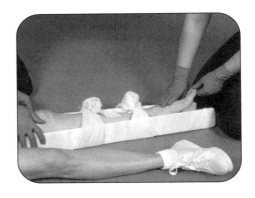

3. Secure the splint to the limb with _____.

4. Assess and record _____ _____ function.

Skill Drill 18-9: Splinting the Hand and Wrist

Test your knowledge of this skill drill by placing the photos below in the correct order. Number the first step with a "1," the second step with at "2," etc.

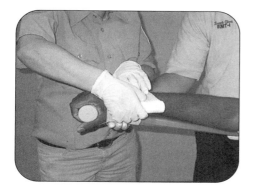

Apply a padded board splint on the palmar side with fingers exposed.

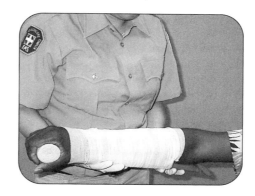

Secure the splint with a roller bandage.

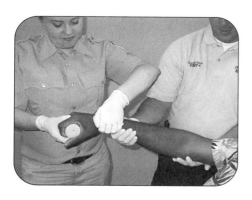

Assess pulse, motor, and sensory functions.

Move the hand into the position of function.

Place a soft roller bandage in the palm.

Workbook Activities

The following activities have been designed to help you. Your instructor may require you to complete some or all of these activities as a regular part of your EMT-I training program. You are encouraged to complete any activity that your instructor does not assign as a way to enhance your learning in the classroom.

Chapter Review

The following exercises provide an opportunity to refresh your knowledge of this chapter.

Matching

Match each of the terms in the left column to the appropriate definition in the right column.

_____ **1.** Asthma

_____ **2.** Pulmonary edema

_____ **3.** Epiglottitis

_____ **4.** Emphysema

_____ **5.** Pleural effusion

_____ **6.** Pneumothorax

_____ **7.** Dyspnea

_____ **8.** Pneumonia

_____ **9.** Hypoxia

_____ **10.** Ventilation

_____ **11.** Hyperventilation

_____ **12.** Allergen

_____ **13.** Embolus

_____ **14.** Wheezing

_____ **15.** Atelectasis

_____ **16.** Hypoxic drive

_____ **17.** CO_2 retention

_____ **18.** Rales

_____ **19.** Stridor

_____ **20.** Carpopedal spasm

_____ **21.** Inspiration

_____ **22.** Ronchi

_____ **23.** COPD

_____ **24.** Subcutaneous emphysema

_____ **25.** Chronic bronchitis

_____ **26.** Pleuritic chest pain

_____ **27.** Respiration

A. movement of air in and out of the lungs

B. acute spasm of the bronchioles associated with excessive mucus production and sometimes spasm of the bronchiolar muscles

C. accumulation of air in the pleural space

D. fluid build-up in the alveoli and lung tissue

E. an infectious disease of the lung that damages lung tissue

F. a substance that causes an allergic reaction

G. difficulty breathing

H. bacterial infection that can produce severe swelling

I. a blood clot or other substance in the circulatory system that travels to a blood vessel where it causes blockage

J. disease of the lungs in which the alveoli stretch, lose elasticity, and are destroyed

K. rapid or deep breathing that lowers blood carbon dioxide levels below normal

L. fluid outside of the lung

M. condition in which the body's cells and tissues do not have enough oxygen

N. chronic obstructive pulmonary disease; the slow degenerative process bringing changes in the alveoli and bronchioles

O. air bubbles trapped underneath the skin

P. tingling spasms of the phalanges resulting from hyperventilation

Q. crackling, moist breath sounds

R. sharp stabbing pain in the chest worsened by a deep breath; caused by inflammation or irritation of the pleura

S. viral infection; swollen nasal mucous membranes and fluid from the nose

T. resulting from respiratory disease, chronically high blood levels of CO_2

Respiratory Emergencies

_____ **28.** Common cold

_____ **29.** Expiration

_____ **30.** Croup

_____ **31.** Perfusion

_____ **32.** Diffusion

_____ **33.** Status asthmaticus

_____ **34.** Diphtheria

_____ **35.** Pulmonary thromboembolism

U. backup system that controls respirations when oxygen levels fall dangerously low

V. act of breathing out or exhaling

W. the movement of gases from higher to lower concentration

X. prolonged exacerbation of asthma that does not respond to conventional therapy

Y. collapse of the alveoli

Z. usually seen in children; barking cough

AA. high-pitched, whistling breath sound

BB. membrane lining of the pharynx that can severely obstruct air passage into the pharynx

CC. gas exchange occurring at the pulmonary and cellular levels

DD. supplying organs and tissues with oxygen

EE. harsh, high-pitched inspiratory barking sound

FF. the act of breathing in or inhaling

GG. irritation and inflammation of major passages

HH. coarse, rattling breath sounds

II. blood clot in blood vessels of the lung causing an obstruction

Multiple Choice

Read each item carefully, then select the best response.

_____ **1.** When treating a patient with dyspnea, you must be prepared to treat:

   A. the symptoms.

   B. the underlying problem.

   C. the patient's anxiety.

   D. all of the above.

_____ **2.** The oxygen–carbon dioxide exchange takes place in the:

   A. trachea.

   B. bronchial tree.

   C. alveoli.

   D. blood.

_____ **3.** Oxygen–carbon dioxide exchange may be hampered if:

    A. the pleural space is filled with air or excess fluid.

    B. the alveoli are damaged.

    C. the air passages are obstructed.

    D. all of the above.

_____ **4.** If carbon dioxide levels drop too low, the body compensates by breathing:

    A. normally.

    B. rapidly and deeply.

    C. slower and less deeply.

    D. fast and shallow.

_____ **5.** If the level of carbon dioxide in the arterial blood rises above normal, the patient breathes:

    A. normally.

    B. rapidly and deeply.

    C. slower and less deeply.

    D. fast and shallow.

_____ **6.** _____ is/are a sign(s) of adequate breathing.

    A. A normal rate and depth

    B. Pale or cyanotic skin

    C. Pursed lips and nasal flaring

    D. Cool, damp skin

_____ **7.** The level of carbon dioxide in the arterial blood can rise because of:

    A. emphysema.

    B. chronic bronchitis.

    C. cardiovascular disease.

    D. all of the above.

_____ **8.** The second stimulus that develops in patients with abnormally high levels of carbon dioxide responds to:

    A. increased oxygen levels.

    B. decreased oxygen levels.

    C. increased carbon dioxide levels.

    D. decreased carbon dioxide levels.

_____ **9.** The level of _____ bathing the brain stem is what stimulates a healthy person to breathe.

    A. oxygen

    B. carbon dioxide

    C. spinal fluid

    D. none of the above

_____ **10.** _____ is a sign of hypoxia to the brain.

    A. Altered mental status

    B. Decreased heart rate

    C. Decreased respiratory rate

    D. Delayed capillary refill time

_____ **11.** An obstruction to the exchange of gases between the alveoli and the capillaries may result from:

    A. epiglottitis.

    B. pneumonia.

    C. colds.

    D. all of the above.

_____ **12.** _____ is the adequate supply of oxygen and nutrients to the body.

    A. Diffusion

    B. The Fick principle

    C. Perfusion

    D. Apnea

_____ **13.** _____ is when the supply of oxygen and nutrients is inadequate. This is also called "shock."

    A. Pulmonary edema

    B. Hypoperfusion

    C. Carbon dioxide retention

    D. Diffusion

_____ **14.** Pulmonary edema can develop quickly after a major:

    A. heart attack.

    B. episode of syncope.

    C. brain injury.

    D. all of the above.

_____ **15.** The _____ is the narrowest point in a child's airway.

    A. carina

    B. trachea

    C. epiglottis

    D. larynx

_____ **16.** In addition to a major heart attack, pulmonary edema can also be produced by:

    A. inhaling large amounts of smoke.

    B. traumatic injuries to the chest.

    C. inhaling toxic chemical fumes.

    D. all of the above.

_____ **17.** Chronic oxygenation problems from bronchitis can lead to:

    A. cerebral edema.

    B. upper airway obstruction.

    C. right-sided heart failure.

    D. fluid retention.

1999 _____ **18.** Management of cardiogenic pulmonary edema includes _____.

    A. IV access.

    B. oxygen.

    C. a diuretic as per protocol.

    D. all of the above.

_____ **19.** Patients with noncardiogenic pulmonary edema tend to have a history of:

    A. hypoxic episode.

    B. hypoperfusion.

    C. recent chest trauma.

    D. all of the above.

_____ **20.** _____ is a loss of the elastic material around the air spaces resulting from chronic stretching of the alveoli when bronchitic airways obstruct easy expulsion of gases.

    A. Emphysema

    B. Bronchitis

    C. Pneumonia

    D. Diphtheria

_____ **21.** Most patients with COPD will:

  A. chronically produce sputum.

  B. have a chronic cough.

  C. have difficulty expelling air from their lungs.

  D. all of the above.

_____ **22.** The patient with COPD usually presents with:

  A. an increased blood pressure.

  B. a productive cough with green or yellow sputum.

  C. a decreased heart rate.

  D. all of the above.

_____ **23.** Management of obstructive lung disease includes:

  A. placing the patient in the left lateral recumbent position.

  B. watching for paroxysmal changes.

  C. none of the above.

  D. all of the above.

1999 _____ **24.** Side effects of beta agonists such as albuterol or epinephrine can include:

  A. increased automaticity

  B. increased contractility.

  C. increased heart rate.

  D. all of the above.

_____ **25.** A pneumothorax caused by a medical condition without any injury is known as:

  A. a tension pneumothorax.

  B. a subcutaneous pneumothorax.

  C. a spontaneous pnemothorax.

  D. none of the above.

_____ **26.** Asthma produces (a) characteristic _____ as patients attempt to exhale through partially obstructed air passages.

  A. rhonchi

  B. stridor

  C. wheezing

  D. rattle

_____ **27.** An allergic response to certain foods or some other allergen may produce an acute:

  A. bronchodilation.

  B. asthma attack.

  C. vasoconstriction.

  D. insulin release.

_____ **28.** Treatment for anaphylaxis and acute asthma attacks includes:

  A. epinephrine.

  B. high-flow oxygen.

  C. antihistamines.

  D. all of the above.

_____ **29.** A collection of fluid outside the lungs on one or both sides of the chest is called a:

  A. spontaneous pneumothorax.

  B. subcutaneous emphysema.

  C. pleural effusion.

  D. tension pneumothorax.

_____ **30.** Always consider _____ in patients who were eating just before becoming short of breath:

    A. upper airway obstruction

    B. anaphylaxis

    C. lower airway obstruction

    D. bronchoconstriction

_____ **31.** Pulmonary emboli may occur as a result of:

    A. damage to the lining of the vessels.

    B. a tendency for blood to clot unusually fast.

    C. slow blood flow in the lower extremity.

    D. all of the above.

_____ **32.** _____ is defined as overbreathing to the point that the level of arterial carbon dioxide falls below normal.

    A. Reactive airway syndrome

    B. Hyperventilation

    C. Tachypnea

    D. Pleural effusion

_____ **33.** In a COPD patient, slowing of respirations after administration of oxygen does not necessarily mean that the patient no longer needs the oxygen; he or she may need:

    A. insulin.

    B. even more oxygen.

    C. mouth-to-mouth resuscitation.

    D. none of the above.

_____ **34.** Aspiration of vomit into the lungs may cause:

    A. croup.

    B. alkalosis.

    C. pneumonia.

    D. bronchitis.

_____ **35.** Questions to ask during the focused history and physical examination include:

    A. What has the patient already done for the breathing problem?

    B. Does the patient use a prescribed inhaler?

    C. Does the patient have any allergies?

    D. all of the above.

_____ **36.** The problem in asthma is getting the air:

    A. to diffuse through mucus.

    B. past the carina.

    C. into the narrowed trachea.

    D. out of the lungs.

_____ **37.** Generic names for popular inhaled medications include:

    A. Ventolin.

    B. Metaprel.

    C. terbutaline.

    D. all of the above.

_____ **38.** Contraindications to helping a patient self-administer any MDI medication include:

    A. not obtaining permission from medical control.

    B. noticing that the inhaler is not prescribed for this patient.

    C. noticing that the patient has already met the maximum prescribed dose.

    D. all of the above.

_____ **39.** Possible side effects of over-the-counter cold medications may include:

    A. agitation.

    B. increased heart rate.

    C. increased blood pressure.

    D. all of the above.

_____ **40.** A prolonged asthma attack that is unrelieved by epinephrine may progress to a condition known as:

    A. pleural effusion.

    B. status epilepticus.

    C. status asthmaticus.

    D. reactive airway disease.

Labeling EMT-I anatomy review web

Label the following diagram with the correct terms.

Upper airway

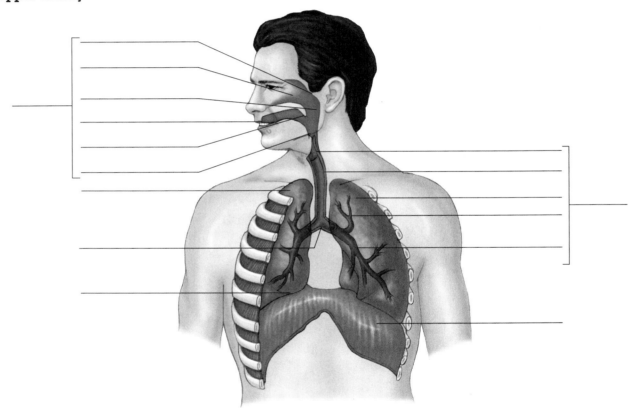

Vocabulary EMT-I vocab explorer web

Define the following terms in the space provided.

1. Stridor:

_____

_____

_____

2. Croup:

_____

_____

_____

3. Rales:

_____

_____

_____

4. Rhonchi:

_____

_____

_____

5. Diphtheria:

_____

_____

_____

6. Chronic obstructive pulmonary disease (COPD):

_____

_____

_____

Fill-in

Read each item carefully, then complete the statement by filling in the missing word(s).

1. The level of _____ bathing the brain stem stimulates respiration.

2. The level of _____ in the blood is a secondary stimulus for respiration.

3. _____ entering the alveoli passes into the capillaries, which carry

   _____ back to the heart.

4. Carbon dioxide and oxygen are exchanged in the _____.

5. _____ _____ is one of the most common causes of hospital admissions

   in the United States.

6. Abnormal breathing is indicated by a rate slower than _____ breaths per minute or

   faster than _____ breaths per minute.

7. During respiration, oxygen is provided to the blood, and _____ is removed from it.

8. Exacerbating factors in asthma tend to be _____ in children and _____

   in adults.

9. Patients with emphysema and asthma are at high risk for _____ when a weakened

   portion of lung ruptures, often during coughing.

1999 10. When performing intubation, _____ both confirms and provides ongoing assessment of

   the endotracheal tube position.

True/False

If you believe the statement to be more true than false, write the letter "T" in the space provided. If you believe the statement to be more false than true, write the letter "F."

_____ 1. Chronic bronchitis is characterized by spasming and narrowing of the bronchioles resulting from exposure to allergens.

_____ 2. With pneumothorax, the lung collapses because the negative vacuum pressure in the pleural space is lost.

_____ 3. Anaphylactic reactions occur only in patients with a previous history of asthma or allergies.

_____ 4. Decreased breath sounds in asthma occur because fluid in the pleural space has moved the lung away from the chest wall.

_____ 5. Pulmonary emboli are difficult to diagnose.

_____ 6. A patient with aspirin poisoning may hyperventilate in response to acidosis.

_____ 7. The distinction between hyperventilation and hyperventilation syndrome is straightforward and should guide the EMT-I's treatment choices.

_____ 8. COPD most often results from cigarette smoking.

_____ 9. Concerning hypoxia-driven patients, never withhold oxygen from a patient exhibiting signs of distress.

_____ 10. You may see frothy pink sputum at the nose and mouth of the most severe cases of pulmonary edema.

Short Answer

Complete this section with short written answers in the space provided.

1. List five characteristics of normal breathing.

_____

_____

_____

2. List three abnormal breath sounds associated with COPD, with a brief description of each one.

_____

_____

_____

3. Under what conditions should you not assist a patient with a metered-dose inhaler?

_____

_____

_____

4. Describe chronic bronchitis.

_____

_____

_____

5. List five signs of inadequate breathing.

_____

_____

_____

6. Explain carbon dioxide retention.

_____

_____

_____

Word Fun EMT-I vocab explorer web

The following crossword puzzle is an activity provided to reinforce correct spelling and understanding of medical terminology associated with emergency care and the EMT-I. Use the clues provided to complete the puzzle.

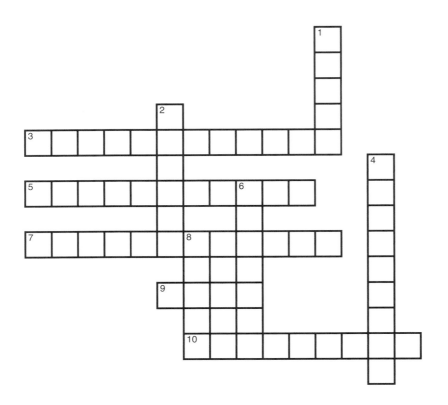

Across

3. bacterial infection of the epiglottis
5. collapsed alveoli
7. secondary drive, based on levels of oxygen
9. chronic obstructive pulmonary disease; emphysema, chronic bronchitis
10. oxygen/waste exchange at the cellular level

Down

1. crackling, moist breath sound; sounds like hairs being rubbed together behind your ear
2. coarse, rattling breath sounds
4. movement of gases from higher concentration to a lower concentration
6. harsh, high pitched barking
8. barking cough sounds, usually in children

Ambulance Calls

The following real case scenarios will give you an opportunity to explore the concerns associated with patient management. Read each scenario, then answer each question in detail.

1999 **1.** You are dispatched to the home of a 56-year-old male complaining of a sudden onset of severe dyspnea with sharp localized chest pain. His history reveals surgery for a hip fracture last week. He has been completely immobile until today.

How would you best manage this patient?

_____

_____

_____

_____

_____

_____

_____

_____

2. You are dispatched to a residence where you find a 24-year-old female who is visibly upset and breathing rapidly. She is complaining of numbness and tingling in her hands and feet, as well as dyspnea. Family members tell you that they found her this way and that she has a history of panic attacks. The patient assures you that this is not a panic attack and that it is hard for her to breathe.

How would you best manage this patient?

_____

_____

_____

_____

_____

_____

_____

_____

1999 **3.** You are called to the home of a 66-year-old male complaining of severe dyspnea. He is sitting in a recliner, smoking a cigarette, and complaining of a recent chest cold. He denies having a productive cough. The patient has a history of COPD and is on home oxygen at 2 L/min via nasal cannula. His family tells you he has a long history of breathing problems and emphysema. He is leaning forward, cyanotic around his lips, and his respirations are 36 and shallow.

How would you best manage this patient?

_____

_____

_____

_____

_____

_____

_____

_____

Skill Drills

Skill Drill 19–1: Assisting a Patient with a Metered-Dose Inhaler

Test your knowledge of this skill drill by filling in the correct words in the photo captions.

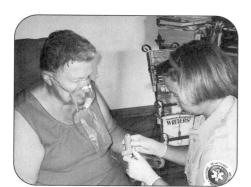

1. Ensure inhaler is at room temperature or _____.

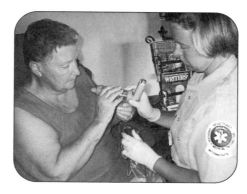

2. Remove oxygen mask. Hand inhaler to patient. Instruct about breathing and _____ _____. Use a _____ if patient has one.

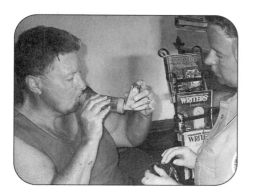

3. Instruct patient to press inhaler and inhale. Give instructions about _____.

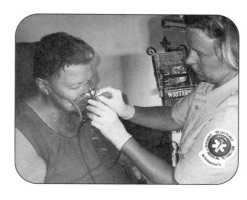

4. Reapply _____. After a few _____, have patient repeat _____ if order/protocol allows.

Workbook Activities

The following activities have been designed to help you. Your instructor may require you to complete some or all of these activities as a regular part of your EMT-I training program. You are encouraged to complete any activity that your instructor does not assign as a way to enhance your learning in the classroom.

Chapter Review

The following exercises provide an opportunity to refresh your knowledge of this chapter.

Matching

Match each of the terms in the left column to the appropriate definition in the right column.

_____ 1. Absolute refractory period

_____ 2. Atherosclerosis

_____ 3. Angina pectoris

_____ 4. Automaticity

_____ 5. Atrioventricular (AV) node

_____ 6. Arteriosclerosis

_____ 7. Bigeminy

_____ 8. Bradycardia

_____ 9. Diastole

_____ 10. Conductivity

_____ 11. Depolarization

_____ 12. CHF

_____ 13. Cardiac output

_____ 14. Ischemia

_____ 15. Escape complex

_____ 16. Mediastinum

_____ 17. Isoelectric line

_____ 18. Quadrigeminy

_____ 19. Polarized state

_____ 20. Perfusion

_____ 21. Repolarization

_____ 22. Premature complex

_____ 23. Sinoatrial (SA) node

_____ 24. Supraventricular

_____ 25. Tachycardia

_____ 26. Ventricular tachycardia

A. premature complex occurring every second beat

B. cholesterol/calcium buildup in blood vessels

C. site in right atrium responsible for slowing electrical conduction

D. period of time in the cell firing cycle at which it's impossible to restimulate the cell into firing an impulse to fire off another impulse

E. Short-lived chest discomfort caused by partial or temporary blockage of blood to the heart muscle

F. thickening of arterial walls

G. the ability of cardiac cells to generate impulse even when there is no external nervous stimulus

H. slow heart rate; less then 60 beats per minute

I. amount of blood pumped through the circulatory system in 1 minute

J. relaxation phase of the heart, when the ventricles are filling with blood

K. state in which the cell becomes more positive; during the latter part of resting state and is completed during activation by the action potential

L. the ability of the cardiac cells to conduct electrical impulses

M. congestive heart failure; usually resulting in backup fluid in the lungs

N. a beat that occurs after a normal pacemaker fails to fire

O. baseline of a tracing on an electrocardiogram (ECG)

P. a lack of oxygen that deprives tissue of necessary nutrients

Q. the area in the chest that lies between the lungs and contains the heart and great vessels

R. the flow of blood through body tissues and vessels

S. process of returning to cardiac cells' resting state

Cardiovascular Emergencies

_____ **27.** Unifocal

_____ **28.** Ventricular fibrillation

_____ **29.** Transcutaneous pacing (TCP)

_____ **30.** Syncope

T. premature complex every 4th beat

U. the state of the resting cell

V. complex that arrives earlier than expected for the cadence of rhythm

W. rapid heart rhythm in which the electrical impulse begins in the ventricle

X. term used to describe singly occurring PVC(S) originating in the same ectopic focus

Y. the normal site of the origin of electrical impulses; located in the right atrium

Z. cardiac rhythm that originates above the ventricles

AA. a system that delivers pacing impulses to the heart through the skin via adhesive cutaneous electrodes

BB. fainting spell

CC. rapid heart rhythm, more that 100 beats per minute

DD. disorganized, ineffective twitching of the ventricles

Multiple Choice

Read each item carefully, then select the best response.

_____ **1.** The _____ is the strongest and largest of the four cardiac chambers.

    A. right atria

    B. left atria

    C. right ventricle

    D. left ventricle

_____ **2.** The aorta receives its blood supply from the:

    A. right atria.

    B. left atria.

    C. right ventricle.

    D. left ventricle.

_____ **3.** Blood enters into the right atrium from the body through the:

    A. vena cava.

    B. aorta.

    C. pulmonary artery.

    D. pulmonary vein.

_____ **4.** The only vein(s) in the body to carry oxygenated blood is (are) the:
   A. external jugular veins.
   B. pulmonary veins.
   C. subclavian veins.
   D. inferior vena cava.

_____ **5.** Normal electrical impulses originate in the sinus node, just above the:
   A. atria.
   B. ventricles.
   C. AV junction.
   D. Bundle of His.

_____ **6.** The "lub" of the "lub-DUB" sound of the heart is caused by:
   A. the sudden closure of the mitral and tricuspid valves.
   B. closure of the aortic and pulmonic valves at the end of ventricular contraction.
   C. gas exchange within the alveoli.
   D. a heart murmur.

_____ **7.** A bruit sound over a main blood vessel indicates:
   A. angina pectoris.
   B. arteriosclerotic disease.
   C. atherosclerosis.
   D. all of the above.

_____ **8.** The _____ are tiny blood vessels about one cell thick.
   A. arterioles
   B. venules
   C. capillaries
   D. ventricles

_____ **9.** Which has the fastest pacer in the heart?
   A. SA node
   B. AV node
   C. Bundle branch
   D. Bachman bundle

_____ **10.** _____ is the maximum pressure exerted by the left ventricle as it contracts.
   A. Cardiac output
   B. Diastolic blood pressure
   C. Systolic blood pressure
   D. Stroke volume

_____ **11.** Atherosclerosis can lead to a complete _____ of a coronary artery.
   A. occlusion
   B. disintegration
   C. dilation
   D. contraction

_____ **12.** Cardiac cells differ from the rest of the cells in the body because:
   A. they can function without insulin.
   B. they can regenerate themselves.
   C. they can generate their own impulse to contract.
   D. none of the above.

_____ **13.** Tissues downstream from a blood clot will suffer from lack of oxygen. If blood flow is resumed in a short time, the _____ tissues will recover.
   A. dead
   B. ischemic
   C. necrosed
   D. dry

_____ **14.** Risk factors for myocardial infarction include all of the following EXCEPT:
  A. male gender.
  B. high blood pressure.
  C. stress.
  D. increased activity level.

_____ **15.** When, for a brief period of time, heart tissues do not get enough oxygen, the pain is called:
  A. AMI.
  B. angina.
  C. ischemia.
  D. CAD.

_____ **16.** Angina pain may be felt in the:
  A. arms.
  B. midback.
  C. epigastrium.
  D. all of the above.

_____ **17.** Angina may be associated with:
  A. shortness of breath.
  B. nausea.
  C. sweating.
  D. all of the above.

_____ **18.** Which of the following assessment findings would best suggest right-sided heart failure?
  A. Orthopnea
  B. Pulmonary edema
  C. Nocturnal dyspnea
  D. Distended jugular veins

_____ **19.** About _____ minutes after blood flow is cut off, some heart muscle cells begin to die.
  A. 10
  B. 20
  C. 30
  D. 40

_____ **20.** An acute myocardial infarction is more likely to occur in the larger, thick-walled left ventricle, which needs more _____ than in the right ventricle.
  A. oxygen and glucose
  B. force to pump
  C. blood and oxygen
  D. electrical activity

_____ **21.** Nitroglycerin is given to patients with suspected cardiac chest pain because of these physiologic effects on smooth muscle:
  A. relaxation and increased preload.
  B. relaxation and decreased preload.
  C. contraction and increased afterload.
  D. contraction and decreased preload.

_____ **22.** Consequences of AMI may include:
  A. cardiogenic shock.
  B. congestive heart failure.
  C. sudden death.
  D. all of the above.

_____ **23.** Sudden death is usually the result of _____, in which the heart fails to generate an effective blood flow.

  A. AMI

  B. atherosclerosis

  C. PVCs

  D. cardiac arrest

_____ **24.** Disorganized, ineffective quivering of the ventricles is known as:

  A. ventricular fibrillation.

  B. asystole.

  C. ventricular stand still.

  D. ventricular tachycardia.

_____ **25.** In _____, often caused by a heart attack, the problem is that the heart lacks enough power to force the proper volume of blood through the circulatory system.

  A. asystole

  B. cardiogenic shock

  C. ventricular fibrillation

  D. angina

_____ **26.** Causes of congestive heart failure include all of the following EXCEPT:

  A. chronic hypotension.

  B. heart valve damage.

  C. a myocardial infarction.

  D. longstanding high blood pressure.

_____ **27.** Signs and symptoms of shock include all of the following EXCEPT:

  A. elevated heart rate.

  B. pale, clammy skin.

  C. air hunger.

  D. elevated blood pressure.

_____ **28.** In patients with CHF, changes in heart function occur, including:

  A. a decrease in heart rate.

  B. enlargement of the left ventricle.

  C. enlargement of the right ventricle.

  D. a decrease in blood pressure.

_____ **29.** Fluid that collects in the feet and legs is called:

  A. pedal edema.

  B. pulmonary edema.

  C. cerebral edema.

  D. tibial edema.

_____ **30.** All patient assessments begin by determining whether or not the patient:

  A. is breathing.

  B. can talk.

  C. is responsive.

  D. has a pulse.

_____ **31.** AEDs are safe to use in children older than:

  A. 10 years.

  B. 8 years.

  C. 5 years.

  D. 1 year.

_____ **32.** To assess chest pain, use the mnemonic:
   A. AVPU.
   B. OPQRST.
   C. SAMPLE.
   D. CHART.

_____ **33.** Nitroglycerin may be in the form of a:
   A. skin patch.
   B. spray.
   C. pill.
   D. all of the above.

_____ **34.** When administering nitroglycerin to a patient, you should check the patient's _____ within 5 minutes after each dose.
   A. level of consciousness
   B. breathing
   C. pulse
   D. blood pressure

_____ **35.** In general, a maximum of _____ dose(s) of nitroglycerin is (are) given for any one episode of chest pain.
   A. one
   B. two
   C. three
   D. four

_____ **36.** _____ are inserted when the electrical control system of the heart is so damaged that it cannot function properly.
   A. Stents
   B. Pacemakers
   C. Balloon angioplasties
   D. Defibrillators

_____ **37.** When the battery wears out in a pacemaker, the patient may experience:
   A. syncope.
   B. dizziness.
   C. weakness.
   D. all of the above.

_____ **38.** The computer inside the AED is specifically programmed to recognize rhythms that require defibrillation to correct, most commonly:
   A. asystole.
   B. ventricular tachycardia.
   C. ventricular fibrillation.
   D. supraventricular tachycardia.

_____ **39.** You should apply the AED only to unresponsive patients with no:
   A. significant medical problems.
   B. cardiac history.
   C. pulse.
   D. brain activity.

_____ **40.** _____ usually refers to a state of cardiac arrest despite an organized electrical complex.
   A. Asystole
   B. Pulseless electrical activity
   C. Ventricular fibrillation
   D. Ventricular tachycardia

_____ **41.** The links in the chain of survival include all of the following EXCEPT:

    A. early access and CPR.

    B. early ACLS.

    C. early administration of nitroglycerin.

    D. early defibrillation.

_____ **42.** An AED may fail to function properly due to:

    A. the batteries not working.

    B. improper maintenance.

    C. operator error.

    D. all of the above.

Labeling EMT-I anatomy review web

Label the following diagrams with the correct terms.

Blood Flow through the Heart

A. _____

B. _____

C. _____

D. _____

E. _____

F. _____

G. _____

H. _____

I. _____

J. _____

K. _____

L. _____

M. _____

N. _____

O. _____   U. _____   AA. _____

P. _____   V. _____   BB. _____

Q. _____   W. _____   CC. _____

R. _____   X. _____   DD. _____

S. _____   Y. _____   EE. _____

T. _____   Z. _____

The Coronary Arteries

A. _____

B. _____

C. _____

D. _____

E. _____

F. _____

G. _____

H. _____

I. _____

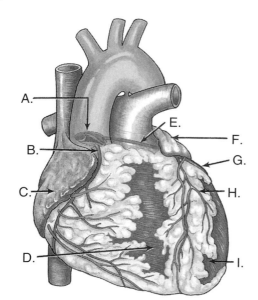

The Cardiovascular System

A. _____

B. _____

C. _____

D. _____

E. _____

F. _____

G. _____

H. _____

I. _____

J. _____

K. _____

L. _____

M. _____

N. _____

O. _____

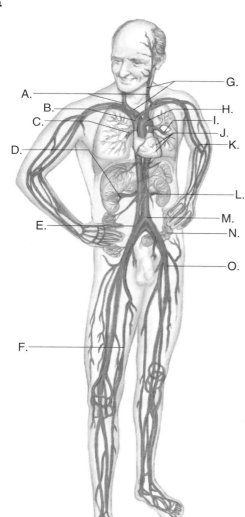

Vocabulary EMT-I vocab explorer web

Define the following terms in the space provided.

1. Angina pectoris:

_____

_____

_____

2. Ventricular fibrillation:

_____

_____

_____

3. Cardiogenic shock:

_____

_____

_____

4. Acute myocardial infarction (AMI):

_____

_____

_____

5. Cardiac arrest:

_____

_____

_____

6. Syncope:

_____

_____

_____

7. Congestive heart failure (CHF):

_____

_____

_____

Fill-in

Read each item carefully, then complete the statement by filling in the missing word(s).

1. The heart is divided down the middle by a wall called the _____.

2. The _____ is the largest artery.

3. The _____ ventricle pumps blood in through the pulmonary circulation.

4. Electrical impulses spread from the _____ node to the ventricles.

5. _____ cells remove carbon dioxide from the body's tissues.

6. The heart has _____ chambers.

7. The _____ side of the heart is more muscular because it must pump blood into the aorta and all the other arteries of the body.

1999 8. _____ are devices that are applied to the skin to detect electrical activity and convey it to a machine for display.

1999 9. One box on the graph paper represents _____ seconds.

1999 10. The QRS interval is normally less than _____ seconds.

1999 11. The normal heart rhythm originates in the _____ _____ and is called a

_____ _____ _____

1999 12. _____ are false abnormalities of baseline present on an ECG due to sources other than the patient's bioelectrical impulses.

True/False

If you believe the statement to be more true than false, write the letter "T" in the space provided. If you believe the statement to be more false than true, write the letter "F."

_____ 1. The right side of the heart pumps oxygen-rich blood to the body.
_____ 2. In the normal heart, the need for increased blood flow to the myocardium is easily met by an increase in heart rate.
_____ 3. Atherosclerosis results in narrowing of the lumen of coronary arteries.
_____ 4. Infarction is a temporary interruption of the blood supply to the tissues.
_____ 5. Angina can result from a spasm of the artery.
_____ 6. The pain of angina and the pain of AMI are easily distinguishable.
_____ 7. Nitroglycerin works in most patients within 5 minutes to relieve the pain of AMI.
_____ 8. If an AED malfunctions during use, you must report that problem to the manufacturer and the Department of Human Resources.
_____ 9. Angina occurs when the heart's need for oxygen exceeds its supply.
_____ 10. White blood cells are the most numerous and help the blood to clot.

1999 _____ **11.** Patients with signs of cardiogenic shock may benefit from the use of inotropic drugs and antiarrhytmics.

1999 _____ **12.** Once CHF develops, it can be treated but not cured.

1999 _____ **13.** Morphine should be considered with the use of furosemide (Lasix) in treatment of CHF.

_____ **14.** The American Heart Association reports cardiovascular disease accounts for 1 out of every 2.6 deaths.

_____ **15.** Artherosclerosis is only found in coronary arteries.

Short Answer

Complete this section with short written answers in the space provided.

1. Name and describe the two basic types of defibrillators.

_____

_____

_____

2. What are the three most common errors of AED use?

_____

_____

_____

3. If ALS is not responding to the scene, what are the three points at which transport should be initiated for a cardiac arrest patient?

_____

_____

_____

4. List six safety considerations for operating an AED.

_____

_____

_____

5. What is the procedure for assisting a patient with nitroglycerin administration?

_____

_____

_____

6. List three ways in which AMI pain differs from angina pain.

_____

_____

_____

7. List three serious consequences of AMI.

_____

_____

_____

8. Name at least five signs and symptoms associated with AMI.

_____

_____

_____

9. Describe the technique for AED pad placement.

_____

_____

_____

10. List the intrinsic rates of the following pacing cells.

SA node   _____ BPM

Atrial cells   _____ BPM

AV node   _____ BPM

His bundle   _____ BPM

Bundle branch   _____ BPM

Purkinje cells   _____ BPM

Myocardial cells   _____ BPM

11. The AED should only be applied to unresponsive patients who are pulseless and apneic. Why?

_____

_____

_____

1999 **12.** State the pharmacologic interventions associated with suspected cardiac chest pain, using the mnemonic "MONA."

M:_____

O:_____

N:_____

A:_____

Rhythm Recognition

Analyze and interpret the following rhythm strips, and complete the tables below.

1999 1.

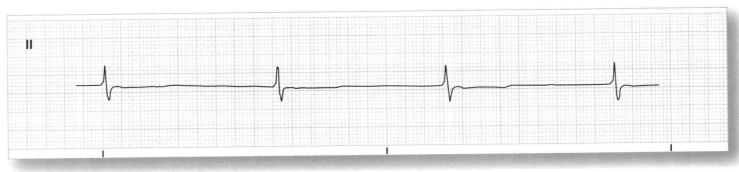

Rate:

Regularity:

P waves:

P:QRS ratio:

P-R intervals:

QRS width:

Grouping:

Dropped beats:

Rhythm:

1999 2.

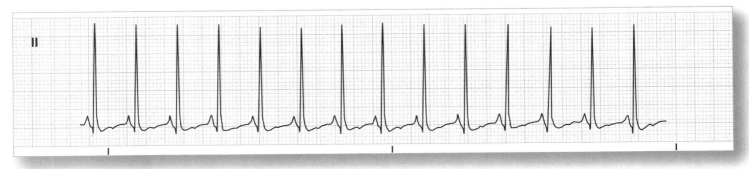

Rate:

Regularity:

P waves:

P:QRS ratio:

P-R intervals:

QRS width:

Grouping:

Dropped beats:

Rhythm:

1999   3.

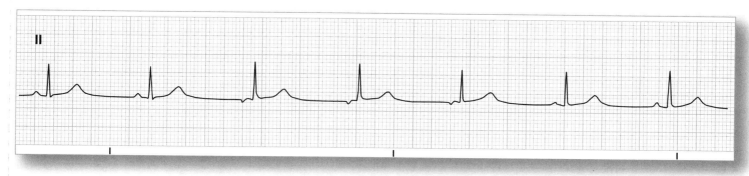

Rate: P-R intervals:

Regularity: QRS width:

P waves: Grouping:

                                Dropped beats:

P:QRS ratio: Rhythm:

1999   4.

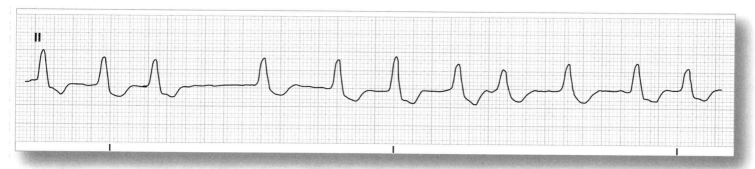

Rate: P-R intervals:

Regularity: QRS width:

P waves: Grouping:

                                Dropped beats:

P:QRS ratio: Rhythm:

1999 **5.**

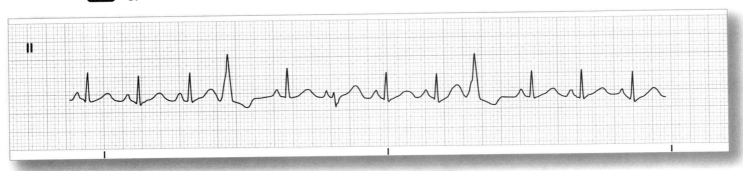

Rate:

Regularity:

P waves:

P:QRS ratio:

P-R intervals:

QRS width:

Grouping:

Dropped beats:

Rhythm:

1999 **6.**

Rate:

Regularity:

P waves:

P:QRS ratio:

P-R intervals:

QRS width:

Grouping:

Dropped beats:

Rhythm:

1999 7.

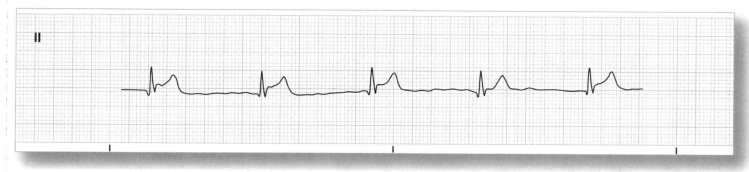

Rate: P-R intervals:

Regularity: QRS width:

P waves: Grouping:

                                           Dropped beats:

P:QRS ratio: Rhythm:

1999 8.

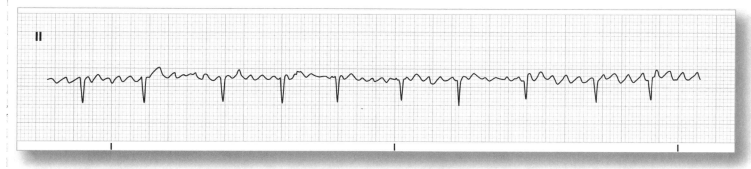

Rate: P-R intervals:

Regularity: QRS width:

P waves: Grouping:

                                           Dropped beats:

P:QRS ratio: Rhythm:

1999 9.

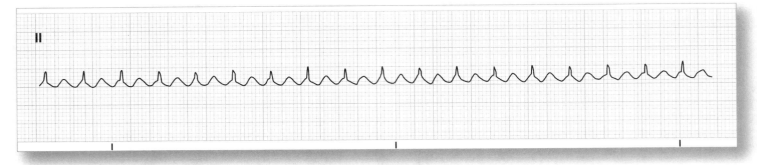

Rate: P-R intervals:

Regularity: QRS width:

P waves: Grouping:

                                   Dropped beats:

P:QRS ratio: Rhythm:

1999 10.

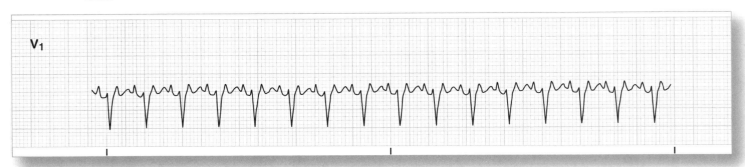

Rate: P-R intervals:

Regularity: QRS width:

P waves: Grouping:

                                   Dropped beats:

P:QRS ratio: Rhythm:

1999 11.

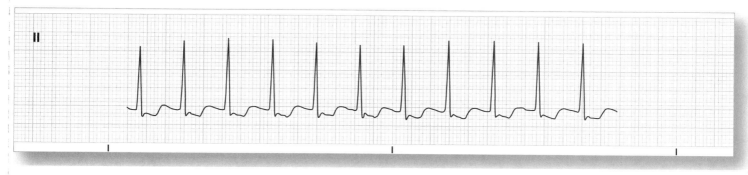

Rate: P-R intervals:

Regularity: QRS width:

P waves: Grouping:

                                         Dropped beats:

P:QRS ratio: Rhythm:

1999 12.

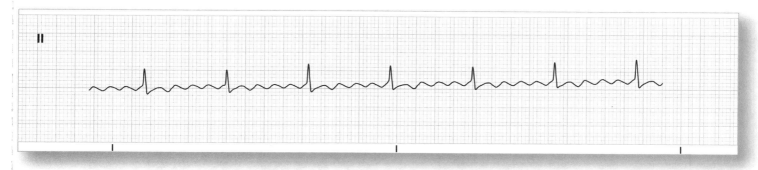

Rate: P-R intervals:

Regularity: QRS width:

P waves: Grouping:

                                         Dropped beats:

P:QRS ratio: Rhythm:

1999 13.

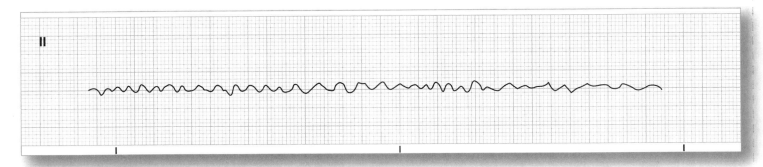

Rate: P-R intervals:

Regularity: QRS width:

P waves: Grouping:

                               Dropped beats:

P:QRS ratio: Rhythm:

1999 14.

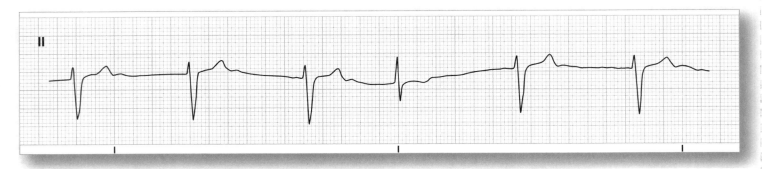

Rate: P-R intervals:

Regularity: QRS width:

P waves: Grouping:

                               Dropped beats:

P:QRS ratio: Rhythm:

1999 15.

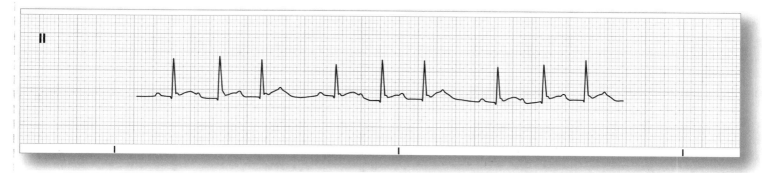

Rate: P-R intervals:

Regularity: QRS width:

P waves: Grouping:

                                   Dropped beats:

P:QRS ratio: Rhythm:

1999 16.

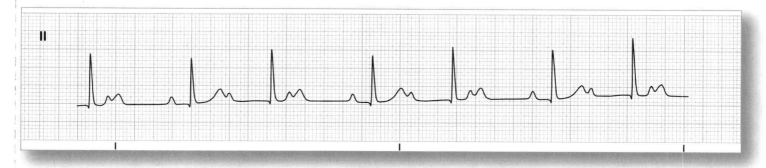

Rate: P-R intervals:

Regularity: QRS width:

P waves: Grouping:

                                   Dropped beats:

P:QRS ratio: Rhythm:

1999 17.

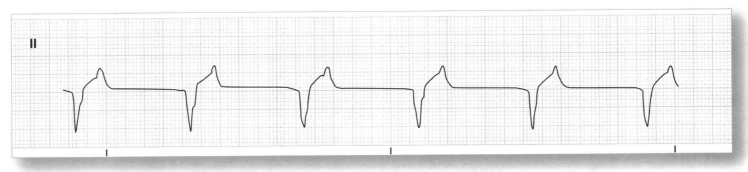

Rate: P-R intervals:

Regularity: QRS width:

P waves: Grouping:

                               Dropped beats:

P:QRS ratio: Rhythm:

1999 18.

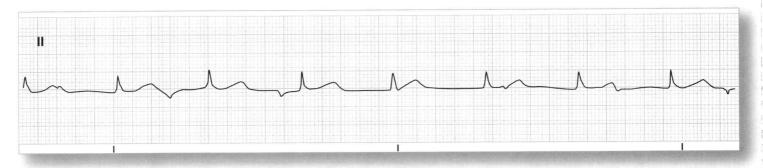

Rate: P-R intervals:

Regularity: QRS width:

P waves: Grouping:

                               Dropped beats:

P:QRS ratio: Rhythm:

1999 19.

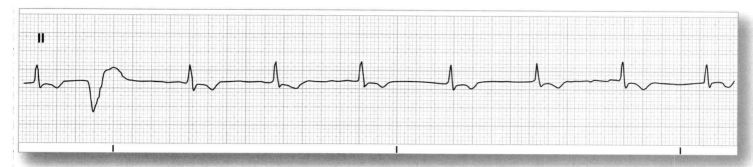

Rate: P-R intervals:

Regularity: QRS width:

P waves: Grouping:

                                   Dropped beats:

P:QRS ratio: Rhythm:

1999 20.

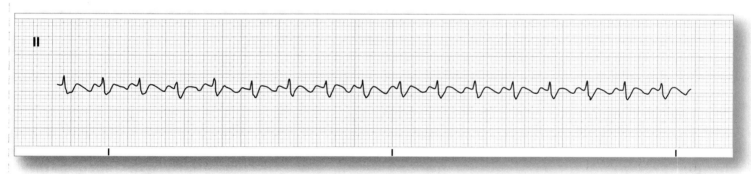

Rate: P-R intervals:

Regularity: QRS width:

P waves: Grouping:

                                   Dropped beats:

P:QRS ratio: Rhythm:

1999 21.

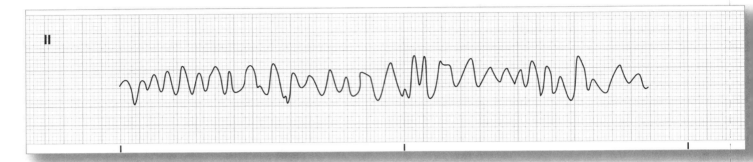

Rate: P-R intervals:

Regularity: QRS width:

P waves: Grouping:

                                Dropped beats:

P:QRS ratio: Rhythm:

1999 22.

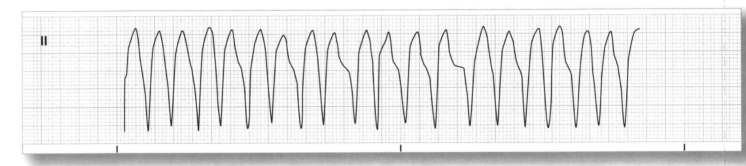

Rate: P-R intervals:

Regularity: QRS width:

P waves: Grouping:

                                Dropped beats:

P:QRS ratio: Rhythm:

1999 23.

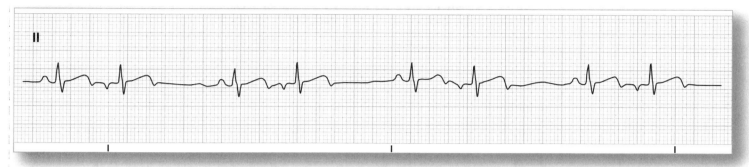

Rate:

Regularity:

P waves:

P:QRS ratio:

P-R intervals:

QRS width:

Grouping:

Dropped beats:

Rhythm:

1999 24.

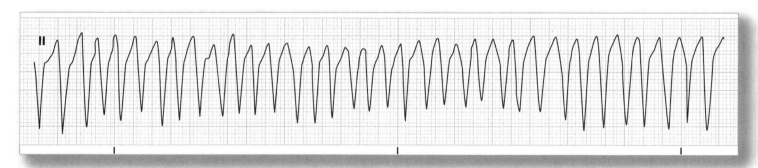

Rate:

Regularity:

P waves:

P:QRS ratio:

P-R intervals:

QRS width:

Grouping:

Dropped beats:

Rhythm:

Word Fun EMT-I vocab explorer web

The following crossword puzzle is an activity provided to reinforce correct spelling and understanding of medical terminology associated with emergency care and the EMT-I. Use the clues in the column to complete the puzzle.

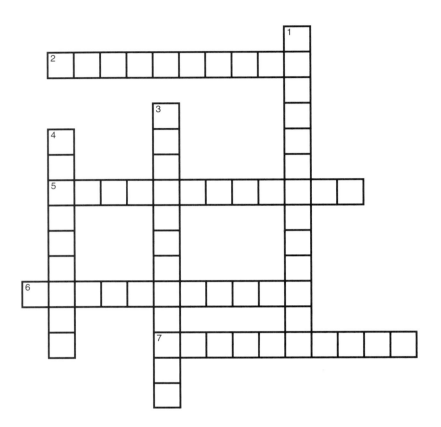

Across

2. Swelling of the feet and ankles; possible sign of CHF

5. One heart beat; a single pulse

6. Separates the the left atrium from the left ventricle

7. Irregular heart rhythm

Down

1. Heart fails to generate effective and detectable blood flow

3. To shock; attempt to restore normal sinus rhythm

4. Blockage

Ambulance Calls

The following real case scenarios provide an opportunity to explore the concerns associated with patient management. Read each scenario, then answer each question in detail.

1. You are dispatched to the residence of a 58-year-old man complaining of chest pain. He states that it feels like "somebody is standing on my chest." He sat down when it started and took a nitroglycerin tablet. He is still a little nauseated and sweaty, but feels better. He is very anxious. The heart monitor shows the following.

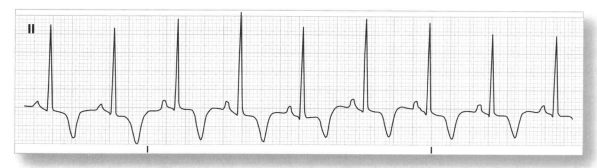

How would you best manage this patient?

_____

_____

_____

_____

_____

_____

_____

_____

1999 **2.** You are called to a business office for a 38-year-old man complaining of indigestion. Coworkers tell you that the pain started suddenly and he clutched his chest and vomited. He insists that he will be all right, and that it is probably something he ate. He is pale and diaphoretic. His heart monitor shows the following.

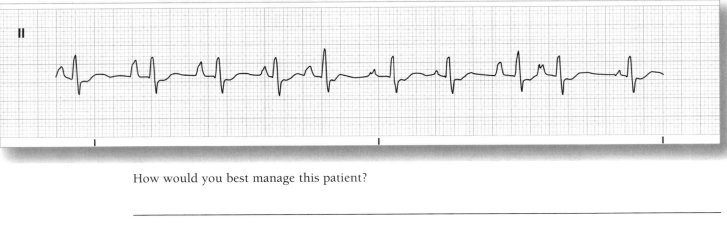

How would you best manage this patient?

_____

_____

_____

_____

_____

_____

_____

_____

1999 **3.** You are dispatched to a local personal care home for an elderly woman complaining of shortness of breath. She is gasping for breath and is extremely anxious. Her legs are very swollen and she says she took her "water pill" this morning. The staff tells you that she has a history of diabetes, congestive heart failure, and hypertension.

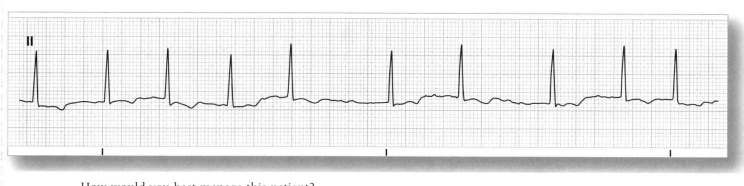

How would you best manage this patient?

_____

_____

_____

_____

_____

_____

_____

_____

Skill Drills

Skill Drill 20-3: Treating a Conscious Patient for Chest Discomfort
Test your knowledge of this skill drill by filling in the correct words in the photo captions.

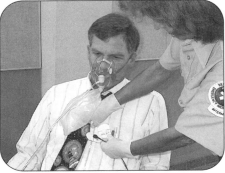

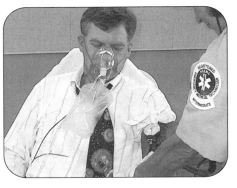

1. _____ the patient, and perform the initial assessment. Apply _____.

2. Apply a _____ _____, and note the presence of any _____. Treat accordingly.

3. _____ the patient. Measure and record the patient's _____ _____. Gain _____ access.

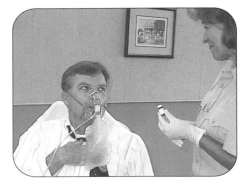

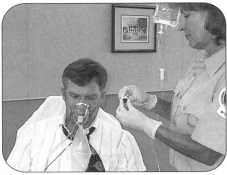

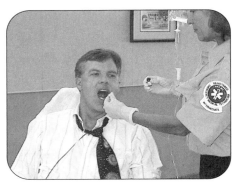

4. Obtain a _____ _____ and physical exam. Ask specific questions about the patient's _____ _____.

5. Prepare to assist with prescribed _____; check the medication and its _____.

6. Help the patient administer the prescribed _____.

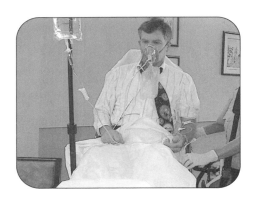

7. _____ the patient.

1999 **Skill Drill 20-4: AED and CPR**

Test your knowledge of this skill drill by placing the photos below in the correct order. Number the first step with a "1," the second step with a "2," and so on.

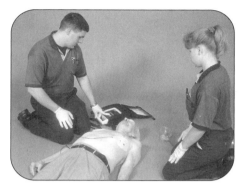

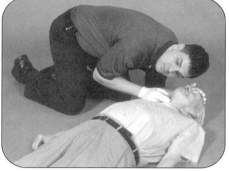

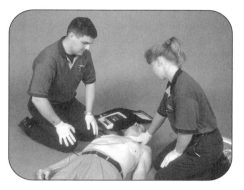

Turn on the AED; begin narrative if needed.

Apply AED pads.

Stop CPR.

Stop CPR if in progress.

Assess responsiveness.

Check breathing and pulse.

If unresponsive, not breathing, or breathing inadequately, give two slow ventilations.

After 2 minutes of CPR, reanalyze the cardiac rhythm. If no shock is advised, check the pulse.

If pulse is absent, continue CPR.

If pulse is present, check breathing.

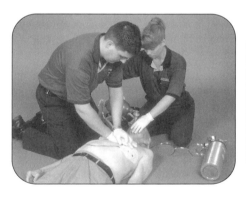

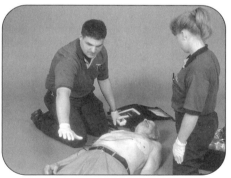

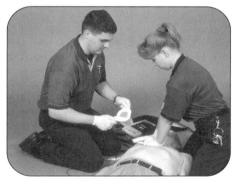

If breathing adequately, give 100% oxygen and transport. If apneic or breathing inadequately, continue rescue breathing at 10 to 12 breaths/min, and transport.

If no pulse, perform five cycles (approximately 2 minutes) of CPR.

Clear the patient, and analyze again.

If necessary, deliver another shock and immediately resume CPR.

Repeat defibrillation every 2 minutes as needed.

Transport the patient, and contact medical control.

Verbally and visually clear the patient.

Push the analyze button if there is one.

If no shock advised, perform five cycles (approximately 2 minutes) of CPR and reassess.

If a shock is advised, recheck that all are clear, and push the shock button.

After the shock is delivered, immediately begin five cycles of CPR, beginning with chest compressions.

After five cycles (approximately 2 minutes) of CPR, reanalyze the patient's rhythm.

If the machine advises a shock, clear the patient, push the shock button, and immediately resume CPR.

If pulseless, begin CPR.

Remove sufficient clothing to gain access to the patient's chest.

Prepare the AED pads.

1999 **Skill Drill 20-6: Defibrillation**

Test your knowledge of this skill drill by filling in the correct words in the photo captions.

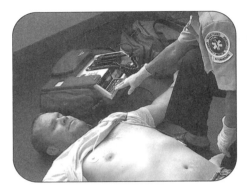

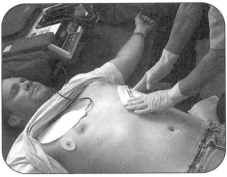

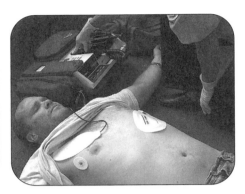

1. Determine the _____

_____ .

2. Apply _____

_____ according to

the manufacturer's recommendation.

(If using _____ , ap-

ply electrode _____

to the paddles before placing them

on the patient's chest.)

3. Continue _____

while charging.

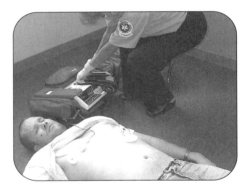

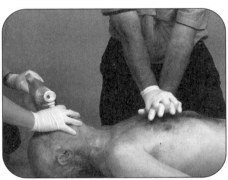

4. Reassess the _____ ,

and clear anyone around the patient.

Deliver the _____ .

5. Resume immediate CPR. Reassess

after _____ .

1999 Skill Drill 20-7: Transcutaneous Pacing

Test your knowledge of this skill drill by placing the photos below in the correct order. Number the first step with a "1," the second step with a "2," and so on.

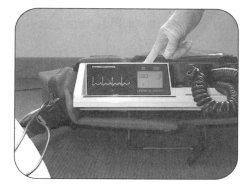

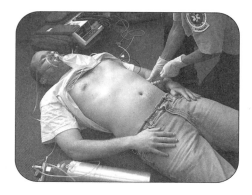

Connect the electrodes to the cardiac monitor, and select desired heart rate.

Slowly adjust the electrical current setting until electrical capture is obtained.

Determine the need for pacing.

Attach the three-lead cables.

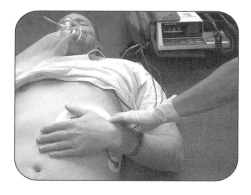

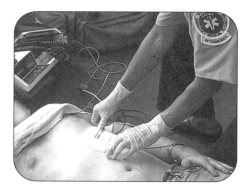

Assess the patient's pulse to ensure mechanical capture.

Apply the pacing electrodes.

Workbook Activities

The following activities have been designed to help you. Your instructor may require you to complete some or all of these activities as a regular part of your EMT-I training program. You are encouraged to complete any activity that your instructor does not assign as a way to enhance your learning in the classroom.

Chapter Review

The following exercises provide an opportunity to refresh your knowledge of this chapter.

Matching

Match each of the terms in the left column to the appropriate definition in the right column.

_____ 1. Hormone

_____ 2. Polydipsia

_____ 3. Hypoglycemia

_____ 4. Type I diabetes

_____ 5. Diabetic ketoacidosis

_____ 6. Insulin

_____ 7. Diabetic coma

_____ 8. Polyuria

_____ 9. Type II diabetes

_____ 10. Polyphagia

_____ 11. Insulin shock

_____ 12. Glucose

_____ 13. Kussmaul respirations

_____ 14. Hyperglycemia

_____ 15. Diabetes mellitus

_____ 16. Glycolysis

_____ 17. Islets of Langerhans

_____ 18. Glucagon

_____ 19. Diabetic ketoacidosis

_____ 20. Glycogenolysis

_____ 21. Gluconeogenesis

A. altered level of consciousness caused by insufficient glucose in the blood

B. diabetes that usually starts in childhood; requires insulin

C. excessive eating

D. deep, rapid breathing

E. excessive urination

F. frequent drinking to satisfy excessive thirst persisting for a long period of time

G. diabetes with onset later in life; can be controlled by diet and oral medication

H. chemical produced by a gland that regulates body organs

I. when blood glucose is below normal

J. a metabolic disorder in which the ability to metabolize carbohydrates is impaired

K. extremely high blood glucose level

L. pathologic condition resulting from the accumulation of acids in the body resulting from uncontrolled diabetes

M. hormone that enables glucose to enter the cells

N. primary fuel, along with oxygen, for cellular metabolism

O. state of unconsciousness resulting from several problems, including ketoacidosis, dehydration, and hyperglycemia

Diabetic Emergencies

_____ **22.** Hyperglycemic hyperosmolar nonketotic coma (HHNC)

P. when new glucose is produced other than through the metabolization of carbohydrates

Q. a form of acidosis in uncontrolled diabetes in which certain acids accumulate when insulin is not available

R. conversion of glucose into energy via metabolic pathways

S. process by which glycogen is converted to glucose; facilitated by glucagon

T. hormone released from alpha cells in the islets of Langerhans; converts glycogen to glucose when blood glucose levels drop

U. pancreas structures composed of four types of cells; beta cell responsible for the production of insulin

V. condition characterized by severe hyperglycemia, hyperosmolality, and dehydration, but no ketoacidosis

Multiple Choice

Read each item carefully, then select the best response.

Questions 1 to 5 pertain to the following scenario:

You are called to the home of a 44-year-old male complaining of an altered mental status, malaise, and feeling flushed. During your focused history, the patient denies any diabetic history, yet his blood glucose level is 456 mg/dL.

_____ **1.** With what type of diabetes is he likely to be diagnosed?

A. Type I

B. Type II

C. Sugar diabetes

D. HHNC

_____ **2.** In what range would you expect to find his blood glucose level?

A. 80 to 120 mg/dL

B. 90 to 140 mg/dL

C. 70 to 110 mg/dL

D. 60 to 100 mg/dL

_____ 3. You would expect the excess glucose to be excreted through:

A. the lymphatic system.

B. sweat.

C. respiratory efforts.

D. urine.

_____ 4. The patient is presenting with deep rapid breathing known as:

A. hyperventilation.

B. stridor.

C. Kussmaul respirations.

D. none of the above.

_____ 5. Your treatment should include:

A. monitoring ABCs.

B. high-flow oxygen.

C. cardiac monitoring.

D. all of the above.

_____ 6. Diabetes is a metabolic disorder in which the hormone _____ is missing or ineffective.

A. estrogen

B. adrenalin

C. insulin

D. epinephrine

_____ 7. The accumulation of ketones and fatty acids in blood tissue can lead to a dangerous condition in diabetic patients known as:

A. diabetic ketoacidosis.

B. insulin shock.

C. HHNC.

D. hypoglycemia.

_____ 8. The term for excessive eating as a result of cellular "hunger" is:

A. polyuria.

B. polydipsia.

C. polyphagia.

D. polyphony.

_____ 9. Insulin is produced by the:

A. adrenal glands.

B. hypothalamus.

C. spleen.

D. pancreas.

_____ 10. Factors that may contribute to diabetic coma include:

A. infection.

B. alcohol consumption.

C. insufficient insulin.

D. all of the above.

_____ 11. The only organ that does not require insulin to allow glucose to enter its cells is the:

A. liver.

B. brain.

C. pancreas.

D. heart.

_____ **12.** The sweet or fruity odor on the breath of a diabetic patient is caused by _____ in the blood.

    A. acetone

    B. ketones

    C. alcohol

    D. insulin

_____ **13.** The term for excessive thirst is:

    A. polyuria.

    B. polydipsia.

    C. polyphagia.

    D. polyphony.

_____ **14.** Oral diabetic medications include:

    A. glyburide (Micronase).

    B. glipizide (Glucotrol).

    C. chlorpropamide (Diabinase).

    D. all of the above.

_____ **15.** _____ is one of the basic sugars in the body.

    A. Dextrose

    B. Sucrose

    C. Fructose

    D. Syrup

_____ **16.** _____ is the hormone that is normally produced by the pancreas that enables glucose to enter the cells.

    A. Insulin

    B. Adrenalin

    C. Estrogen

    D. Epinephrine

_____ **17.** The term for excessive urination is:

    A. polyuria.

    B. polydipsia.

    C. polyphagia.

    D. polyphony.

_____ **18.** When fat is used as an immediate energy source, _____ and fatty acids are formed as waste products.

    A. dextrose

    B. sucrose

    C. ketones

    D. bicarbonate

_____ **19.** Excess glucose in stored in the liver and skeletal muscle as:

    A. glucagon.

    B. islets of Langerhans.

    C. insulin.

    D. excess glucose is not stored in the liver.

_____ **20.** The onset of hypoglycemia can occur within:

    A. seconds.

    B. minutes.

    C. hours.

    D. days.

_____ **21.** Without _____, or with very low levels, brain cells rapidly suffer permanent damage.
   A. epinephrine
   B. ketones
   C. bicarbonate
   D. glucose

_____ **22.** _____ is/are a potentially life-threatening complication of insulin shock.
   A. Kussmaul respirations
   B. Hypotension
   C. Seizures
   D. Polydipsia

_____ **23.** Your patient is presenting with signs of dehydration. What should you administer?
   A. Oral glucose
   B. A 20-mL/kg bolus of an isotonic crystalloid
   C. Dextrose 50% wide open until patient reaches a blood level of 150 mg/dL
   D. Full-flow oxygen

_____ **24.** Diabetic coma may develop as a result of:
   A. too little insulin.
   B. too much insulin.
   C. overhydration.
   D. metabolic alkalosis.

_____ **25.** Always suspect hypoglycemia in any patient with:
   A. Kussmaul respirations.
   B. an altered mental status.
   C. nausea and vomiting.
   D. all of the above.

_____ **26.** The most important step in caring for the unresponsive diabetic patient is to:
   A. give oral glucose immediately.
   B. perform a focused assessment.
   C. open the airway.
   D. obtain a SAMPLE history.

_____ **27.** Determination of diabetic coma or insulin shock should:
   A. be made before transport of the patient.
   B. be made before administration of oral glucose.
   C. be determined by a urine glucose test.
   D. be based on your knowledge of the signs and symptoms of each condition.

_____ **28.** An unresponsive patient involved in a motor vehicle crash with a diabetic identification bracelet should be suspected to be _____ until proven otherwise.
   A. hypoglycemic
   B. hyperglycemic
   C. intoxicated
   D. in shock

_____ **29.** Contraindications for the use of oral glucose include:
   A. unconsciousness.
   B. known alcoholism.
   C. insulin shock.
   D. all of the above.

_____ **30.** The medication of choice to treat an unconscious adult experiencing hypoglycemia is:
   A. 1 g of glucagon.
   B. 500 mL of D_5W.
   C. 25 g of D_{25}.
   D. 25 g of D_{50}.

_____ **31.** Signs and symptoms associated with hypoglycemia include:
  A. warm dry skin.
  B. rapid weak pulse.
  C. Kussmaul respirations.
  D. anxious or combative behavior.

_____ **32.** The patient in insulin shock is experiencing:
  A. hyperglycemia.
  B. hypoglycemia.
  C. diabetic ketoacidosis.
  D. a low production of insulin.

_____ **33.** Signs of dehydration include:
  A. good skin turgor.
  B. elevated blood pressure.
  C. sunken eyes.
  D. all of the above.

_____ **34.** Diabetic patients who complain of "not feeling so well" should:
  A. have their glucose level checked.
  B. have a rapid trauma assessment completed.
  C. be rapidly transported to the closest medical facility.
  D. immediately be given oral glucose.

_____ **35.** Causes of insulin shock include:
  A. taking too much insulin.
  B. vigorous exercise without sufficient glucose intake.
  C. nausea, vomiting, and/or anorexia.
  D. all of the above.

_____ **36.** Insulin shock can develop more often and more severely in children than in adults because of their:
  A. high activity level and failure to maintain a strict schedule of eating.
  B. genetic makeup.
  C. smaller body size.
  D. all of the above.

_____ **37.** Because diabetic coma is a complex metabolic condition that usually develops over time and involves all the tissues of the body, correcting this condition may:
  A. be accomplished quickly through the use of oral glucose.
  B. require rapid infusion of IV fluid to prevent permanent brain damage.
  C. take many hours in a hospital setting.
  D. include a reduction in the amount of insulin normally taken by the patient.

_____ **38.** A patient in insulin shock or a diabetic coma may appear to be:
  A. having a heart attack.
  B. perfectly normal.
  C. intoxicated.
  D. having a stroke.

_____ **39.** When dealing with a diabetic patient who has an altered mental status, you should:
  A. place oral glucose gel under the tongue of the unresponsive patient.
  B. only place sugar under the tongue of the unresponsive patient.
  C. give a small dose of insulin to the unresponsive patient.
  D. not attempt to give anything by mouth to an unresponsive patient.

_____ **40.** Be careful when administering any type of sugar/glucose to patients in insulin shock. They usually only require:
  A. 1 teaspoon.
  B. a few sips of a sweetened drink.
  C. ¼ of a candy bar.
  D. none of the above.

Labeling EMT-I

The following table will give you an opportunity to review the characteristics of diabetic emergencies. In each box, fill in the characteristic of the emergency based on the given condition.

Characteristics of hyperglycemia and hypoglycemia

TABLE 21-1 Characteristics of Diabetic Emergencies	Hyperglycemia	Hypoglycemia
History		
Food intake		
Insulin dose		
Onset		
Skin		
Infection		
Gastrointestinal Tract		
Thirst		
Hunger		
Vomiting		
Respiratory System		
Breathing		
Odor of breath		
Cardiovascular System		
Blood pressure		
Pulse		
Nervous System		
Consciousness		
Urine		
Sugar		
Acetone		
Treatment		
Response		

Vocabulary EMT-I vocab explorer web

Define the following terms in the space provided.

1. Diabetes mellitus:

_____

_____

_____

2. Kussmaul respirations:

_____

_____

_____

3. Glucagon:

_____

_____

_____

4. Insulin:

_____

_____

_____

5. Ketoacidosis:

_____

_____

_____

Fill-in

Read each item carefully, then complete the statement by filling in the missing word(s).

1. The full name of diabetes is _____ _____.

2. Diabetes is considered to be a(n) _____ _____ in which the body's

ability to metabolize simple carbohydrates is impaired.

3. Diabetes is defined as a lack of or _____ action of insulin.

4. Too much blood glucose by itself does not always cause _____ _____,

but on some occasions, it can lead to it.

5. A patient in insulin shock needs _____ immediately, and a patient in a diabetic coma needs _____ and IV fluid therapy.

6. To differentiate if the patient is intoxicated or having a diabetic emergency, it may be necessary to perform a _____ _____ _____.

True/False

If you believe the statement to be more true than false, write the letter "T" in the space provided. If you believe the statement to be more false than true, write the letter "F."

_____ 1. When patients use fat for energy, the fat waste products increase the amount of acid in the blood and tissue.

_____ 2. It is possible to have sufficient glucose in the bloodstream and yet not have it reach inside the cell.

_____ 3. If blood glucose levels remain low, a patient may lose consciousness or have permanent brain damage.

_____ 4. Signs and symptoms can develop quickly in children because their level of activity can exhaust their glucose levels.

_____ 5. Diabetic emergencies can occur when a patient's blood glucose level gets too high or when it drops too low.

_____ 6. Diabetes is caused by the lack of adequate amounts of insulin.

_____ 7. Diabetic patients may require insulin to control their blood glucose.

_____ 8. Glucose is a hormone that enables insulin to enter the cells of the body.

_____ 9. Insulin is one of the basic sugars essential for cell metabolism in humans.

_____ 10. Diabetes can cause kidney failure, blindness, and damage to blood vessels.

_____ 11. Most children with diabetes are insulin dependent.

_____ 12. Getting oral glucose into the unconscious patient is better than the patient receiving nothing.

1999 _____ 13. Intubation should not be used in diabetic emergencies because it could prevent the use of oral glucose.

_____ 14. Dehydration is a concern for patients experiencing a diabetic emergency.

Short Answer

Complete this section with short written answers in the space provided.

1. What is the role of insulin in metabolism?

_____

_____

_____

2. What are two trade names for oral glucose?

_____

_____

_____

3. When should you not give oral glucose to a patient experiencing a suspected diabetic emergency?

_____

_____

_____

4. List the trade names of three oral medications used by diabetics.

_____

_____

_____

5. What are the three problems associated with the development of diabetic coma?

_____

_____

_____

6. List the physical signs of diabetic coma.

_____

_____

_____

7. If a diabetic patient was fine 2 hours ago and now is unconscious and unresponsive, which diabetes-related condition would you suspect and why?

_____

_____

_____

8. Why should oral glucose be given to any diabetic patient with an altered level of consciousness?

_____

_____

_____

9. Intracranial pressure and possible intracranial bleeding is a contraindication to D_5W. What are their signs/symptoms?

_____

_____

_____

Word Fun EMT-I vocab explorer web

The following crossword puzzle is an activity provided to reinforce correct spelling and understanding of medical terminology associated with emergency care and the EMT-I. Use the clues in the column to complete the puzzle.

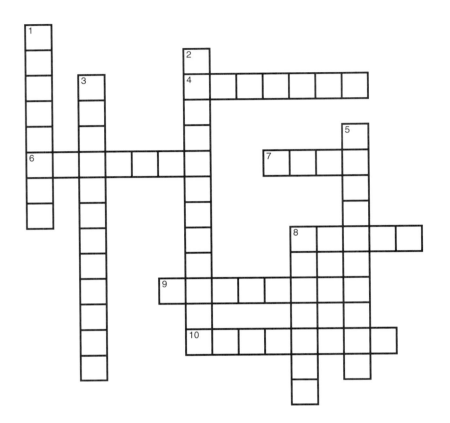

Across

4. Hormone produced in the pancreas
6. Fuel for cellular metabolism
7. Prefex meaning "low"
8. Prefex meaning "high"
9. Passage of unusually large volume of urine
10. The accumulation of acids in the body

Down

1. Converts glycogen into glucose when the body's glucose levels drop
2. Unresponsiveness caused by dehydration; very high blood glucose level; ketoacidosis
3. Significant hypoglycemia; unresponsive or altered mental status
5. Excessive eating
8. Chemical substance produced by a gland

Ambulance Calls

The following real case scenarios provide an opportunity to explore the concerns associated with patient management. Read each scenario, then answer each question in detail.

1. You are called to a local residence where you find a 22-year-old female supine in bed, unresponsive to your attempts to rouse her. She is cold and clammy with gurgling respirations. Her mother tells you that her only history is diabetes, which she has had since she was a small child. What steps would you take in managing this patient?

_____

_____

_____

_____

_____

_____

_____

_____

2. You are dispatched to a minor motor vehicle crash. The police officer on scene tells you it is a one-car wreck involving a tree, and the driver is "not acting right." The driver, a 33-year-old male, appears intoxicated, but there is no smell of alcohol. He has no visible injuries. How would you best manage this patient?

_____

_____

_____

_____

_____

_____

_____

3. You are called to a personal care home where the staff tells you that one of their residents does not feel well. They take you to the room of a 76-year-old male, a known diabetic patient, who is slumped over in a recliner. He has a fruity smell to his breath and is hot to the touch. His mental status is extremely altered. How would you best manage this patient?

_____

_____

_____

_____

_____

_____

_____

Skill Drills

Skill Drill 21-1: Administering Glucose
Test your knowledge by placing the photos below in the correct order. Number the first step with a "1," the second step with a "2," etc.

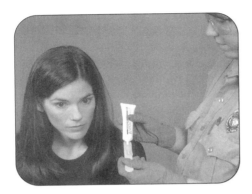

_____

Squeeze the entire tube of oral glucose onto the bottom third of a bite stick or tongue depressor.

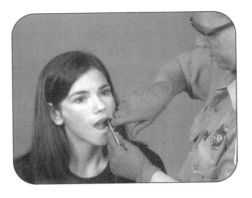

_____

Open the patient's mouth.

Place the tongue depressor on the mucous membranes between the cheek and the gum with the gel side next to the cheek.

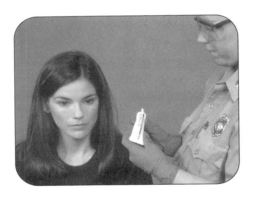

_____

Make sure that the tube of glucose is intact and has not expired.

Skill Drill 21-2: Administration of D₅₀

Test your knowledge by filling in the correct words in the photo captions.

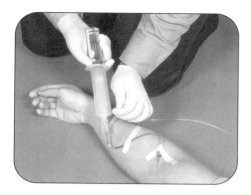

1. Ensure the IV line is patent by pulling back on the plunger to see if _____ returns through the IV tubing.

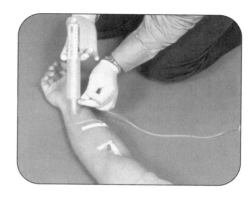

2. Crimp the IV tubing _____ to the injection port. Depress the plunger _____ to avoid rupturing the vein.

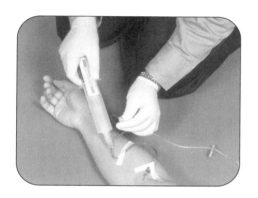

3. Recheck after _____ of the dose has been given by pulling back on the plunger again to check for _____.

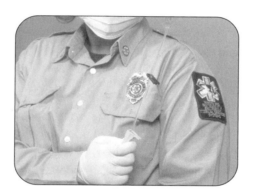

4. _____ the IV line by opening the line for a few seconds.

Workbook Activities

The following activities have been designed to help you. Your instructor may require you to complete some or all of these activities as a regular part of your EMT-I training program. You are encouraged to complete any activity that your instructor does not assign as a way to enhance your learning in the classroom.

Chapter Review

The following exercises provide an opportunity to refresh your knowledge of this chapter.

Matching

Match each of the terms in the left column to the appropriate definition in the right column.

_____ **1.** Allergic reaction

_____ **2.** Leukotrienes

_____ **3.** Wheezing

_____ **4.** Anaphylaxis

_____ **5.** Urticaria

_____ **6.** Stridor

_____ **7.** Allergen

_____ **8.** Wheal

_____ **9.** Antivenin

_____ **10.** Toxin

_____ **11.** Hypersensitivity

_____ **12.** Epinephrine

_____ **13.** Histamines

_____ **14.** Rabid

_____ **15.** Angiodema

_____ **16.** Envenomation

A. substance that counteracts the effect of venom from a bite or sting

B. substance made by the body; released in anaphylaxis

C. harsh, high-pitched inspiratory sound, usually resulting from upper airway obstruction

D. raised, swollen area on the skin resulting from an insect bite or allergic reaction

E. an exaggerated immune response to any substance

F. multiple raised areas on the skin that itch or burn

G. a poison or harmful substance

H. substance that causes an allergic reaction

I. a high-pitched, whistling breath sound, usually resulting from blockage of the airway, typically heard on expiration

J. extreme allergic reaction; an overreaction to a toxin

K. plasma seepage out of the capillaries into the surrounding tissue

L. describes an animal that is infected with rabies

M. act of injecting venom

N. released by the immune system in allergic reactions

O. the drug of choice for an anaphylactic reaction

P. abnormal sensitivity

Allergic Reactions and Envenomations

Multiple Choice

Read each item carefully, then select the best response.

_____ 1. It is important to provide prompt transport for any patient who may be having an allergic reaction and to continue to reassess the patient's vital signs en route because:

  A. you can only administer epinephrine once.

  B. the oxygen level may be too high.

  C. signs and symptoms may change rapidly.

  D. all of the above.

_____ 2. Side effects of the administration of epinephrine include:

  A. tachycardia.

  B. chest pain.

  C. nausea.

  D. all of the above.

_____ 3. Black widow spiders may be found in:

  A. New Hampshire.

  B. woodpiles.

  C. Georgia.

  D. all of the above.

_____ 4. Steps for assisting a patient with administration of an EpiPen include:

  A. taking BSI precautions.

  B. placing the tip of the auto-injector against the medial part of the patient's thigh.

  C. recapping the injector before placing it in the trash.

  D. all of the above.

_____ 5. Coral snakes may be found in:

  A. Florida.

  B. Kansas.

  C. New Jersey.

  D. all of the above.

_____ 6. The venom of the brown recluse spider is cytotoxic. It causes severe:

  A. nausea and vomiting.

  B. local tissue damage.

  C. headaches.

  D. all of the above.

_____ 7. Since ticks are only a fraction of an inch long and their bite is not painful, they can easily be mistaken for:

   A. dirt.

   B. a freckle.

   C. acne.

   D. all of the above.

_____ 8. Rocky Mountain spotted fever and Lyme disease are both spread through the tick's:

   A. saliva.

   B. blood.

   C. hormones.

   D. all of the above.

_____ 9. Signs of envenomation by a pit viper include:

   A. swelling.

   B. severe burning pain at the site of the injury.

   C. ecchymosis.

   D. all of the above.

_____ 10. Removal of a tick should be accomplished by:

   A. suffocating it with gasoline.

   B. burning it with a lighted match to cause it to release its grip.

   C. using fine tweezers to pull it straight out of the skin.

   D. suffocating it with Vaseline.

_____ 11. Allergens may include:

   A. food.

   B. animal bites.

   C. semen.

   D. all of the above.

_____ 12. The wasp's stinger is unbarbed, meaning that it can:

   A. be removed easily.

   B. inflict multiple stings.

   C. inject more venom with each sting.

   D. penetrate deeper.

_____ 13. Anaphylaxis is not always life threatening, but it typically involves:

   A. multiple organ systems.

   B. wheezing.

   C. urticaria.

   D. wheals.

_____ 14. Signs and symptoms of insect stings or bites include:

   A. swelling.

   B. wheals.

   C. localized heat.

   D. all of the above.

_____ 15. Prolonged respiratory difficulty can cause _____, shock, and even death.

   A. tachypnea

   B. pulmonary edema

   C. tachycardia

   D. airway obstruction

_____ 16. Speed is essential because more than two thirds of patients who die of anaphylaxis do so within the first:

    A. 10 minutes.

    B. 30 minutes.

    C. hour.

    D. 3 hours.

_____ 17. Questions to ask when obtaining a history from a patient appearing to have an allergic reaction include:

    A. whether the patient has a history of allergies.

    B. what the patient was exposed to.

    C. how the patient was exposed.

    D. all of the above.

_____ 18. Systemic symptoms from envenomation by a coelenterate may include:

    A. muscle cramps.

    B. headache.

    C. dizziness.

    D. all of the above.

_____ 19. Treatment for a black widow spider bite consists of maintaining:

    A. the airway.

    B. breathing.

    C. circulation.

    D. all of the above.

_____ 20. Treatment of a snake bite from a pit viper includes:

    A. calming the patient.

    B. providing BLS as needed if the patient shows no sign of envenomation.

    C. marking the skin with a pen over the swollen area to note whether swelling is spreading.

    D. all of the above.

_____ 21. The dosage of epinephrine in an adult EpiPen is:

    A. 0.10 mg.

    B. 0.15 mg.

    C. 0.30 mg.

    D. 0.50 mg.

_____ 22. Epinephrine, whether made by the body or by a drug manufacturer, works rapidly to:

    A. raise the pulse rate and blood pressure.

    B. inhibit an allergic reaction.

    C. dilate the bronchioles.

    D. all of the above.

_____ 23. A bite in the abdomen from a black widow spider may cause muscle spasms so severe that the patient may be thought to have:

    A. peritonitis.

    B. gastrointestinal bleeding.

    C. a stomach virus.

    D. all of the above.

_____ 24. If a patient suspected of having an allergic reaction has no signs of respiratory distress or shock, you should:

    A. place the patient in a supine position.

    B. continue with the focused assessment.

    C. administer epinephrine via an EpiPen auto-injector before signs and symptoms develop.

    D. all of the above.

_____ **25.** Systemic signs of envenomation by a pit viper may include:

 A. localized swelling.

 B. ecchymosis.

 C. shock.

 D. all of the above.

_____ **26.** Often, there is/are limited or no _____ associated with a coral snake bite.

 A. respiratory problems

 B. local symptoms

 C. bizarre behavior

 D. paralysis of the nervous system

_____ **27.** Because the stinger of the honeybee is barbed and remains in the wound, it can continue to inject venom for up to:

 A. 1 minute.

 B. 15 minutes.

 C. 20 minutes.

 D. several hours.

_____ **28.** You should not use tweezers or forceps to remove an embedded stinger because:

 A. squeezing may cause the stinger to inject more venom into the wound.

 B. the stinger may break off in the wound.

 C. the tweezers are not sterile and may cause infection.

 D. removing the stinger may cause bleeding.

_____ **29.** Your assessment of the patient experiencing an allergic reaction should include evaluations of the:

 A. respiratory system.

 B. circulatory system.

 C. skin.

 D. all of the above.

_____ **30.** Eating certain foods, such as shellfish or nuts, may result in a relatively _____ reaction that can still be quite severe.

 A. mild

 B. fast

 C. slow

 D. rapid

_____ **31.** In dealing with allergy-related emergencies, you must be aware of the possibility of acute _____ and cardiovascular collapse.

 A. hypotension

 B. tachypnea

 C. airway obstruction

 D. shock

_____ **32.** Wheezing occurs because excessive _____ and mucus are secreted into the bronchial passages.

 A. fluid

 B. carbon dioxide

 C. blood

 D. all of the above

_____ **33.** A patient suffering from an anaphylactic reaction should be placed in the:

 A. position of comfort.

 B. sitting position.

 C. Trendelenburg's position.

 D. supine position with head and shoulders elevated.

Vocabulary EMT-I vocab explorer web

Define the following terms in the space provided.

1. Anaphylaxis:

_____

_____

_____

2. Histamine:

_____

_____

_____

3. Epinephrine:

_____

_____

_____

4. Envenomation:

_____

_____

_____

5. Rabies:

_____

_____

_____

Fill-in

Read each item carefully, then complete the statement by filling in the missing word(s).

1. Wheezing occurs because excessive fluid and mucus are secreted into the _____

_____.

2. Small areas of generalized itching or burning that appear as multiple small raised areas on the skin are

called _____.

3. The stinger of the honeybee is _____ so that the bee cannot withdraw it.

4. A reaction involving the entire body is called _____.

5. The presence of _____ or respiratory distress indicates that the patient is having a severe enough allergic reaction to lead to death.

6. The patient in anaphylaxis with dyspnea should be placed in the _____ position with the head and shoulders elevated.

7. Epinephrine inhibits the allergic reaction and dilates the _____.

8. Your ability to recognize and manage the many signs and symptoms of allergic reactions may be the only thing standing between a patient and _____ _____.

9. The rabies virus is in the saliva of a _____, or infected, animal and is transmitted through biting or licking an open wound.

10. Two of the most common signs of anaphylaxis are _____ and _____.

True/False

If you believe the statement to be more true than false, write the letter "T" in the space provided. If you believe the statement to be more false than true, write the letter "F."

_____ **1.** Ice should be promptly applied to any insect sting or snake bite with swelling.

_____ **2.** The most common type of pit viper is the copperhead.

_____ **3.** Cottonmouths are known for aggressive behavior.

_____ **4.** Ticks should be removed by firmly grasping them with tweezers while rotating them counterclockwise.

_____ **5.** The pain of coelenterate stings may respond to flushing with cold water.

_____ **6.** Allergic reactions can occur in response to almost any substance.

_____ **7.** An allergic reaction occurs when the body has an immune response to a substance.

_____ **8.** Wheezing is a high-pitched breath sound, usually resulting from blockage of the airway and heard on expiration.

_____ **9.** For a patient appearing to have an allergic reaction, give 100% oxygen via nasal cannula.

_____ **10.** Systemic symptoms of envenomation by coelenterates include headache, dizziness, and hypotension.

_____ **11.** The human mouth contains more bacteria and viruses than even a dog's, so the EMT-I should consider penetrating human bites very serious and in need of medical treatment.

1999 _____ **12.** When treating an envenomation patient, monitor cardiac rhythm and treat arrhythmias according to standard ACLS protocols.

Short Answer

Complete this section with short written answers in the space provided.

1. What are some of the common side effects of epinephrine?

_____

_____

_____

2. What are the five stimuli that most often cause allergic reactions?

_____

_____

_____

3. What are the steps for administering or assisting with administration of an epinephrine auto-injector?

_____

_____

_____

4. What are the common respiratory and circulatory signs or symptoms of an allergic reaction?

_____

_____

_____

5. What treatments for a snake bite assist with slowing and monitoring the spread of venom?

_____

_____

_____

6. What are the two most common poisonous spiders in the United States and how do their bites differ?

_____

_____

_____

7. Dog and human bites, however minor, must be evaluated by a physician if the skin is broken. Why?

_____

_____

_____

8. What are the steps in treating a coelenterate envenomation?

_____

_____

_____

1999 **9.** In some areas of the country, EMT-I squads can administer epinephrine for anaphylaxis. What dosage would you use for adults and children?

_____

_____

_____

Word Fun EMT-I vocab explorer web

The following crossword puzzle is an activity provided to reinforce correct spelling and understanding of medical terminology associated with emergency care and the EMT-I. Use the clues in the column to complete the puzzle.

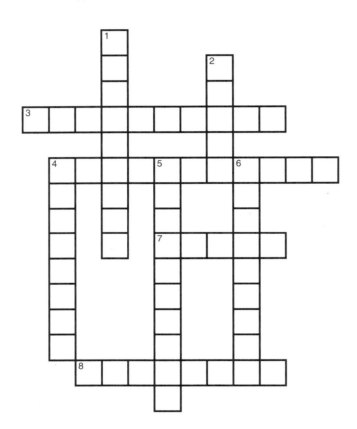

Across

3. May cause airway swelling/closure during anaphylaxis

4. An extreme, over-reaction to an allergen

7. A poisonous or harmful substance

8. High pitched breath sound caused by bronchoconstriction

Down

1. Hives

2. A raised, swollen, well defined area on the skin

4. A substance that causes an allergic reaction

5. Immune response to allergen; the release of

6. Serum that counteracts the effect of venom

Ambulance Calls

The following real case scenarios provide an opportunity to explore the concerns associated with patient management. Read each scenario, then answer each question in detail.

1. You are dispatched to the scene of a dog bite where you find a 7-year-old male complaining of several puncture wounds to his left calf. He is visibly upset, but bleeding is controlled. The dog, a family pet, is locked inside the house.

   How would you best manage this patient?

   _____

   _____

   _____

   _____

   _____

   _____

   _____

2. You are called to a possible allergic reaction from the sting of a jellyfish. Your patient, a 32-year-old female, is having difficulty breathing, has weak radial pulses, and is covered in hives.

   How would you manage this patient?

   _____

   _____

   _____

   _____

   _____

   _____

   _____

3. You are dispatched to a local seafood restaurant for a person who is having difficulty breathing. Upon arrival you find a 22-year-old female with facial edema, cyanosis around the lips, audible wheezing, and urticaria on her face and upper body. Her boyfriend tells you she ate shrimp and she is allergic to them. He also tells you she has some medicine in her purse and hands you an EpiPen prescribed for her. How would you best manage this patient?

_____

_____

_____

_____

_____

_____

_____

_____

Skill Drills

Skill Drill 22-1: Using an Auto-Injector
Test your knowledge by filling in the correct words in the photo captions.

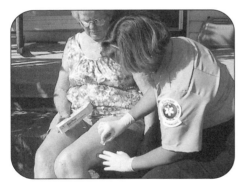
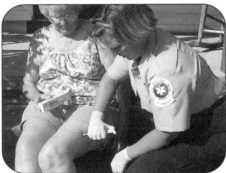
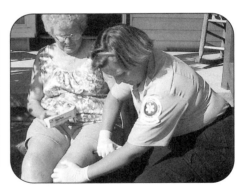

1. Remove the auto-injector's

_____

_____, and quickly

wipe the thigh with

_____.

2. Place the tip of the auto-injector

against the _____

thigh.

3. Push the _____

firmly against the

_____ and hold it

in place until all the medication is

injected.

Skill Drill 22-2: Using an AnaKit
Test your knowledge of this skill drill by placing the following photos in the correct order. Number the first step with a "1," the second step with a "2," etc.

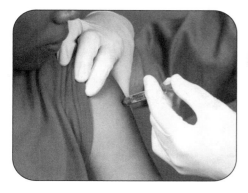

Hold the syringe steady and push the plunger until it stops.

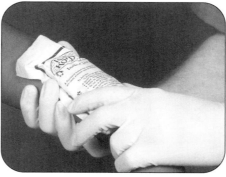

If available, apply a cold pack to the sting site.

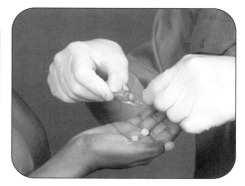

Have the patient chew and swallow the Chlo-Amine antihistamine tablets provided in the kit.

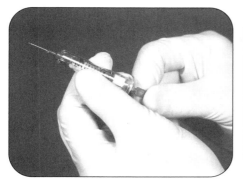

Turn the plunger one-quarter turn.

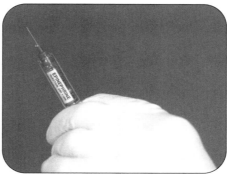

Hold the syringe upright and carefully depress the plunger to remove air.

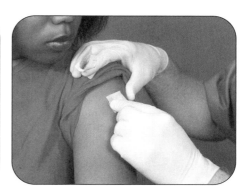

Prepare the injection site with antiseptic and remove the needle cover.

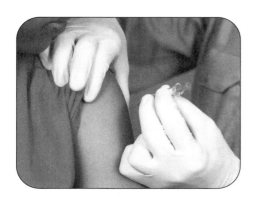

Quickly insert the needle into the muscle.

Workbook Activities

The following activities have been designed to help you. Your instructor may require you to complete some or all of these activities as a regular part of your EMT-I training program. You are encouraged to complete any activity that your instructor does not assign as a way to enhance your learning in the classroom.

Chapter Review

The following exercises provide an opportunity to refresh your knowledge of this chapter.

Matching

Match each of the terms in the left column to the appropriate definition in the right column.

_____ **1.** Poison

_____ **2.** Substance abuse

_____ **3.** Antidote

_____ **4.** Tolerance

_____ **5.** Addiction

_____ **6.** Ingestion

_____ **7.** Hematemesis

_____ **8.** Stimulant

_____ **9.** Opioid

_____ **10.** Sedative

_____ **11.** Hallucinogens

_____ **12.** Toxin

_____ **13.** Vomitus

_____ **14.** Delirium tremens

_____ **15.** Emesis

A. agent(s) producing false perceptions

B. drug or agent with actions similar to morphine

C. poison or harmful substance produced from bacteria, animals, or plants

D. may result from eating improperly canned food

E. need for increasing amounts of a drug to obtain the same effect

F. agent that produces an excited state

G. any substance whose chemical action can damage body structures or impair body functions

H. a substance that will counteract the effects of a particular poison

I. the misuse of any substance to produce a desired effect

J. taking a substance by mouth

K. overwhelming obsession to continue use of a drug or agent

L. vomiting blood

M. vomiting

N. vomited material

O. severe withdrawal syndrome in people deprived of ethyl alcohol

Multiple Choice

Read each item carefully, then select the best response.

_____ **1.** Activated charcoal is in the form of a(n):

  A. elixir.

  B. suspension.

  C. syrup.

  D. emulsion.

Poisonings and Overdose Emergencies

_____ **2.** The presence of burning or blistering of the mucous membranes suggests:

A. ingestion of depressants.

B. ingestion of poison.

C. overdose of heroin.

D. the patient may be a heavy smoker.

_____ **3.** Treatment for ingestion of poisonous plants includes:

A. assessing the ABCs.

B. taking the plant to the emergency department.

C. prompt transport.

D. all of the above.

_____ **4.** The most important consideration in caring for a patient who has been exposed to an organophosphate insecticide or some other cholinergic agent is to:

A. maintain the airway.

B. apply high-flow oxygen.

C. avoid exposure yourself.

D. initiate CPR.

_____ **5.** Objects that may provide clues to the nature of the poison include:

A. a needle or syringe.

B. scattered pills.

C. chemicals.

D. all of the above.

_____ **6.** The most worrisome avenue of poisoning is:

A. ingestion.

B. inhalation.

C. injection.

D. absorption.

_____ **7.** The major side effect of ingesting activated charcoal is:

A. depressed respirations.

B. overproduction of stomach acid.

C. black stools.

D. increased blood pressure.

_____ **8.** Alcohol is a powerful CNS depressant. It:

    A. sharpens the sense of awareness.

    B. slows reflexes.

    C. increases reaction time.

    D. all of the above.

_____ **9.** Frequently abused synthetic opioids include:

    A. heroin.

    B. morphine.

    C. Demerol.

    D. all of the above.

_____ **10.** Treatment of patients who have overdosed with sedative-hypnotics and have respiratory depression is to:

    A. provide airway clearance.

    B. provide ventilatory assistance.

    C. provide prompt transport.

    D. all of the above.

_____ **11.** Anticholinergic medications have properties that block the _____ nerves.

    A. parasympathetic

    B. sympathetic

    C. adrenergic

    D. parasympatholytic

_____ **12.** _____ crack produces the most rapid means of absorption and therefore the most potent effect.

    A. Injected

    B. Absorbed

    C. Smoked

    D. Ingested

_____ **13.** "Nerve gases" overstimulate normal body functions that are controlled by parasympathetic nerves causing:

    A. increased salivation.

    B. increased heart rate.

    C. increased urination.

    D. all of the above.

_____ **14.** Medicine containers can provide critical information such as:

    A. the number of pills originally in the bottle.

    B. the prescribed dose.

    C. the name and concentration of the drug.

    D. all of the above.

_____ **15.** Signs and symptoms of staphylococcal food poisoning include:

    A. difficulty in speaking.

    B. nausea, vomiting, and diarrhea.

    C. blurred vision.

    D. all of the above.

_____ **16.** Inhalant effects range from mild drowsiness to coma, but unlike most other sedative-hypnotics, these agents may often cause:

    A. seizures.

    B. vomiting.

    C. swelling of the tongue.

    D. all of the above.

_____ **17.** Cocaine may be taken via:

    A. inhalation.

    B. injection.

    C. absorption.

    D. all of the above.

_____ **18.** Abusable substances include:

    A. vitamins.

    B. nasal decongestants.

    C. food.

    D. all of the above.

_____ **19.** Charcoal is not indicated for patients who:

    A. have ingested an acid, alkali, or petroleum product.

    B. have a decreased level of consciousness.

    C. are unable to swallow.

    D. all of the above.

_____ **20.** A person who has been using marijuana rarely needs transport to the hospital. Exceptions may include someone who is:

    A. hallucinating.

    B. very anxious.

    C. paranoid.

    D. all of the above.

_____ **21.** Halogenated hydrocarbon solvents can make the heart supersensitive to the patient's own _____, putting the patient at high risk for sudden cardiac death from ventricular fibrillation.

    A. blood

    B. electrical activity

    C. adrenalin

    D. antibodies

_____ **22.** Sympathomimetics are CNS stimulants that frequently cause:

    A. hypotension.

    B. tachycardia.

    C. pinpoint pupils.

    D. all of the above.

_____ **23.** Carbon monoxide:

    A. is odorless.

    B. produces severe hypoxia.

    C. does not damage or irritate the lungs.

    D. all of the above.

_____ **24.** Chlorine:

    A. is odorless.

    B. does not damage or irritate the lungs.

    C. causes pulmonary edema.

    D. all of the above.

_____ **25.** Localized signs and symptoms of absorbed poisoning include:

    A. history of exposure.

    B. burns and/or irritation of the skin.

    C. dyspnea.

    D. all of the above.

_____ **26.** Poisoning by injection is almost always the result of:

    A. repetitive bee stings.

    B. pit viper envenomation.

    C. deliberate drug overdose.

    D. homicide.

_____ **27.** When dealing with substances such as phosphorous and elemental sodium, you should:

    A. brush the chemical off the patient.

    B. remove contaminated clothing.

    C. apply a dry dressing to the burn area.

    D. all of the above.

_____ **28.** Injected poisons are impossible to dilute or remove because they are usually _____ and/or cause intense local tissue destruction.

    A. absorbed quickly into the body

    B. bound to hemoglobin

    C. large compounds

    D. combined with the cerebrospinal fluid

_____ **29.** Medical problems that may cause the patient to present as intoxicated include:

    A. head trauma.

    B. toxic reactions.

    C. uncontrolled diabetes.

    D. all of the above.

_____ **30.** Signs and symptoms of alcohol withdrawal include:

    A. agitation and restlessness.

    B. fever, sweating.

    C. seizures.

    D. all of the above.

_____ **31.** Treatments for inhaled poisons include:

    A. moving the patient into fresh air.

    B. applying an SCBA to the patient.

    C. covering the patient to prevent spread of the poison.

    D. all of the above.

_____ **32.** Signs and symptoms of chlorine exposure include:

    A. cough.

    B. chest pain.

    C. wheezing.

    D. all of the above.

_____ **33.** Ingested poisons include:

    A. contaminated food.

    B. household cleaners.

    C. plants.

    D. all of the above.

_____ **34.** The majority of poisoning is through:

    A. ingestion.

    B. inhalation.

    C. injection.

    D. absorption.

_____ **35.** Ingestion of an opiate, sedative, or barbituate can cause depression of the CNS and:

    A. paralysis of the extremities.

    B. dilation of the pupils.

    C. carpopedal spasms.

    D. slow breathing.

_____ **36.** Inhaled poisons include:

    A. chlorine.

    B. venom.

    C. dieffenbachia.

    D. all of the above.

_____ **37.** Activated charcoal works by _____ the stomach.

    A. binding with the poison in

    B. creating turbulence in

    C. flushing the acid out of

    D. pushing the toxin down into

_____ **38.** The most important treatment for poisoning is _____ and/or physically removing the poisonous agent.

    A. administering a specific antidote

    B. high-flow oxygen

    C. diluting

    D. syrup of ipecac

_____ **39.** Delirium tremens may develop _____ after a person stops drinking or when consumption levels are decreased suddenly.

    A. 6 to 48 hours

    B. 6 to 72 hours

    C. 1 to 7 days

    D. 6 to 12 days

1999 _____ **40.** Patients who have taken opioids will respond to naloxone (Narcan) within _____ when given intravenously.

    A. 30 to 60 seconds

    B. 2 minutes

    C. 5 minutes

    D. Naloxone is not used in conjunction with an opioid overdose.

_____ **41.** Halogenated hydrocarbon solvents used in inhalants can make the heart highly sensitive to the patient's own adrenalin, putting the patient at high risk for sudden cardiac death from:

    A. ventricular fibrillation.

    B. wondering pacemaker.

    C. heart blocks.

    D. PVCs.

1999 _____ **42.** The EMT-I should consider giving a patient who has abused anticholinergic agents:

    A. Narcan.

    B. epinephrine.

    C. sodium bicarbonate.

    D. activated charcoal.

1999 _____ **43.** Management for the patient who has come into contact with cholinergic agents may include:

    A. atropine.

    B. diazepam.

    C. monitoring cardiac rhythm.

    D. all of the above.

Vocabulary EMT-I

Define the following terms in the space provided.

1. Sedative-hypnotic:

_____

_____

_____

2. Anticholinergic:

_____

_____

_____

3. Delirium tremens:

_____

_____

_____

4. Hallucinogen:

_____

_____

_____

5. Addiction:

_____

_____

_____

6. Substance abuse:

_____

_____

_____

7. Hypnotic:

_____

_____

_____

Fill-in

Read each item carefully, then complete the statement by filling in the missing word(s).

1. When dealing with exposure to chemicals, treatment focuses on support: assessing and maintaining the patient's _____.

2. The most commonly abused drug in the United States is _____.

3. Activated charcoal works by _____, or sticking to, many commonly ingested poisons, preventing the toxin from being absorbed into the body.

4. If the patient has a chemical agent in the eyes, you should irrigate them quickly and thoroughly, at least _____ for acid substances and _____ for alkalis.

5. Opioid analgesics are CNS depressants and can cause severe _____ _____.

6. Severe acute alcohol ingestion may cause _____.

7. Your primary responsibility to the patient who has been poisoned is to _____ that a poisoning occurred.

8. The usual dosage for activated charcoal for an adult or child is _____ of activated charcoal per _____ of body weight.

9. As you irrigate the eyes, make sure that the fluid runs from the bridge of the nose _____.

10. Approximately 80% of all poisoning is by _____, including plants, contaminated food, and most drugs.

11. Patients experiencing alcohol withdrawal may develop _____ _____ if they no longer have their daily source of alcohol.

12. Phosphorus and elemental sodium _____ when they come in contact with water.

13. Increasing tolerance of a substance can lead to _____.

14. _____ may develop from sweating, fluid loss, insufficient fluid intake, or vomiting associated with delirium tremens.

15. If you have even the slightest suspicion that a patient has taken a _____ _____, you should notify medical control and begin emergency treatment at once.

1999 16. When treating a patient who has abused sympathomimetics, the EMT-I's care should include _____ the cardiac rhythm and treating _____ following standard ACLS protocols.

1999 17. When treating patients who have come into contact with cholinergic agents such as "nerve gas," consider giving _____ to dry up secretions.

1999 **18.** When placing patients on a cardiac monitor, arrhythmias should be treated according to standard

_____ protocols.

True/False

If you believe the statement to be more true than false, write the letter "T" in the space provided. If you believe the statement to be more false than true, write the letter "F."

_____ **1.** The usual adult dose of activated charcoal is 25 to 50 g.

_____ **2.** The general treatment for a poisoned patient is to induce vomiting.

_____ **3.** Activated charcoal is a standard of care in all ingestions.

_____ **4.** Inhaled chlorine produces profound hypoxia without lung irritation.

_____ **5.** Shaking activated charcoal decreases its effectiveness.

_____ **6.** A patient with an opioid overdose typically presents with pinpoint pupils.

_____ **7.** Cholinergics are chemicals such as nerve gases, organophosphate insecticides, or certain wild mushrooms.

_____ **8.** Alcohol is a stimulant.

_____ **9.** Demerol, Dilaudid, and Vicodin are all examples of opioids.

_____ **10.** Cocaine is one of the most addicting substances known.

_____ **11.** The telephone number for the National Poison Control Center is 1-800-222-1222.

_____ **12.** In the past, syrup of ipecac was used to induce vomiting, but it is no longer recommended.

_____ **13.** You should assume all intoxicated patients are experiencing a drug overdose and will require a thorough examination by a physician.

_____ **14.** A patient taking opiods (narcotics) will likely have dilated pupils.

1999 _____ **15.** When treating a patient who has abused inhalants, the EMT-I's care should include cardiac monitoring, treating arrhythmias according to ACLS protocols, and being prepared to intubate.

Short Answer

Complete this section with short written answers in the space provided.

1. How does activated charcoal work to counteract ingested poison?

_____

_____

_____

2. What are the four routes of contact for poisoning?

_____

_____

_____

3. List the typical signs and symptoms of an overdose of sympathomimetics.

_____

_____

_____

4. What are the two main mechanisms of food poisoning?

_____

_____

_____

5. What differentiates the presentation of acetaminophen poisoning from that of other substances? What does this mean to the prehospital caregiver?

_____

_____

_____

6. To what condition do the mnemonics DUMBELS and SLUDGE pertain, and what do they mean?

_____

_____

_____

7. In addition to alcohol and marijuana, what are the seven categories of drugs seen in overdoses/ poisoning?

_____

_____

_____

8. What five questions should you ask a possible poisoning victim?

_____

_____

_____

9. Why should phosphorous or elemental sodium poisoning victims not be irrigated?

_____

_____

_____

1999 **10.** When giving naloxone (Narcan) to a patient, what should the EMT-I be on the alert for?

_____

_____

Word Fun EMT-I vocab explorer web

The following crossword puzzle is an activity provided to reinforce correct spelling and understanding of medical terminology associated with emergency care and the EMT-I. Use the clues in the column to complete the puzzle.

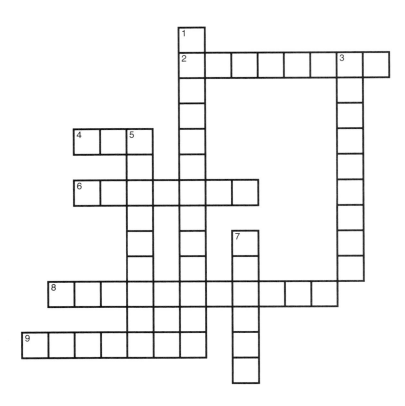

Across

2. Substance used to neutralize or counteract a poison

4. Delirium tremens

6. Drugs with actions similar to morphine

8. Vomiting blood

9. Vomited material

Down

1. An agent that produces false perceptions of the senses

3. The need for increasing amounts of a drug to obtain the same effect

5. An agent producing an excited state

7. Vomiting

Ambulance Calls

The following real case scenarios provide an opportunity to explore the concerns associated with patient management. Read each scenario, then answer each question in detail.

1. You are dispatched to a scene where a 42-year-old male was found face down in an alley. Police tell you he is a known alcoholic and probably just "fell out" again. He is pain responsive and has blood trickling from his nose where he struck the asphalt.

How would you best manage this patient?

_____

_____

_____

_____

_____

_____

_____

_____

2. You are called to a local child care center where a toddler has been found chewing on the leaves of an unknown plant. The supervisor tells you she thinks the plant may be poisonous and they were not sure what they should do. His mother has been called and will meet you at the hospital.

How would you best manage this patient?

_____

_____

_____

_____

_____

_____

_____

3. You are called to a possible suicide attempt. You arrive on the scene to find police and a neighbor in the home of a 25-year-old female who is unresponsive, supine on her bed. The neighbor tells you that the patient recently broke up with her boyfriend and has been very distraught. There is an empty pill bottle on the nightstand. When you look at the label you see that the prescription was filled yesterday and there were 30 tablets dispensed. There is also an empty liquor bottle on the floor.

How would you best manage this patient?

_____

_____

_____

_____

_____

_____

_____

Workbook Activities

The following activities have been designed to help you. Your instructor may require you to complete some or all of these activities as a regular part of your EMT-I training program. You are encouraged to complete any activity that your instructor does not assign as a way to enhance your learning in the classroom.

Chapter Review

The following exercises provide an opportunity to refresh your knowledge of this chapter.

Matching

Match each of the terms in the left column to the appropriate definition in the right column.

_____ **1.** Syncope

_____ **2.** Hemiparesis

_____ **3.** Postictal state

_____ **4.** Ischemic cells

_____ **5.** Absence seizure

_____ **6.** TIA

_____ **7.** Infarcted cells

_____ **8.** Clonic phase

_____ **9.** Status epilepticus

_____ **10.** Hypoglycemia

_____ **11.** Aphasia

_____ **12.** Tonic phase

_____ **13.** Dysarthria

_____ **14.** Atherosclerosis

_____ **15.** Cerebral embolism

_____ **16.** Incontinence

_____ **17.** Ischemic stroke

_____ **18.** Cerebrovascular accident

_____ **19.** Febrile seizures

_____ **20.** Hemorrhagic stroke

_____ **21.** Thrombus

_____ **22.** Stroke

_____ **23.** Generalized seizure

_____ **24.** Seizure

_____ **25.** Arterial rupture

A. slurred, hard to understand speech

B. cells receiving sufficient blood after an event to stay alive but not enough to function properly

C. seizure movement; muscle contractions and relaxations in rapid succession

D. temporary loss of consciousness; fainting

E. period following a seizure, typically lasting 5 to 30 minutes

F. transient ischemic attack; "small stroke"

G. weakness on one side of the body

H. low blood glucose

I. seizure characterized by a brief lapse of attention; formerly known as petit mal seizure

J. cells that die as a result of loss of blood flow

K. in a seizure, steady, rigid muscle contraction with no relaxation

L. inability to produce or understand speech

M. seizures lasting more than 10 minutes or two or more seizures in a row without a return to consciousness

N. loss of brain function in certain brain cells not getting enough oxygen during a CVA

O. generalized, uncoordinated muscular activity associated with loss of consciousness; a convulsion

P. resulting from sudden high fever, particularly in children

Q. local clotting of blood in the cerebral arteries that may result in a subsequent stroke

R. a buildup of cholesterol and calcium inside the walls of blood vessels

S. occurs when blood flow to a particular part of the brain is cut off by a blockage

CHAPTER 24

Neurologic Emergencies

T. seizure characterized by severe twitching; formerly known as grand mal seizure

U. loss of bowel and bladder control

V. occurs as a result of bleeding inside the brain

W. interruption of blood flow to the brain resulting in the loss of brain function; CVA

X. when a clot travels to the brain and obstructs a cerebral artery

Y. rupture of an artery

Multiple Choice
Read each item carefully, then select the best response.

_____ **1.** Seizures may occur as a result of:

A. metabolic problems.

B. a brain tumor.

C. a recent or old head injury.

D. all of the above.

_____ **2.** The _____ controls the most basic functions of the body, such as breathing, blood pressure, swallowing, and pupil constriction.

A. brain stem

B. cerebellum

C. cerebrum

D. spinal cord

_____ **3.** At each vertebra in the neck and back, _____ nerves called spinal nerves branch out from the spinal cord and carry signals to and from the body.

A. two

B. three

C. four

D. five

_____ **4.** Brain disorders include all of the following EXCEPT:

A. coma.

B. infection.

C. hypoglycemia.

D. tumor.

_____ **5.** When blood flow to a particular part of the brain is cut off by a blockage inside a blood vessel, the result is:

    A. a hemorrhagic stroke.

    B. atherosclerosis.

    C. an ischemic stroke.

    D. a cerebral embolism.

_____ **6.** Patients who are at the highest risk of hemorrhagic stroke are those who have:

    A. untreated hypertension.

    B. an aneurysm.

    C. a berry aneurysm.

    D. atherosclerosis.

_____ **7.** Patients with a subarachnoid hemorrhage typically complain of a sudden severe:

    A. bout of dizziness.

    B. headache.

    C. altered mental status.

    D. thirst.

_____ **8.** The plaque that builds up in atherosclerosis obstructs blood flow and interferes with the vessel's ability to:

    A. constrict.

    B. dilate.

    C. diffuse.

    D. exchange gases.

_____ **9.** A TIA, or small stroke, is the name given to a stroke when symptoms go away on their own in less than:

    A. half an hour.

    B. 1 hour.

    C. 12 hours.

    D. 24 hours.

_____ **10.** Seizures characterized by unconsciousness and a generalized severe twitching of all the body's muscles that lasts several minutes or longer is called a:

    A. generalized seizure.

    B. petit mal seizure.

    C. focal motor seizure.

    D. febrile seizure.

_____ **11.** Metabolic seizures may be due to:

    A. epilepsy.

    B. a brain tumor.

    C. high fevers.

    D. hypoglycemia.

_____ **12.** When assessing a patient with a history of seizure activity, it is important to:

    A. determine whether this episode differs from any previous ones.

    B. recognize the postictal state.

    C. look for other problems associated with the seizure.

    D. all of the above.

_____ **13.** Signs and symptoms of possible seizure activity include:

    A. altered mental status.

    B. incontinence.

    C. rapid and deep respirations.

    D. all of the above.

_____ **14.** Common causes of altered mental status include all of the following EXCEPT:

A. body temperature abnormalities.

B. hypoxemia.

C. unequal pupils.

D. hypoglycemia.

_____ **15.** The principle difference between a patient who has had a stroke and a patient with hypoglycemia almost always has to do with the:

A. pupillary response.

B. mental status.

C. blood pressure.

D. capillary refill time.

_____ **16.** Consider the possibility of _____ in a patient who has had a seizure.

A. brain injury

B. hyperglycemia

C. hypoglycemia

D. hypertension

_____ **17.** Individuals with chronic alcoholism can have abnormalities in liver function and in their blood-clotting and immune systems, which can predispose them to:

A. intracranial bleeding.

B. brain and bloodstream infections.

C. hypoglycemia.

D. all of the above.

_____ **18.** Low oxygen levels in the bloodstream will affect the entire brain, causing:

A. anxiety.

B. restlessness.

C. confusion.

D. all of the above.

_____ **19.** Patients with _____ may have trouble understanding speech but can speak clearly.

A. aphasia

B. receptive aphasia

C. expressive aphasia

D. dysarthria

_____ **20.** High blood pressure in stroke patients should not be treated in the field because:

A. the brain is raising the blood pressure in an attempt to force more oxygen into its injured parts.

B. quite often, blood pressure will return to normal or may drop significantly on its own.

C. many times it is a response to bleeding in the brain.

D. all of the above.

_____ **21.** All of the following conditions may simulate a stroke EXCEPT:

A. hyperglycemia.

B. a postictal state.

C. hypoglycemia.

D. subdural bleeding.

_____ **22.** When assessing a patient with a possible CVA, you should check the _____ first.

A. pulse

B. airway

C. pupils

D. blood pressure

_____ **23.** Indications that the patient can understand you include:

    A. pressure of the hand.

    B. efforts to speak.

    C. nodding the head.

    D. all of the above.

_____ **24.** Key physical tests for patients suspected of having a stroke include tests of:

    A. speech.

    B. neck movement.

    C. leg movement.

    D. all of the above.

_____ **25.** A patient with a GCS of 12 has:

    A. no dysfunction.

    B. mild dysfunction.

    C. moderate to severe dysfunction.

    D. severe dysfunction.

_____ **26.** To transport the suspected stroke patient, the patient should be placed in which position?

    A. Trendelenburg's

    B. Fowler's

    C. Comfortable

    D. Lithotomy

_____ **27.** Following a major seizure, you should anticipate:

    A. a decreased heart rate.

    B. rapid, deep respirations.

    C. respiratory arrest.

    D. a return to their normal mental status within 5 to 10 minutes.

_____ **28.** Assess mental status with the mnemonic:

    A. OPQRST.

    B. SAMPLE.

    C. AVPU.

    D. PEARL.

_____ **29.** Even a patient who has a history of chronic epilepsy that is controlled with medications may have an occasional seizure, commonly referred to as a(n) _____ seizure.

    A. chronic

    B. generalized

    C. absence

    D. breakthrough

_____ **30.** Patients experiencing an aneurysm in the brain frequently describe their symptom as:

    A. lightheadedness.

    B. "the worst headache of my life."

    C. dizziness.

    D. feeling like they might faint.

_____ **31.** TIAs may be a warning sign of/that:

    A. a larger permanent stroke is imminent.

    B. a seizure.

    C. an aneurysm.

    D. a syncopal episode.

_____ **32.** In the postictal state, breathing becomes fast and deep. Why?

    A. It's the body's attempt to balance the pH in the bloodstream.

    B. They're simply out of breath at the end of a seizure.

    C. They've converted over to the hypoxic drive.

    D. It's an unknown mystery that will take care of itself.

_____ **33.** A person who appears intoxicated may instead be experiencing:
   A. intracranial bleeding.
   B. brain and bloodstream infections.
   C. hypoglycemia.
   D. all of the above.

Labeling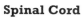

Label the following diagrams with the correct terms.

Brain

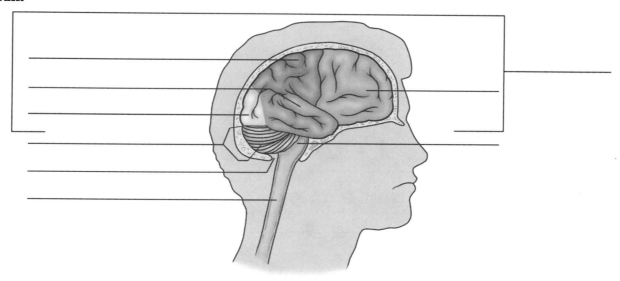

Spinal Cord

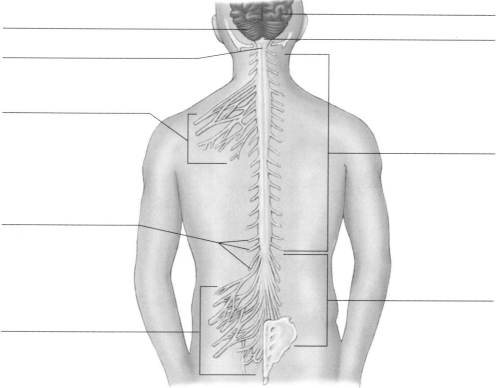

Vocabulary EMT-I [vocab explorer | web]

Define the following terms in the space provided.

1. Cerebrovascular accident (CVA):

_____

_____

_____

2. Ischemic stroke:

_____

_____

_____

3. Transient ischemic attack (TIA):

_____

_____

_____

4. Hemorrhagic stroke:

_____

_____

_____

5. Generalized seizure:

_____

_____

_____

6. Absence seizure:

_____

_____

_____

7. Atherosclerosis:

_____

_____

_____

8. Cerebral embolism:

_____

_____

_____

9. Febrile seizure:

_____

_____

_____

10. Thrombosis:

_____

_____

_____

Fill-in

Read each item carefully, then complete the statement by filling in the missing word(s).

1. There are _____ cranial nerves.

2. Playing the piano is coordinated by the _____.

3. The front part of the cerebrum controls _____ and _____.

4. The cranial nerves run to the _____.

5. The brain is divided into _____ major parts.

6. All messages traveling to and from the brain travel along _____.

7. Each hemisphere of the cerebrum controls activities on the _____ side of the body and

the _____ side of the face.

8. The _____ is the largest part of the brain.

9. _____ is a loss of bowel and bladder control and can result from a generalized seizure.

10. The _____ is the body's computer.

11. The onset of _____ bleeding is usually very rapid after injury.

12. Weakness on one side of the body is known as _____.

13. No matter what the cause, you should consider _____ _____

_____ to be an emergency that requires immediate attention, even when it appears that

the cause may simply be alcohol intoxication or a minor car crash or fall.

14. _____ _____, commonly referred to as "clot busters," have been shown

to reverse symptoms of stroke if given within _____ after the onset of symptoms.

15. Make a special effort to determine when the patient last appeared to be _____. This will

tell physicians in the emergency department whether it is safe to begin certain treatments.

1999 **16.** If the patient is actively seizing, consider the use of _____ or _____

_____.

True/False

If you believe the statement to be more true than false, write the letter "T" in the space provided. If you believe the statement to be more false than true, write the letter "F."

_____ **1.** The postictal state following a seizure commonly lasts only about 3 to 5 minutes.

_____ **2.** Metabolic seizures result from an area of abnormality in the brain.

_____ **3.** Febrile seizures result from sudden high fevers and are generally well tolerated by children.

_____ **4.** Hemiparesis is the inability to speak or understand speech.

_____ **5.** The dura covers the brain.

_____ **6.** Unconscious stroke patients are usually unable to speak or hear.

_____ **7.** Right-sided facial droop is most likely an indication of a problem in the right cerebral hemisphere.

_____ **8.** Stroke is the third most common cause of death in the United States after heart disease and cancer.

_____ **9.** Chronic or poorly controlled hypotensive patients are at high risk for hemorrhagic stroke.

_____ **10.** Patients with right hemisphere strokes may be completely oblivious to their problem.

_____ **11.** Friends and family members may think a patient has had a stroke when he or she is actually in cardiac arrest.

Short Answer

Complete this section with short written answers in the space provided.

1. List and describe the three key tests for assessing stroke.

_____

_____

_____

2. Why is prompt transport of stroke patients critical?

_____

_____

_____

3. What are some techniques for cooling a child with a febrile seizure?

_____

_____

_____

4. Describe the characteristics of a postictal state.

_____

_____

_____

5. What is the difference between infarcted and ischemic cells?

_____

_____

_____

6. List three conditions that may simulate stroke.

_____

_____

_____

Word Fun EMT-I

The following crossword puzzle is an activity provided to reinforce correct spelling and understanding of medical terminology associated with emergency care and the EMT-I. Use the clues in the column to complete the puzzle.

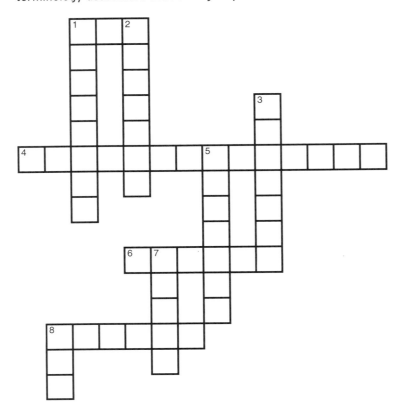

Across

1. Mini stroke

4. Results from sudden high fever, particularly in children

6. Cells not getting enough oxygen during a CVA

8. Repetitive muscle contractions and relaxations; seizure movement

Down

1. Local clotting of blood in the cerebral arteries

2. Inability to understand or produce speech

3. Uncoordinated muscular activity associated with loss of consciousness; a convulsion

5. To faint

7. Steady, rigid muscle contraction without relaxation during a seizure

8. Cerebrovascular accident; stoke

Ambulance Calls

The following real case scenarios will give you an opportunity to explore the concerns associated with patient management. Read each scenario, then answer each question in detail.

1. You are called to a residence for an 18-month-old girl who experienced seizure-like activity approximately 15 minutes prior to your arrival. The only history is a recent upper respiratory infection, but the mother forgot to give the child her medication for 3 days. The patient is lethargic, flushed, and very hot to the touch. The mother does not have a thermometer.

How would you best manage this patient?

_____

_____

_____

_____

_____

_____

_____

_____

1999 **2.** You are dispatched to a 36-year-old male who had seizure activity at least an hour ago. The patient is incontinent, cold, clammy, and unresponsive. His friends tell you that the "shaking" stopped, and he has not woken up. They thought he might just be tired until they discovered they could not wake him. He has no history of seizure activity. He has diabetes for which he takes medication.

How would you best manage this patient?

_____

_____

_____

_____

_____

_____

_____

_____

3. You are dispatched to the residence of a 77-year-old male complaining of possible CVA. He presents with facial drooping on his left side as well as left-sided weakness. He appears to be in no apparent distress. His blood pressure is 190/110, pulse is 84, and respirations are 16 and nonlabored. He has no history of strokes.

How would you best manage this patient?

_____

_____

_____

_____

_____

_____

_____

Workbook Activities

The following activities have been designed to help you. Your instructor may require you to complete some or all of these activities as a regular part of your EMT-I training program. You are encouraged to complete any activity that your instructor does not assign as a way to enhance your learning in the classroom.

Chapter Review

The following exercises provide an opportunity to refresh your knowledge of this chapter.

Matching

Match each of the terms in the left column to the appropriate definition in the right column.

_____ **1.** Aneurysm

_____ **2.** Colic

_____ **3.** Peristalsis

_____ **4.** Ulcer

_____ **5.** Hernia

_____ **6.** Ileus

_____ **7.** Guarding

_____ **8.** Anorexia

_____ **9.** Emesis

_____ **10.** Referred pain

_____ **11.** Acute abdomen

_____ **12.** Pancreatitis

_____ **13.** Strangulation

_____ **14.** Peritonitis

_____ **15.** Peritoneum

_____ **16.** Diverticulitis

_____ **16.** Cholecystitis

_____ **17.** Appendicitis

A. paralysis of the bowel

B. pain felt in an area of the body other than at the actual source

C. protective involuntary abdominal muscle contractions

D. acute intermittent cramping abdominal pain

E. waves of alternate circular contraction and relaxation of the intestines

F. vomiting

G. sudden onset of pain within the abdomen

H. a membrane lining the abdomen

I. swelling or enlargement of a weakened arterial wall

J. loss of hunger or appetite

K. protrusion of a loop of an organ or tissue through an abnormal body opening

L. obstruction of blood circulation resulting from compression or entrapment of organ tissue

M. abrasion of the stomach or small intestine

N. inflammation of the pancreas

O. inflammation of the peritoneum

P. inflammation of the gallbladder

Q. inflammation of a diverticulum, usually in the colon

R. inflammation of the appendix

Nontraumatic Abdominal Emergencies

Multiple Choice

Read each item carefully, then select the best response.

_____ **1.** Peritonitis, with associated fluid loss, may lead to _____ shock.

　　A. hemorrhagic

　　B. septic

　　C. hypovolemic

　　D. metabolic

_____ **2.** Distention of the abdomen is gauged by:

　　A. visualization.

　　B. auscultation.

　　C. palpation.

　　D. the patient's complaint of pain around the umbilicus.

_____ **3.** A hernia that returns to its proper body cavity is said to be:

　　A. reducible.

　　B. extractable.

　　C. incarcerated.

　　D. replaceable.

_____ **4.** Sensory nerves from the spinal cord to the skin and muscles are part of the:

　　A. somatic nervous system.

　　B. peripheral nervous system.

　　C. autonomic nervous system.

　　D. sympathetic nervous system.

_____ **5.** When an organ of the abdomen is enlarged, rough palpation may cause _____ of the organ.

　　A. distention

　　B. nausea

　　C. swelling

　　D. rupture

_____ **6.** Severe back pain may be associated with which condition?

　　A. Abdominal aortic aneurysm

　　B. PID

　　C. Appendicitis

　　D. Mittelschmerz

_____ **7.** The _____ are found in the retroperitoneal space.

   A. stomach and gallbladder

   B. kidneys, genitourinary structures, and large vessels

   C. liver and pancreas

   D. adrenal glands and uterus

_____ **8.** A(n) _____ may occur as a result of a surgical wound that has failed to heal properly.

   A. ectopic pregnancy

   B. strangulation

   C. hernia

   D. ulcer

_____ **9.** The peritoneal membrane that can perceive the sensations of pain, pressure, and cold is the:

   A. meningeal.

   B. parietal.

   C. retroperitoneal.

   D. visceral.

_____ **10.** Common disease(s) that produce(s) signs of an acute abdomen include:

   A. diverticulitis.

   B. cholecystitis.

   C. acute appendicitis.

   D. all of the above.

_____ **11.** A patient with peritonitis may present with rapid, shallow breaths resulting from:

   A. hypovolemia.

   B. ileus.

   C. pain.

   D. inflammation.

_____ **12.** Common signs and symptoms of irritation or inflammation of the peritoneum may include:

   A. a quiet patient who is resting comfortably.

   B. hypertension and tachycardia.

   C. rebound tenderness and fever.

   D. Kussmaul respirations.

_____ **13.** In the patient with peritonitis, the degree of pain and tenderness is usually related directly to the severity of the:

   A. fever.

   B. distention.

   C. peritoneal inflammation.

   D. bleeding.

_____ **14.** Pain associated with diverticulitis is usually felt in the:

   A. right upper quadrant.

   B. left upper quadrant.

   C. right lower quadrant.

   D. left lower quadrant.

_____ **15.** When assessing a patient with severe abdominal pain, you should anticipate the development of _____ and treat the patient when it is evident.

   A. fever

   B. appendicitis

   C. hypovolemic shock

   D. pancreatitis

———— **16.** Peritonitis is associated with:

    A. an overabundance of body fluid in the abdominal cavity.

    B. a loss of body fluid into the abdominal cavity.

    C. a rupture within the abdominal cavity.

    D. the lack of an abdominal cavity.

1999 ———— **17.** Which analgesics (pain medication) should be considered for the acute abdomen?

    A. Morphine

    B. Aspirin

    C. Demerol

    D. None of the above

———— **18.** Geriatric patients may have different signs and symptoms of an acute abdomen. Why?

    A. They have altered pain sensations.

    B. They may not feel discomfort.

    C. They may describe severe conditions as a "mild" discomfort.

    D. All of the above

Labeling **EMT-I** anatomy review web

Label the following diagrams with the correct terms.

Solid Organs

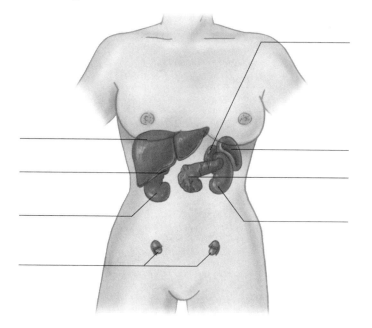

Hollow Organs

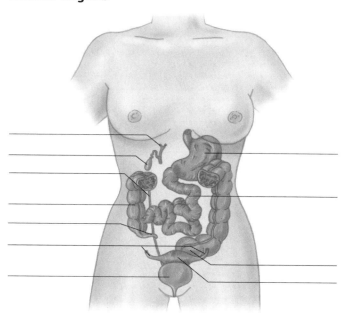

Vocabulary EMT-I [vocab explorer] web

Define the following terms in the space provided.

1. Acute abdomen:

_____

_____

_____

2. Diverticulitis:

_____

_____

_____

3. Ectopic pregnancy:

_____

_____

_____

4. Cholecystitis:

_____

_____

_____

5. Mittelschmertz:

_____

_____

_____

True/False

If you believe the statement to be more true than false, write the letter "T" in the space provided. If you believe the statement to be more false than true, write the letter "F."

_____ **1.** Referred pain is a result of connection between ligaments in the abdominal and chest cavities.

_____ **2.** Abdominal pain in women is usually related to the menstrual cycle and is rarely serious.

_____ **3.** A leading aorta, being retroperitoneal, will not cause peritonitis.

_____ **4.** It is important to accurately diagnose the cause of acute abdominal pain in order to properly treat the patient.

_____ **5.** The parietal peritoneum lines the walls of the abdominal cavity.

_____ **6.** The patient with peritonitis usually reports relief of pain when lying left lateral recumbent with the knees pulled in.

_____ **7.** When palpating the abdomen, always start with the quadrant where the patient complains of the most severe pain.

_____ **8.** Massive hemorrhaging is associated with rupture of an abdominal aortic aneurysm.

_____ **9.** Pneumonia may cause abdominal pain.

_____ **10.** Normal saline is an example of an isotonic crystalloid the EMT-I may use in a 20-mL/kg bolus for hypotension.

1999 _____ **11.** Shock-induced hypoxia can cause cardiac arrhythmias with abdominal pain.

Short Answer

Complete this section with short written answers in the space provided.

1. Explain the phenomenon of referred pain.

_____

_____

_____

2. Should an EMT-I attempt to diagnose the cause of abdominal pain? Why or why not?

_____

_____

_____

3. Why does abdominal distention accompany ileus?

_____

_____

_____

4. What two conditions may result in hypovolemic shock in the patient with an acute abdomen?

_____

_____

_____

5. List the general EMT-I emergency care for patients with acute abdomen.

_____

_____

_____

Word Fun EMT-I vocab explorer web

The following crossword puzzle is an activity provided to reinforce correct spelling and understanding of medical terminology associated with emergency care and the EMT-I. Use the clues in the column to complete the puzzle.

Across

1. An effort to protect the inflamed abdomen

4. Lack of appetite for food

5. Acute, intermittent, cramping abdominal pain

7. Abrasion of the stomach or small intestine

8. Inflammation of the peritoneum

9. Protrusion of an organ or tissue through an abnormal body opening

Down

2. Inflammation of a diverticulum creating abdominal discomfort

3. Inflammation of the pancreas

6. Paralysis of the bowel; stops contractions that move material through the intestine

Ambulance Calls

The following real case scenarios provide an opportunity to explore the concerns associated with patient management. Read each scenario, then answer each question in detail.

1. You are called to the local high school nurse's office for a 16-year-old female complaining of severe, abrupt abdominal pain. She is pale, cool, and clammy with absent radial pulses. The school nurse tells you that the patient found out 4 weeks ago that she is pregnant.

How would you best manage this patient?

_____

_____

_____

_____

_____

_____

_____

_____

2. You are dispatched to a restaurant where a 28-year-old female is complaining of a sudden onset of nausea and vomiting with severe right lower quadrant pain. The patient is doubled over in pain, pale, and clammy. What problem would you suspect and how would you treat this patient?

_____

_____

_____

_____

_____

_____

_____

3. You are called to a residence for a 45-year-old male who has a "lump" in his lower abdomen. Upon inspection, you note a mass protruding from his lower abdomen that has a blue discoloration to the area and is tender on palpation. He tells you he first noticed it several days ago after doing some heavy lifting. How would you best manage this patient?

_____

_____

_____

_____

_____

_____

_____

Workbook Activities

The following activities have been designed to help you. Your instructor may require you to complete some or all of these activities as a regular part of your EMT-I training program. You are encouraged to complete any activity that your instructor does not assign as a way to enhance your learning in the classroom.

Chapter Review

The following exercises provide an opportunity to refresh your knowledge of this chapter.

Matching

Match each of the terms in the left column to the appropriate definition in the right column.

_____ 1. Conduction

_____ 2. Air embolism

_____ 3. Evaporation

_____ 4. Hyperthermia

_____ 5. Diving reflex

_____ 6. Core temperature

_____ 7. Convection

_____ 8. Laryngospasm

_____ 9. Electrolytes

_____ 10. Radiation

_____ 11. Hypothermia

_____ 12. Ambient temperature

_____ 13. Heat cramps

_____ 14. Drowning

_____ 15. Bends

_____ 16. Heat exhaustion

_____ 17. Bradycardia

_____ 18. Heat stroke

_____ 19. Breath-holding syncope

_____ 20. Hyperbaric chamber

_____ 21. Decompression sickness

_____ 22. Near drowning

_____ 23. Environmental emergency

_____ 24. Respiration

_____ 25. Frostbite

_____ 26. Reverse triage

A. slowing of the heart rate caused by sudden immersion in cold water

B. salts and other chemicals dissolved in body fluids

C. severe constriction of the larynx and vocal cords

D. death from suffocation after submersion in water

E. heat loss resulting from standing in a cold room

F. core temperature greater than 101°F

G. condition when the entire body temperature falls

H. condition caused by air bubbles in the blood vessels

I. heat loss that occurs from helicopter rotor blade downwash

J. heat loss resulting from sitting on snow

K. heat loss resulting from sweating

L. painful muscle spasms that occur after vigorous exercise

M. temperature of the surrounding environment

N. temperature of the central part of the body

O. the process of heat loss

P. damage to tissue from cold exposure; frozen body parts

Q. medical condition caused or exacerbated by the weather

R. the physiologic process of heat production in the body

S. self-contained underwater breathing apparatus

T. painful condition when divers ascend too quickly

U. a triage process focused on respiratory and cardiac arrest first, rather than last

V. loss of consciousness caused by a decreased breathing stimulus

W. the loss of body heat as warm air is exhaled and cooler air is inhaled

Environmental Emergencies

_____ **27.** Thermolysis

_____ **28.** Scuba

_____ **29.** Thermogenesis

X. slow heart rate, less than 60 bpm

Y. survival after suffocation in water

Z. common name for decompression sickness

AA. a chamber pressurized to more than atmospheric pressure

BB. life-threatening severe hyperthermia

CC. heat injury when the body loses significant amounts of fluid due to heavy sweating

Multiple Choice

Read each item carefully, then select the best response.

_____ **1.** _____ causes body heat to be lost as warm air in the lungs is exhaled into the atmosphere and cooler air is inhaled.

A. Convection

B. Conduction

C. Radiation

D. Respiration

_____ **2.** Evaporation, the conversion of any liquid to a gas, is a process that requires:

A. energy.

B. circulating air.

C. a warmer ambient temperature.

D. all of the above.

_____ **3.** The rate and amount of heat loss by the body can be modified by:

A. increasing heat production.

B. moving to an area where heat loss is decreased.

C. wearing insulated clothing.

D. all of the above.

_____ **4.** The characteristic appearance of blue lips and/or fingertips seen in hypothermia is the result of:

A. lack of oxygen in venous blood.

B. frostbite.

C. constriction of blood vessels.

D. bruising.

_____ 5. Signs and symptoms of severe systemic hypothermia include all of the following EXCEPT:

   A. weak pulse.

   B. coma.

   C. confusion.

   D. very slow respirations.

_____ 6. Hypothermia is more common among:

   A. elderly individuals.

   B. infants and children.

   C. those who are already ill.

   D. all of the above.

_____ 7. To assess a patient's general temperature, pull back your glove and place the back of your hand on the patient's:

   A. abdomen, underneath the clothing.

   B. forehead.

   C. forearm, on the inside of the wrist.

   D. neck, at the area where you check the carotid pulse.

_____ 8. To protect itself against heat loss, the body normally:

   A. has a parasympathetic response.

   B. constricts blood vessels.

   C. goes into Kussmaul respirations.

   D. none of the above.

_____ 9. Management of hypothermia in the field consists of all of the following EXCEPT:

   A. stabilizing vital functions.

   B. removing wet clothing.

   C. preventing further heat loss.

   D. massaging the cold extremities.

_____ 10. It is necessary to assess the pulse of a hypothermic patient for at least _____, especially before considering CPR.

   A. 10 to 20 seconds

   B. 30 to 45 seconds

   C. 60 to 75 minutes

   D. 2 full minutes

_____ 11. When exposed parts of the body become very cold but not frozen, the condition is called:

   A. frostnip.

   B. chilblains.

   C. immersion foot.

   D. all of the above.

_____ 12. Important factors in determining the severity of a local cold injury include all of the following EXCEPT:

   A. the temperature to which the body part was exposed.

   B. a previous history of frostbite.

   C. the wind velocity during exposure.

   D. the duration of the exposure.

_____ 13. Signs and symptoms of systemic hypothermia include:

   A. blisters and swelling.

   B. hard and waxy skin.

   C. altered mental status.

   D. local tissue damage.

_____ **14.** When the body is exposed to more heat energy than it loses, _____ results.

    A. hyperthermia

    B. heat cramps

    C. heat exhaustion

    D. heatstroke

_____ **15.** Contributing factors to the development of heat illnesses include:

    A. high air temperature.

    B. vigorous exercise.

    C. high humidity.

    D. all of the above.

_____ **16.** Keeping yourself hydrated while on duty is very important. Drink at least _____ of water per day and more when exertion or heat is involved.

    A. 8 glasses

    B. 1 liter

    C. 2 liters

    D. 3 liters

_____ **17.** All of the following statements concerning heat cramps are true EXCEPT:

    A. they only occur when it is hot outdoors.

    B. they may be seen in well-conditioned athletes.

    C. the exact cause of heat cramps is not well understood.

    D. dehydration may play a role in the development of heat cramps.

_____ **18.** Signs and symptoms of heat exhaustion and associated hypovolemia include:

    A. cold clammy skin with ashen pallor.

    B. dizziness, weakness, or faintness.

    C. normal vital signs.

    D. all of the above.

_____ **19.** Be prepared to transport the patient to the hospital for aggressive treatment of hyperthermia if:

    A. the symptoms do not clear up promptly.

    B. the level of consciousness improves.

    C. the temperature drops.

    D. all of the above.

_____ **20.** Often, the first sign of heatstroke is:

    A. a change in behavior.

    B. an increase in pulse rate.

    C. an increase in respirations.

    D. hot, dry, flushed skin.

_____ **21.** The least common but most serious illness caused by heat exposure, occurring when the body is subjected to more heat than it can handle and normal mechanisms for getting rid of the excess heat are overwhelmed, is:

    A. hyperthermia.

    B. heat cramps.

    C. heat exhaustion.

    D. heatstroke.

_____ **22.** _____ is the body's attempt at self-preservation by preventing water from entering the lungs.

    A. Bronchoconstriction

    B. Laryngospasm

    C. Esophageal spasms

    D. Swelling in the oropharynx

_____ **23.** Treatment of drowning/near drowning begins with:

   A. opening the airway.

   B. ventilation with 100% oxygen via BVM device.

   C. suctioning the lungs to remove the water.

   D. rescue and removal from the water.

_____ **24.** If you are unsure whether or not a spinal injury has occurred, you should:

   A. stabilize and protect the patient's spine.

   B. provide mouth-to-mouth ventilation as you would in any other situation.

   C. ascertain whether or not there is a spinal injury.

   D. all of the above.

_____ **25.** After removing a near-drowning patient from the water, it may be difficult to find a pulse because of:

   A. dilation of peripheral blood vessels.

   B. body temperature at the core.

   C. low cardiac output.

   D. all of the above.

_____ **26.** If the near-drowning victim has evidence of upper airway obstruction by foreign matter, attempt to clear it by:

   A. removing the obstruction manually.

   B. suction.

   C. using abdominal thrusts.

   D. all of the above.

_____ **27.** Management of mildly hypothermic patients should include all the following EXCEPT:

   A. managing the ABCs.

   B. having them drink warm coffee or tea if available.

   C. assessing the patient's pulse for 30 to 45 seconds.

   D. handling the patient gently.

_____ **28.** You should never give up on resuscitating a cold-water drowning victim because:

   A. when the patient is submerged in water colder than body temperature, heat is maintained in the body.

   B. the resulting hypothermia can protect vital organs from the lack of oxygen.

   C. the resulting hypothermia raises the metabolic rate.

   D. all of the above.

_____ **29.** Causes of children drowning include:

   A. child abuse.

   B. lack of adult supervision.

   C. pool was not surrounded by a 6′ high fence.

   D. all of the above.

_____ **30.** Areas usually affected by descent problems include:

   A. the lungs.

   B. the skin.

   C. the joints.

   D. vision.

_____ **31.** Potential problems associated with rupture of the lungs include:

   A. air emboli.

   B. pneumomediastinum.

   C. pneumothorax.

   D. all of the above.

_____ **32.** The organs most severely affected by air embolism are the:

    A. brain and spinal cord.

    B. brain and heart.

    C. heart and lungs.

    D. brain and lungs.

1999 _____ **33.** The cardiac rhythm most often seen with hypothermic patients is:

    A. A-fib.

    B. V-fib.

    C. idoventricular rhythms.

    D. atrioventricular blocks.

_____ **34.** The most common illness caused by heat is:

    A. heat exhaustion.

    B. heat collapse.

    C. heat prostration.

    D. all of the above.

_____ **35.** Signs and symptoms of heat exhaustion and those associated with hypovolemia are:

    A. cool clammy skin.

    B. dry tongue and thirst.

    C. dizziness, weakness, or faintness with nausea or headache.

    D. all of the above.

Vocabulary EMT-I

Define the following terms in the space provided.

1. Hyperbaric chamber:

_____

_____

_____

2. Decompression sickness:

_____

_____

_____

3. Heat exhaustion:

_____

_____

_____

4. Frostbite:

_____

_____

_____

5. Near drowning:

_____

_____

_____

6. Pneumomediastinum:

_____

_____

_____

Fill-in

Read each item carefully, then complete the statement by filling in the missing word(s).

1. Do not attempt to rewarm patients who have _____ to _____ hypothermia because they are prone to developing arrhythmias unless handled very carefully.

2. Most significant diving injuries occur during _____.

3. When treating a patient with frostbite, never attempt _____ if there is any chance that the part may freeze again before the patient reaches the hospital.

4. As with so many hazards, you cannot help others if you do not practice _____.

5. _____, a common effect of hypothermia, is the body's attempt to maintain heat.

6. Whenever a person dives or jumps into very cold water, the _____ _____ may cause immediate bradycardia.

7. If the patient is alert and responds appropriately, the hypothermia is _____.

8. Oxygen and IV packs both may be warmed by _____ _____ _____ to the tubing.

9. Oxygen and IV packs both may be cooled by _____ _____ _____ to the tubing.

1999 **10.** _____ _____ exposed to very low temperatures may be less effective, and the hypothermic patient's _____ _____ is typically to slow to effectively process them.

1999 **11.** Due to the potential for _____, always monitor the cardiac status of a lightning strike victim.

12. Do not perform abdominal thrusts unless a foreign body airway obstruction is present. Doing so will increase the risk of _____ of water and _____.

13. You should never _____ _____ on resuscitating a cold-water drowning victim.

True/False

If you believe the statement to be more true than false, write the letter "T" in the space provided. If you believe the statement to be more false than true, write the letter "F."

_____ **1.** Normal body temperature is 98.6°F (37°C).

_____ **2.** To assess the skin temperature in a patient experiencing a generalized cold emergency, you should feel the patient's skin.

_____ **3.** Mild hypothermia occurs when the core temperature drops to 85°F.

_____ **4.** The body's most efficient heat-regulating mechanisms are sweating and dilation of skin blood vessels.

_____ **5.** People who are at greatest risk for heat illnesses are the elderly and children.

_____ **6.** The signs and symptoms of exposure to heat can include moist pale skin.

_____ **7.** The strongest stimulus for breathing is an elevation of oxygen in the blood.

_____ **8.** Immediate bradycardia after jumping in cold water is called the diving reflex.

_____ **9.** The signs and symptoms of exposure to heat can include hot, dry skin.

1999 _____ **10.** Because cold muscle is a poor conductor of electricity, the cardiac monitor may show asystole, but the patient may indeed have a cardiac rhythm.

_____ **11.** During vigorous exercise, the body can lose more than 1 L of sweat per hour.

_____ **12.** Heat cramps usually occur in the legs or abdominal muscles.

_____ **13.** In heat exhaustion, there is typically a neurologic deficit.

_____ **14.** When confronted with multiple lighting strike victims, the EMT-Is should focus their efforts on those who appear dead.

_____ **15.** Air embolism may occur on a dive as shallow as 6′.

_____ **16.** Emergency treatment is the same for both air embolism and decompression sickness.

1999 _____ **17.** Any patient with suspected hypoxia following a water-related incident should be placed on a cardiac monitor and observed for arrhythmias.

Short Answer

Complete this section with short written answers in the space provided.

1. What are three ways to modify heat loss? Give an example of each.

_____

_____

_____

2. What are the steps in treating heatstroke?

_____

_____

_____

3. What is an air embolism and how does it occur?

_____

_____

_____

4. For what diving emergencies are hyperbaric chambers used?

_____

_____

_____

5. How should a frostbitten foot be treated?

_____

_____

_____

6. What are the four "Do Nots" in relation to local cold injuries?

_____

_____

_____

7. What are the potential signs and symptoms of an air embolism?

_____

_____

_____

8. Describe laryngospasm and its effects on the near-drowning patient.

_____

_____

_____

Word Fun EMT-I vocab explorer web

The following crossword puzzle is an activity provided to reinforce correct spelling and understanding of medical terminology associated with emergency care and the EMT-I. Use the clues in the column to complete the puzzle.

Across

2. The loss of heat by direct contact

5. The loss of body heat caused by air movement

7. Air bubbles in the blood vessels

8. Severe constriction of the larynx and vocal cords

9. The direct loss of body heat to colder objects, or heat gained from warmer objects

10. Salts and other chemicals that are dissolved in body fluids

Down

1. Heat injury due to loss of fluids and electrolytes because of heavy sweating

3. The process of heat loss

4. Common name for decompression sickness

6. A life threatening condition of severe hyperthermia

Ambulance Calls

The following real case scenarios provide an opportunity to explore the concerns associated with patient management. Read each scenario, then answer each question in detail.

1. You are called to the local airport for a 52-year-old male who is the pilot of his own aircraft. He tells you he is having severe abdominal pain and joint pain. History reveals that the patient is returning from a dive trip off the coast. He says he has had "the bends" before and this feels similar.

How would you best manage this patient?

_____

_____

_____

_____

_____

_____

_____

_____

2. You are called to the residence of a 74-year-old female. Neighbors tell you that she was found this morning sitting on her porch. The temperature was below freezing. She went outside because she had no heat in her house anyway. She is cold to the touch but responds appropriately to your questions. How would you best manage this patient?

_____

_____

_____

_____

_____

_____

_____

3. You are dispatched to the local high school for a 15-year-old female complaining of a sudden onset of abdominal cramps. It is very hot inside the gym, and she was exercising vigorously. She is sitting on the bleachers, doubled over and crying. How would you best manage this patient?

_____

_____

_____

_____

_____

_____

_____

1999 **4.** You are called to the local outdoor swimming pool for a lifeguard who has been struck by lighting. As you approach the scene you notice a young male, unconscious, leaning back over the lifeguard chair. How would you best manage this patient?

_____

_____

_____

_____

_____

_____

_____

_____

Skill Drills

Skill Drill 26-1: Treating for Heat Exhaustion
Test your knowledge by filling in the correct words in the photo captions.

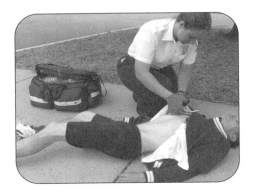

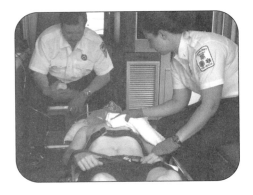

1. Remove _____

_____.

2. Move the patient to a

_____

_____. Give

_____. Place the

patient in a _____

position, elevate the legs, and

_____ the patient.

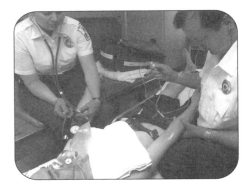

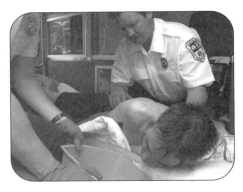

3. Establish _____

_____. Give normal

_____ fluid boluses

of 20 mL/kg as needed if the patient

is _____ or unable

to take _____ by

mouth.

4. If nausea develops,

_____ the patient on

his or her side.

Skill Drill 26-2: Stabilizing a Suspected Spinal Injury in the Water

Test your knowledge by placing the photos below in the correct order. Number the first step with a "1," the second step with a "2," etc.

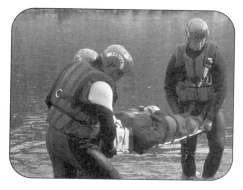

Remove the patient from the water.

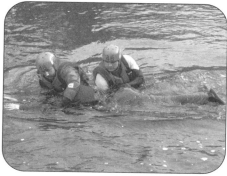

Turn the patient to a supine position by rotating the entire upper half of the body as a single unit.

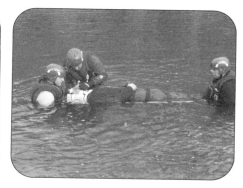

Secure the patient to the backboard.

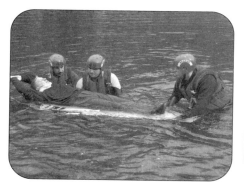

Float a buoyant backboard under the patient.

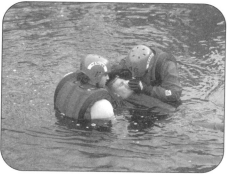

As soon as the patient is turned, begin artificial ventilation using the mouth-to-mouth method or a pocket mask.

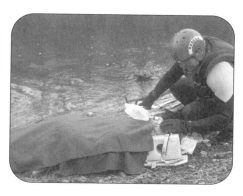

Cover the patient with a blanket, and apply oxygen if breathing.

Begin CPR if breathing and pulse are absent.

Workbook Activities

The following activities have been designed to help you. Your instructor may require you to complete some or all of these activities as a regular part of your EMT-I training program. You are encouraged to complete any activity that your instructor does not assign as a way to enhance your learning in the classroom.

Chapter Review

The following exercises provide an opportunity to refresh your knowledge of this chapter.

Matching

Match each of the terms in the left column to the appropriate definition in the right column.

_____ 1. Behavioral crisis

_____ 2. Psychogenic

_____ 3. Organic brain syndrome

_____ 4. Depression

_____ 5. Functional disorder

_____ 6. Behavior

_____ 7. ADL

_____ 8. Altered mental status

_____ 9. Mental disorder

A. what you can see of a person's response to the environment; his or her actions

B. temporary or permanent dysfunction of the brain caused by a disturbance in brain tissue function

C. any reaction to events that interferes with activities of daily living or is unacceptable to the patient or others

D. a persistent mood of sadness, despair, or discouragement

E. abnormal operation of an organ that cannot be traced to an obvious change in the structure or the physiology of the organ

F. a symptom or illness caused by mental factors as opposed to physical ones

G. a change in the way a person thinks and behaves

H. an illness with psychological or behavioral symptoms

I. activities of daily living; basic activities a person usually accomplishes during a normal day

Multiple Choice

Read each item carefully, then select the best response.

_____ 1. A psychological or behavioral crisis may be the result of:

A. mind-altering substances.

B. the emergency situation.

C. stress.

D. all of the above.

CHAPTER 27

Behavioral Emergencies

_____ **2.** A normal reaction to a crisis situation would be:

A. Monday morning blues that last until Friday.

B. feeling "blue" after the break up of a long-term relationship.

C. feeling depressed week after week with no discernible cause.

D. all of the above.

_____ **3.** The cause of a behavioral crisis experienced by an unmanageable patient may be:

A. drug use.

B. a history of mental illness.

C. alcohol abuse.

D. all of the above.

_____ **4.** An altered mental status can arise from:

A. hypoglycemia.

B. hypoxia.

C. exposure to excessive heat or cold.

D. all the above.

_____ **5.** If the interruption of daily routine tends to recur on a regular basis, the behavior is also considered a _____ problem.

A. mental health

B. functional disorder

C. behavioral

D. psychogenic

_____ **6.** If an abnormal or disturbing pattern of behavior lasts for at least _____, it is regarded as a matter of concern from a mental health standpoint.

A. 6 weeks

B. a month

C. 6 months

D. a year

_____ **7.** A person who is no longer able to respond appropriately to the environment may be having what is called a psychological or _____ emergency.

A. psychiatric

B. behavioral

C. functional

D. adjustment

_____ **8.** Mental disorders may be caused by a:

    A. social disturbance.

    B. chemical disturbance.

    C. biological disturbance.

    D. all of the above.

_____ **9.** An altered mental status may arise from:

    A. an oxygen saturation of 98%.

    B. moderate temperatures.

    C. an inadequate blood flow to the brain.

    D. adequate glucose levels in the blood.

_____ **10.** Organic brain syndrome may be caused by:

    A. hypoglycemia.

    B. excessive heat or cold.

    C. lack of oxygen.

    D. all of the above.

_____ **11.** An example of a functional disorder would be:

    A. schizophrenia.

    B. organic brain syndrome.

    C. Alzheimer's.

    D. all of the above.

_____ **12.** When documenting abnormal behavior, it is important to:

    A. record detailed, subjective findings.

    B. avoid judgmental statements.

    C. avoid quoting the patient's own words.

    D. all of the above.

_____ **13.** Safety guidelines for behavioral emergencies include:

    A. assessing the scene.

    B. being prepared to spend extra time.

    C. encouraging purposeful movement.

    D. all of the above.

_____ **14.** In evaluating a situation that is considered a behavioral emergency, the first things to consider are:

    A. airway and breathing.

    B. scene safety and patient response.

    C. history of medications.

    D. respiratory and circulatory status.

_____ **15.** Psychogenic circumstances may include:

    A. severe depression.

    B. death of a loved one.

    C. a history of mental illness.

    D. all of the above.

_____ **16.** Risk factors for suicide may include:

    A. denial of alcohol use.

    B. recent marriage.

    C. holidays.

    D. all of the above.

_____ **17.** Suicidal patients may also be:

   A. homicidal.

   B. hypoxic.

   C. joking.

   D. seeking attention.

_____ **18.** Causes of altered behavior in geriatric patients may include:

   A. constipation.

   B. diabetes.

   C. stroke.

   D. all of the above.

_____ **19.** Restraint of a person must be ordered by:

   A. a physician.

   B. a court order.

   C. a law enforcement officer.

   D. all of the above.

_____ **20.** When restraining a patient without an appropriate order, legal actions may involve charges of:

   A. abandonment.

   B. negligence.

   C. battery.

   D. breach of duty.

_____ **21.** When restraining a patient face down on a stretcher, it is necessary to constantly reassess the patient's:

   A. level of consciousness.

   B. airway.

   C. emotional status.

   D. pulse rate.

_____ **22.** A patient in a mentally unstable condition:

   A. is always violent.

   B. can refuse to consent to treatment.

   C. should never be left alone.

   D. all of the above.

_____ **23.** Which statement is true concerning the use of restraints?

   A. At least four people should be present to carry out the restraint.

   B. Somebody should continue to talk to the patient throughout the process.

   C. Never place your patient face down.

   D. All of the above.

_____ **24.** Reflective listening is a technique that:

   A. requires more time to be effective than is usually available in an EMS setting.

   B. is frequently used by mental health professionals to gain insight into a patient's thinking.

   C. may be a helpful tool to use when other techniques are unsuccessful.

   D. all of the above.

Vocabulary EMT-I [vocab explorer web]

Define the following terms in the space provided.

1. Mental disorder:

_____

_____

_____

2. Activities of daily living (ADL):

_____

_____

_____

3. Altered mental status:

_____

_____

_____

4. Implied consent:

_____

_____

_____

Fill-in

Read each item carefully, then complete the statement by filling in the missing word(s).

1. _____ is what you can see of a person's response to the environment; his or her actions.

2. A _____ or emergency is any reaction to events that interferes with the activities of daily living or has become unacceptable to the patient, family, or community.

3. Chronic _____, or a persistent feeling of sadness or despair, may be a symptom of a mental or physical disorder.

4. _____ is a temporary or permanent dysfunction of the brain, caused by a disturbance in the physical or physiologic functioning of the brain.

5. _____, _____, and _____ may be of great help in answering questions during a behavioral emergency.

6. Any time you encounter an emotionally depressed patient, you must consider the possibility

of _____.

7. At one time or another, one in five Americans have some type of _____

_____.

8. When examining a patient during a behavioral emergency, you should _____ physical

contact in order to minimize patient apprehension.

True/False

If you believe the statement to be more true than false, write the letter "T" in the space provided. If you believe the statement to be more false than true, write the letter "F."

_____ **1.** Depression lasting 2 to 3 weeks after being fired from a job is a normal mental health response.

_____ **2.** Low blood glucose or lack of oxygen to the brain may cause behavioral changes, but not to the degree that a psychiatric emergency could exist.

_____ **3.** From a mental health standpoint, a pattern of abnormal behavior must last at least 3 months to be a matter of concern.

_____ **4.** A disturbed patient should always be transported with restraints.

_____ **5.** It is sometimes helpful to allow a patient with a behavioral emergency some time alone to calm down and collect their thoughts.

_____ **6.** It is important to avoid looking directly at the patient when dealing with a behavioral crisis.

_____ **7.** A patient should never be asked if he or she is considering suicide.

_____ **8.** Urinary tract infections can cause behavioral changes in elderly patients.

_____ **9.** All individuals with mental health disorders are dangerous, violent, or otherwise unmanageable.

_____ **10.** When completing the documentation, it is important to record detailed, subjective findings that support the conclusion of abnormal behavior.

_____ **11.** When restraining a patient, at least four people should be present to carry out the restraint.

_____ **12.** The first thing to consider when evaluating a behavioral emergency is the patients ABCs.

_____ **13.** The EMT-I may only use reasonable force as necessary to control the patient from causing bodily harm to either himself or others.

_____ **14.** Depression accounts for 20% of violent attacks.

Short Answer

Complete this section with short written answers in the space provided.

1. What is the distinction between a behavioral crisis and a mental health problem?

_____

_____

_____

2. What three major areas should be considered in evaluating the possible source of a behavioral crisis?

_____

_____

_____

3. What are three factors to consider in determining the level of force required to restrain a patient?

_____

_____

_____

4. List ten safety guidelines for dealing with behavioral emergencies.

_____

_____

_____

5. List ten risk factors for suicide.

_____

_____

_____

6. Discuss the misconceptions relating to mental disorders. How can these misconceptions be corrected?

_____

_____

_____

Word Fun EMT-I vocab explorer web

The following crossword puzzle is an activity provided to reinforce correct spelling and understanding of medical terminology associated with emergency care and the EMT-I. Use the clues in the column to complete the puzzle.

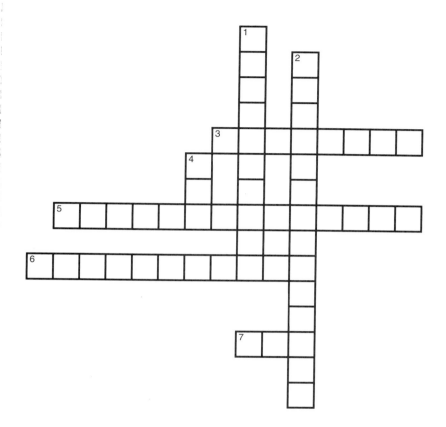

Across

3. How a person functions in response to their environment

5. Caused by a social, psychological, genetic, physical, chemical or biologic disturbance

6. Symptom or illness cause by mental factors

7. Organic brain syndrome; dysfunction of the brain

Down

1. A persistent mood of sadness, despair, and discouragement

2. The point when a person's reactions to events interfere with activities of daily living

4. Activities of daily living

Ambulance Calls

The following real case scenarios provide an opportunity to explore the concerns associated with patient management. Read each scenario, then answer each question in detail.

1. You are dispatched to the residence of a 27-year-old man. Family members called because he has become increasingly more confused and agitated as a result of excessive street drug use. They tell you he has had a large quantity of alcohol and crack cocaine over the past 24 hours. The patient has violent tattoos covering both forearms and is pacing back and forth across the room, clenching and unclenching his fists. He is yelling obscenities at anyone who comes near.

   How would you best manage this patient?

   _____

   _____

   _____

   _____

   _____

   _____

   _____

   _____

2. You are called to the scene of a personal care home where you find a 73-year-old woman with erratic behavior. Staff reports that the patient has a history of mild dementia and hypertension. Her mental status is quite altered from normal. Her ABCs are normal.

   How would you best manage this patient?

   _____

   _____

   _____

   _____

   _____

   _____

   _____

   _____

3. You are dispatched to the residence of a 40-year-old woman who is upset over the loss of her mother 5 weeks ago. She tells you that she has no family and has cared for her elderly mother for the past 7 years. She has not eaten in several days and is severely depressed.

How would you best manage this patient?

_____

_____

_____

_____

_____

_____

_____

_____

Workbook Activities

The following activities have been designed to help you. Your instructor may require you to complete some or all of these activities as a regular part of your EMT-I training program. You are encouraged to complete any activity that your instructor does not assign as a way to enhance your learning in the classroom.

Chapter Review

The following exercises provide an opportunity to refresh your knowledge of this chapter.

Matching

Match each of the terms in the left column to the appropriate definition in the right column.

_____ 1. Cervix

_____ 2. Perineum

_____ 3. Fundus

_____ 4. Fallopian tubes

_____ 5. Hymen

_____ 6. Endometrium

_____ 7. Uterus

_____ 8. Ectopic pregnancy

_____ 9. Vagina

_____ 10. Labia majora

_____ 11. Dysmenorrhea

_____ 12. Labia minora

_____ 13. Clitoris

_____ 14. Menarche

_____ 15. Anus

_____ 16. Abortion

_____ 17. Placenta abruptio

_____ 18. Placenta previa

_____ 19. Ovaries

_____ 20. Prepuce

_____ 21. Oocyte

_____ 22. Urethra

_____ 23. Myometrium

_____ 24. Vaginal orifice

_____ 25. Mons pubis

_____ 26. Vestibule

A. small erectile body partially hidden by the labia minora

B. tubes or ducts extending from near the ovaries

C. the area of skin between the vagina and the anus

D. the neck of the uterus

E. pregnancy that develops outside the uterus, typically in the fallopian tube

F. the outermost part of a woman's reproductive system

G. the initial onset of menstruation occurring during puberty

H. the inner layer of the uterine wall

I. inner lip-shaped structure of the vagina

J. the outlet of the rectum

K. painful menstruation

L. uppermost part of the uterus, farthest from the cervical opening

M. the hollow organ inside the female pelvis where the fetus grows

N. the membrane partially covering the entrance to the vagina

O. outer lip-shaped structure of the vagina

P. foreskin covering the clitoris

Q. canal for the discharge of urine from the bladder to the outside of the body

R. condition in which the placenta develops over the cervix

S. premature separation of the placenta from the wall of the uterus

T. opening of the vagina

U. small space at the beginning of an opening

V. almond-shaped bodies on either side of the pelvic cavity that producing ova

W. the female sex cell

X. the visible external female genitalia

CHAPTER 28

Gynecologic Emergencies

_____ **27.** Menstruation

_____ **28.** Vulva

_____ **29.** Menopause

Y. the muscular wall of the uterus

Z. pad of fatty tissue and coarse skin that lies over the pubic symphysis

AA. cyclic shedding of uterine lining that occurs approximately every 28 days

BB. the cessation of the menstrual cycle and ovarian function

CC. delivery of fetus and placenta before 20 weeks

Multiple Choice

Read each item carefully, then select the best response.

_____ **1.** Your first priority when dealing with a sexual assault victim is to:
   A. manage the airway.
   B. preserve all evidence.
   C. not allow the patient to bathe or brush his or her teeth.
   D. control any bleeding.

_____ **2.** You should consider the possibility of a(n) _____ in women who have missed a menstrual cycle and complain of a sudden stabbing and usually unilateral pain in the lower abdomen.
   A. PID
   B. ectopic pregnancy
   C. miscarriage
   D. placenta abruptio

_____ **3.** Appropriate care for traumatic gynecological emergencies includes:
   A. packing or placing dressings in the vagina.
   B. removing foreign bodies from the vagina as necessary.
   C. all the above.
   D. none of the above.

_____ **4.** When using SAMPLE to determine the nature of a suspected gynecological emergency, which question is not correct?
   A. What medications are you currently taking?
   B. When was your last menstrual cycle?
   C. What events have led up to this?
   D. None of the above.

_____ **5.** Which statement is not correct?
   A. Some women will continue to have menstrual cycles even though they are pregnant.
   B. The genital parts have a rich nerve supply, making injuries very painful.
   C. The absence of the hymen does not denote virginity.
   D. None of the above.

_____ **6.** Care for the patient with an ectopic pregnancy includes:
   A. taking orthostatic vital signs.
   B. noting the presence and volume of blood.
   C. establishing a second IV line with a large-bore catheter.
   D. all the above.

_____ **7.** Causes of vaginal bleeding include:
   A. onset of labor.
   B. PID.
   C. trauma.
   D. all the above.

Labeling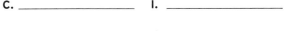

Anatomy of the Female Reproductive System

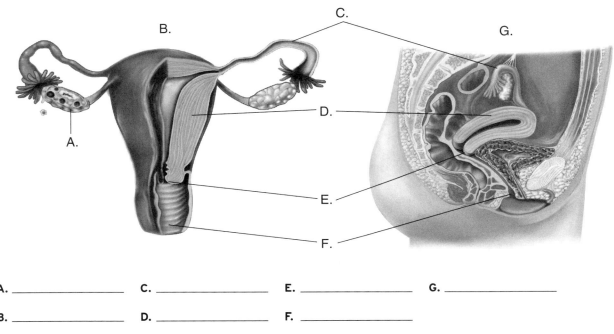

A. _____   C. _____   E. _____   G. _____

B. _____   D. _____   F. _____

A. _____   G. _____

B. _____   H. _____

C. _____   I. _____

D. _____   J. _____

E. _____   K. _____

F. _____   L. _____

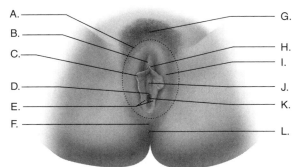

Vocabulary EMT-I

Define the following terms in the space provided.

1. Ectopic pregnancy:

_____

_____

_____

2. Pelvic inflammatory disease (PID):

_____

_____

_____

3. Fallopian tubes:

_____

_____

_____

4. Placenta abruptio:

_____

_____

_____

5. Placenta previa:

_____

_____

_____

Fill-in

Read each item carefully, then complete the statement by filling in the missing word(s).

1. The EMT-I should determine whether the patient has a history of gynecologic problems and whether she

   has had any _____.

2. If the patient is currently bleeding, _____ the amount of blood loss.

3. If there is any evidence of _____ and/or _____, be sure to take it with

   the patient to the hospital.

1999 4. Place the patient on a cardiac monitor and be alert for any _____

   _____.

1999 5. _____ may mask signs and symptoms, making diagnosis difficult.

True/False

If you believe the statement to be more true than false, write the letter "T" in the space provided. If you believe the statement to be more false than true, write the letter "F."

_____ 1. The chief symptoms of PID are pelvic pain and fever.

_____ 2. An ovarian cyst is a fluid-filled sac attached to the inside of the uterus.

_____ 3. Never assume that your emergency call for vaginal hemorrhage is due to normal menstruation.

_____ 4. Any vaginal bleeding during the third trimester of pregnancy is a serious emergency.

_____ 5. Do not examine the genitalia of a victim of sexual assault unless obvious bleeding requires you to apply dressing.

_____ 6. The EMT-I should not offer to call the local rape crisis center for the patient, as it is a violation of patient confidentiality.

Short Answer

Complete this section with short written answers in the space provided.

1. When would it become necessary to initiate an IV during a gynecologic emergency?

   _____

   _____

   _____

2. How should the IV be accomplished?

   _____

   _____

   _____

3. List the causes of vaginal bleeding due to trauma.

_____

_____

_____

Word Fun EMT-I vocab explorer web

The following crossword puzzle is an activity provided to reinforce correct spelling and understanding of medical terminology associated with emergency care and the EMT-I. Use the clues in the column to complete the puzzle.

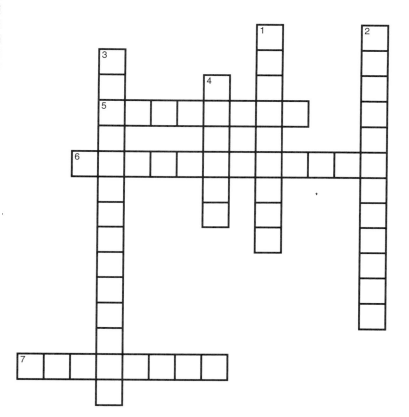

Across

5. Delivery of the fetus and placenta before 20 weeks

6. The cyclic shedding of the uterine lining; occurs approximately every 28 days

7. Area of skin between the vagina and the anus

Down

1. Cessation of the menstrual cycle and ovarian function

2. Painful menstruation

3. Placenta either partially or completely covers the cervix

4. Muscular organ where the fetus grows

Ambulance Calls

The following real case scenarios provide an opportunity to explore the concerns associated with patient management. Read each scenario, then answer each question in detail.

1. You are called to a bar where a 27-year-old woman has been sexually assaulted. When you arrive, you find the woman, the police, and several of her friends in the restroom.

   How would you best manage this call?

   _____

   _____

   _____

   _____

   _____

   _____

   _____

2. If she is refusing care, how would you best manage this patient?

_____

_____

_____

_____

_____

_____

_____

_____

Workbook Activities

The following activities have been designed to help you. Your instructor may require you to complete some or all of these activities as a regular part of your EMT-I training program. You are encouraged to complete any activity that your instructor does not assign as a way to enhance your learning in the classroom.

Chapter Review

The following exercises provide an opportunity to refresh your knowledge of this chapter.

Matching

Match each of the terms in the left column to the appropriate definition in the right column.

_____ 1. Cervix

_____ 2. Perineum

_____ 3. Placenta

_____ 4. Nullipara

_____ 5. Fetus

_____ 6. Birth canal

_____ 7. Uterus

_____ 8. Umbilical cord

_____ 9. Vagina

_____ 10. Breech presentation

_____ 11. Limb presentation

_____ 12. Multipara

_____ 13. Nuchal cord

_____ 14. Presentation

_____ 15. Abruptio placentae

_____ 16. Fallopian tube

_____ 17. Ectopic pregnancy

_____ 18. Amniotic sac

_____ 19. Crowning

_____ 20. Eclampsia

_____ 21. Zygote

_____ 22. Preeclampsia

_____ 23. Gestational diabetes

_____ 24. Meconium

_____ 25. Para

_____ 26. Trimester

A. an umbilical cord that is wrapped around the infant's neck

B. a fluid-filled, bag-like membrane inside the uterus that grows around the developing fetus

C. the area of skin between the vagina and the anus

D. the neck of the uterus

E. connects mother and infant

F. the outermost part of a woman's reproductive system

G. the part of the infant that appears first

H. the vagina and lower part of the uterus

I. a woman who has had more than one live birth

J. premature separation of the placenta from the uterus wall

K. delivery in which the presenting part is a single arm, leg, or foot

L. tissue that develops on the wall of the uterus and is connected to the fetus

M. the hollow organ inside the female pelvis where the fetus grows

N. the developing baby in the uterus

O. delivery in which the buttocks come out first

P. a woman who has never delivered a viable infant

Q. the viewing of the infant's head at the vaginal opening during labor

R. seizures resulting from severe hypertension in the pregnant woman

S. a pregnancy that develops outside the uterus, typically in the fallopian tube

T. two hollow tubes that extend from the uterus to the region of the ovary

U. condition in which progesterone makes the cells resistant to insulin

CHAPTER 29

Obstetric Emergencies

_____ **27.** Grand multipara	**V.** a woman who has delivered seven or more viable infants
_____ **28.** Primigravida	**W.** pregnant
_____ **29.** Uterine rupture	**X.** term to describe the number of times a woman as been pregnant
_____ **30.** Gravid	**Y.** dark green material inside the amniotic fluid
_____ **31.** Gravida	**Z.** a woman who has been pregnant more than once
_____ **32.** Multigravida	**AA.** term to describe the number of times a woman has delivered a viable (live) infant
_____ **33.** Placenta previa	**BB.** condition in which the placenta develops over the cervix
_____ **34.** Term	**CC.** hypertension during pregnancy, protein in urine, and edema; precursor to eclampsia
_____ **35.** Supine hypotensive syndrome	**DD.** a woman's first pregnancy
_____ **36.** Prolapsed umbilical cord	**EE.** situation in which the umbilical cord presents outside the vagina before the infant
	FF. low blood pressure resulting from the compression of the inferior vena cava by the fetus when the mother is supine
	GG. a full 40 week pregnancy
	HH. three segments at time each made up of approximately 3 months
	II. rupture of the uterus
	JJ. a fertilized egg

Multiple Choice

Read each item carefully, then select the best response.

_____ **1.** In the event of a nuchal cord, proper procedure is to:

    A. gently slip the cord over the infant's head or shoulder.

    B. clamp the cord and cut it before delivering the infant.

    C. clamp the cord and cut it, then gently unwind it from around the neck if wrapped around more than once.

    D. all of the above.

_____ **2.** If the amniotic fluid is greenish instead of clear or has a foul odor, this is called:

    A. nuchal rigidity.

    B. meconium staining.

    C. placenta previa.

    D. bloody show.

_____ **3.** Meconium can cause all of the following, except:
- **A.** a depressed newborn.
- **B.** rapid pulse rate.
- **C.** airway obstruction.
- **D.** aspiration.

_____ **4.** You may help control bleeding by massaging the _____ after delivery of the placenta.
- **A.** perineum
- **B.** fundus
- **C.** lower back
- **D.** inner thighs

_____ **5.** You cannot successfully deliver a _____ presentation in the field.
- **A.** limb
- **B.** breech
- **C.** vertex
- **D.** all of the above

_____ **6.** Care for a mother with a prolapsed cord includes:
- **A.** positioning the mother to keep the weight of the infant off the cord.
- **B.** high-flow oxygen and rapid transport.
- **C.** using your hand to hold the infant's head off the cord.
- **D.** all of the above.

_____ **7.** The stages of labor include:
- **A.** dilation of the cervix.
- **B.** expulsion of the baby.
- **C.** delivery of the placenta.
- **D.** all of the above.

_____ **8.** The first stage of labor begins with the onset of contractions and ends when:
- **A.** the infant is born.
- **B.** the cervix is fully dilated.
- **C.** the water breaks.
- **D.** the placenta is delivered.

_____ **9.** Signs of the beginning of labor include:
- **A.** bloody show.
- **B.** contractions of the uterus.
- **C.** rupture of the amniotic sac.
- **D.** all of the above.

_____ **10.** The second stage of labor begins when the cervix is fully dilated and ends when:
- **A.** the infant is born.
- **B.** the water breaks.
- **C.** the placenta delivers.
- **D.** the uterus stops contracting.

_____ **11.** The third stage of labor begins with the birth of the infant and ends with the:
- **A.** release of milk from the breasts.
- **B.** cessation of uterine contractions.
- **C.** delivery of the placenta.
- **D.** cutting of the umbilical cord.

_____ **12.** The difference between preeclampsia and eclampsia is the onset of:
- **A.** seeing spots.
- **B.** seizures.
- **C.** swelling in the hands and feet.
- **D.** headaches.

_____ **13.** You should consider the possibility of a(n) _____ in women who have missed a menstrual cycle and complain of a sudden stabbing and usually unilateral pain in the lower abdomen.

A. PID

B. ectopic pregnancy

C. miscarriage

D. abruptio placentae

_____ **14.** _____ is a condition of late pregnancy that also involves headache, visual changes, and swelling of the hands and feet.

A. Pregnancy-induced hypertension

B. Placenta previa

C. Abruptio placentae

D. Supine hypotensive syndrome

_____ **15.** Low blood pressure resulting from compression of the inferior vena cava by the weight of the fetus when the mother is supine is called:

A. pregnancy-induced hypertension.

B. placenta previa.

C. abruptio placentae.

D. supine hypotensive syndrome.

_____ **16.** _____ is a situation in which the umbilical cord comes out of the vagina before the infant.

A. Eclampsia

B. Placenta previa

C. Abruptio placentae

D. Prolapsed cord

_____ **17.** Premature separation of the placenta from the wall of the uterus is known as:

A. eclampsia.

B. placenta previa.

C. abruptio placentae.

D. prolapsed cord.

_____ **18.** _____ is a condition in which the placenta develops over and covers the cervix.

A. Eclampsia

B. Placenta previa

C. Abruptio placentae

D. Prolapsed cord

_____ **19.** _____ is heralded by the onset of convulsions, or seizures, resulting from severe hypertension in the pregnant woman.

A. Eclampsia

B. Placenta previa

C. Abruptio placentae

D. Supine hypotensive syndrome

_____ **20.** From the time of fertilization to then end of the _____ week, the developing zygote is referred to as an embryo.

A. 2nd

B. 8th

C. 16th

D. none of the above

_____ **21.** After assisting the mother in her delivery and cutting the umbilical cord, you note that the infant is need of an IV, and you've decided to infuse the solution through the umbilical cord itself. Where will you insert the catheter?

A. In one of the two arteries within the cord

B. In one of the two veins within the cord

C. One should not infuse through the umbilical cord.

D. None of the above

_____ **22.** Once the amniotic sac has ruptured, the fetus must be delivered within _____ because of the risk of infection.

    A. 12 hours

    B. 24 hours

    C. 36 hours

    D. 48 hours

_____ **23.** In an emergency prior to delivery, the best way to promote a healthy infant is to:

    A. maintain oxygenation.

    B. maintain ventilation.

    C. maintain perfusion.

    D. all the above.

_____ **24.** The most common cause of vaginal bleeding during the first and second trimesters is:

    A. abortion.

    B. placenta previa.

    C. abruptio placentae.

    D. uterine rupture.

1999 _____ **25.** You arrive at the home of an eclamptic woman. Part of her treatment is likely to include:

    A. oxygen at 2 L/min via nasal cannula.

    B. 8 g of magnesium sulfate IM.

    C. 8 mg via IM.

    D. 2 g of magnesium sulfate via IV bolus over 5 minutes.

Labeling EMT-I anatomy review web

Label the following diagram with the correct terms.

Female Reproductive Tract

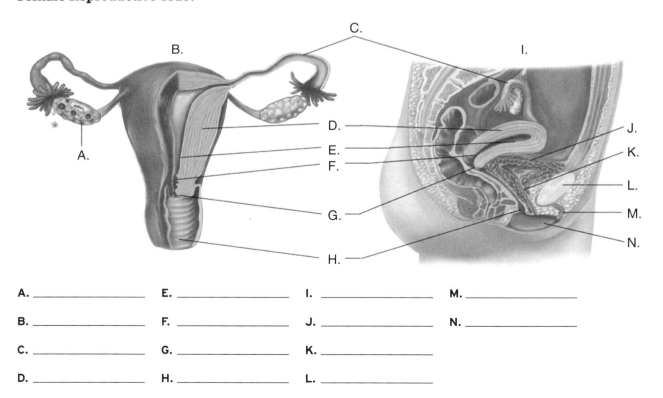

A. _____	E. _____	I. _____	M. _____
B. _____	F. _____	J. _____	N. _____
C. _____	G. _____	K. _____	
D. _____	H. _____	L. _____	

Female External Genitalia

A. _____

B. _____

C. _____

D. _____

E. _____

F. _____

G. _____

H. _____

I. _____

J. _____

K. _____

L. _____

Anatomic Structures of the Pregnant Woman

A. _____

B. _____

C. _____

D. _____

E. _____

F. _____

G. _____

H. _____

I. _____

Vocabulary EMT-I [vocab explorer] [web]

Define the following terms in the space provided.

1. Primigravida:

_____

_____

_____

2. Multigravida:

_____

_____

_____

3. Ectopic pregnancy:

_____

_____

_____

4. Crowning:

_____

_____

_____

5. Eclampsia:

_____

_____

_____

6. Uterine rupture:

_____

_____

_____

7. Supine hypotensive syndrome:

_____

_____

_____

Fill-in

Read each item carefully, then complete the statement by filling in the missing word(s).

1. After delivery, the _____, or afterbirth, separates from the uterus and is delivered.

2. The umbilical cord contains two _____ and one _____.

3. The amniotic sac contains about _____ of amniotic fluid, which helps to insulate and protect the floating fetus as it develops.

4. A full-term pregnancy is from _____ to _____ weeks, counting from the first day of the last menstrual cycle.

5. The pregnancy is divided into three _____ of about 3 months each.

6. The leading cause of maternal death in the first trimester is internal hemorrhage into the abdomen following rupture of an _____.

7. During the delivery, be careful that you do not poke your fingers into the infant's eyes or into the two soft spots, called _____, on the head.

8. The total blood volume increases about _____ by 40 weeks of pregnancy.

9. The heart rate elevates by _____ to _____ beats/min for the mother during pregnancy.

10. The cardiac output rises _____ by the third trimester to compensate for the extra volume in the system caused by the _____ of the _____.

11. The systolic and diastolic blood pressures drop by _____ to _____ by the second trimester and return to near normal by full term.

True/False

If you believe the statement to be more true than false, write the letter "T" in the space provided. If you believe the statement to be more false than true, write the letter "F."

_____ **1.** Crowning occurs when the baby's head obstructs the birth canal, preventing normal delivery.

_____ **2.** Labor begins with the rupture of the amniotic sac and ends with the delivery of the baby's head.

_____ **3.** A woman who is having her first baby is called a multigravida.

_____ **4.** Once labor has begun, it can be slowed by holding the patient's legs together.

_____ **5.** Delivery of the buttocks before the baby's head is called a breech delivery.

_____ **6.** The umbilical cord may be gently pulled to aid in delivery of the placenta.

_____ **7.** A limb presentation occurs when the baby's arm, leg, or foot emerges from the vagina first.

_____ **8.** Dizziness and shortness of breath may be due to the amount of increased CO_2 the patient exhales.

_____ **9.** Morning sickness most commonly occurs between the 8th and 14th week.

_____ **10.** Pain, cramping, and vaginal bleeding are normally present in an ectopic pregnancy.

_____ **11.** Preeclampsia is an increase in blood pressure after the 20th week of gestation.

_____ **12.** With a prolapsed uterus, appropriate care includes one attempt at replacement by pushing it back inside the body.

Short Answer

Complete this section with short written answers in the space provided.

1. What are some possible causes of vaginal hemorrhage in early and late pregnancy?

_____

_____

_____

2. In what position should pregnant patients who are not delivering be transported and why?

_____

_____

_____

3. List three signs that indicate the beginning of labor.

_____

_____

_____

4. Under what three circumstances should you consider delivering the infant at the scene?

_____

_____

_____

5. Why is it important to avoid pushing on the fontanelles?

_____

_____

_____

6. How can you help decrease perineal tearing?

_____

_____

_____

7. What are the two situations in which an EMT-I may insert his or her fingers into a patient's vagina?

_____

_____

_____

Word Fun EMT-I vocab explorer web

The following crossword puzzle is an activity provided to reinforce correct spelling and understanding of medical terminology associated with emergency care and the EMT-I. Use the clues in the column to complete the puzzle.

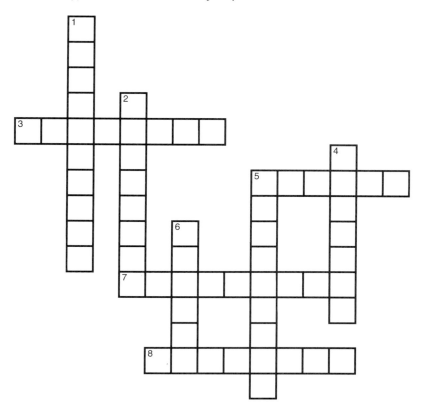

Across

3. Tissue that nourishes the fetus through the umbilical cord

5. Pregnant

7. The ending of the menstrual cycle (menses)

8. Hormone released from the ovaries that stimulates the uterine lining during the menstrual cycle

Down

1. A substance that coats the alveoli in the lungs

2. Area of skin between the urethral opening and the anus

4. The female reproductive organs

5. The process of fetal development following fertilization of an egg

6. The top portion of the uterus

Ambulance Calls

The following real case scenarios provide an opportunity to explore the concerns associated with patient management. Read each scenario, then answer each question in detail.

1. You are called to a 27-year-old woman, primigravida, in her 28th week of gestation. Her husband tells you that she has a history of preeclampsia and that she suddenly started having convulsions. She is voice responsive and very lethargic. Her blood pressure is 230/180 mm Hg.

How would you best manage this patient?

_____

_____

_____

_____

_____

_____

_____

_____

2. You are dispatched to the residence of a 24-year-old woman who is 12 weeks pregnant and complaining of "spotting." The patient tells you that her last pregnancy ended in a miscarriage at 8 weeks. This is her second pregnancy. She denies any pain and vital signs are within normal limits.

How would you best manage this patient?

_____

_____

_____

_____

_____

_____

_____

3. You are on the scene with a 32-year-old woman who is 38 weeks pregnant, and delivery is imminent. As the infant starts to crown, you notice that the amniotic sac is still intact.

How would you best manage this patient?

_____

_____

_____

_____

_____

_____

_____

Skill Drills

Skill Drill 29-1: Delivering the Infant

Test your knowledge of this skill drill by placing the photos below in the correct order. Number the first step with a "1," the second step with a "2," and so on. Also, fill in the correct words in the photo captions.

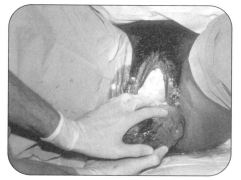

As the upper shoulder appears, guide the head down slightly, if needed, to help deliver the shoulder.

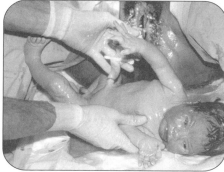

Place the first clamp 7″ from the infant's body and the second 3″ farther and cut between them.

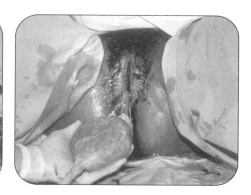

Allow the placenta to deliver itself. Never pull on the cord to speed up placental delivery.

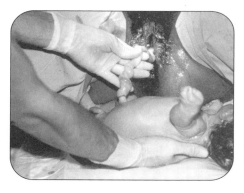

Handle the slippery delivered infant firmly but gently, keeping the neck in neutral position to maintain the airway.

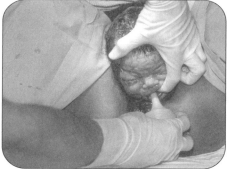

Support the bony parts of the head with your hands as it emerges. Suction fluid from the mouth, then the nostrils.

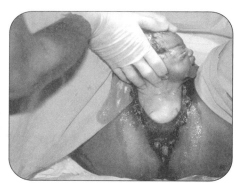

Support the head and upper body as the shoulders deliver. Guide the head up slightly if needed to deliver the lower shoulder.

Workbook Activities

The following activities have been designed to help you. Your instructor may require you to complete some or all of these activities as a regular part of your EMT-I training program. You are encouraged to complete any activity that your instructor does not assign as a way to enhance your learning in the classroom.

Chapter Review

The following exercises provide an opportunity to refresh your knowledge of this chapter.

Matching

Match each of the terms in the left column to the appropriate definition in the right column.

_____ 1. Acidosis

_____ 2. Barotrauma

_____ 3. Fetal alcohol syndrome

_____ 4. Gestational period

_____ 5. Meconium

_____ 6. Newborn

_____ 7. Peripheral cyanosis

_____ 8. Secondary apnea

_____ 9. Vernix caseosa

_____ 10. Acrocyanosis

_____ 11. Central cyanosis

_____ 12. Fetal transition

_____ 13. Infant

_____ 14. Meconium aspirator

_____ 15. Orogastric (OG) tube

_____ 16. Portal venous system

_____ 17. Tactile stimulation

_____ 18. Vocal cord guide

_____ 19. Antepartum

_____ 20. Diaphragmatic hernia

_____ 21. Foramen ovale

_____ 22. Intrapartum

_____ 23. Neonate

_____ 24. Premature

_____ 25. Umbilical vein catheter

_____ 26. Apgar score

A. the accumulation of lactic acid in the blood

B. cyanosis of the hands and feet

C. the phase before delivery of the newborn

D. scoring assessment of the newborn; done at 1 and 5 minutes after birth

E. auscultating the heart rate through the chest wall

F. damage to a newborn's lungs resulting from excessive ventilatory pressure

G. cyanosis to the infant's face and trunk

H. a hole or defect in the diaphragm in which a portion of the bowel herniates into the thoracic cavity

I. the small artery that connects the left pulmonary artery to the aorta

J. a condition in infants who are born to women who are addicted to alcohol

K. when the fluid of the lungs is filled with air

L. opening between the right and left atria, through which the blood passes

M. period of fetal development from fertilization until birth

N. a baby in the first 12 months of life

O. the phase that occurs during delivery

P. the newborn's first bowel movement

Q. device used with an ET tube to suction meconium from the newborn's airway

R. phase of life that occurs during the first 28 days of life

S. phase of life from the first few minutes to the first hours after birth

T. tube that is inserted through the mouth and into the stomach

CHAPTER 30

Neonatal Resuscitation

_____ **27.** Ductus arteriosus

_____ **28.** Primary apnea

_____ **29.** Apical pulse

U. cyanosis of the hands and feet

V. special venous drainage system that takes blood from the intestines to the liver

W. newborn that delivers before 37 weeks gestation or weighs less than 5.5 lbs at birth

X. apnea that can often be reversed with tactile stimulation and suctioning

Y. apnea that is not reversed with tactile stimulation or suctioning

Z. method of stimulation a newborn; flicking the feet or rubbing the lateral thorax

AA. catheter designed to be inserted into the umbilical vein

BB. slippery, cheesy-like substance that covers the newborn at birth

CC. black line on the distal end of the ET tube

Multiple Choice

Read each item carefully, then select the best response.

_____ **1.** Normally, the major physiologic change occurring in the fetus within seconds after birth is:

A. fluid in the alveoli is absorbed into the lung tissue and replaced by air.

B. the umbilical cord is clamped, causing increased blood pressure for the newborn.

C. the alveoli become distended and are able to hold oxygen.

D. all the above.

_____ **2.** Newborn bradycardia (heart rate less than 100 beats/min) is almost always the result of:

A. intracranial pressure (ICP).

B. hypoxia.

C. acidosis.

D. all the above.

_____ **3.** During birth and resuscitation of the newborn, minimum BSI protection includes:

A. gloves.

B. goggles or face shield.

C. gown.

D. all the above.

1999 _____ 4. Medications that can be given via the ET tube include:

    A. No medication can be given to the newborn via the ET tube.

    B. epinephrine.

    C. diazepam.

    D. both B and C.

_____ 5. Vernix caseosa:

    A. must be quickly removed to prevent hypothermia.

    B. should be left on as long as possible to prevent hypothermia.

    C. is seldom present.

    D. is nature's chemical to help stimulate breathing.

_____ 6. Suctioning the newborn:

    A. should be done as soon as the head is delivered.

    B. The mouth is suctioned before the nose.

    C. can produce a vagal response in the first few minutes after birth.

    D. all the above.

_____ 7. Acceptable safe methods for providing tactile stimulation to the newborn include:

    A. gently rubbing the extremities.

    B. holding the newborn upside down.

    C. a light slap on the bottom.

    D. slightly shaking the infant.

_____ 8. Continued use of tactile stimulation in an apneic newborn:

    A. should be performed repeatedly.

    B. is a waste of time.

    C. should be varied to different areas of the body.

    D. is likely to be the basis of litigation.

_____ 9. Most newborns will have an Apgar score of _____ at 1 minute.

    A. 8–10

    B. 7 or 8

    C. 5 or 6

    D. 4 or 5

_____ 10. Most newborns will have an Apgar score of _____ at 5 minutes.

    A. 8–10

    B. 7 or 8

    C. 5 or 6

    D. 4 or 5

_____ 11. Signs of _____ indicate increased work of breathing and respiratory distress.

    A. gasping

    B. grunting

    C. nasal flaring

    D. all of the above

_____ 12. Ventilations in the neonate are provided at a rate of _____ breaths/min.

    A. 80–100

    B. 60–80

    C. 40–60

    D. None of the above

_____ 13. Which statement is most correct concerning oropharyngeal airways and the newborn?

    A. They are second in choice to the nasopharyngeal.

    B. They are routinely needed to maintain a patent airway.

    C. They may be needed to keep the mouth open during ventilations.

    D. They should not be used on the newborn.

_____ **14.** Peripheral cyanosis:

    A. is a life-threatening emergency.

    B. is rare.

    C. is common through the first 24–48 hours of life.

    D. requires aggressive therapy.

1999 _____ **15.** Newborns who require positive pressure ventilation for longer than _____ minutes should have an orogastric tube inserted.

    A. 1

    B. 2

    C. 3

    D. 4

1999 _____ **16.** Problems associated with gastric distention can be reduced by:

    A. inserting an OG tube.

    B. suctioning gastric contents.

    C. leaving the tube in place as a vent for air entering the stomach.

    D. all the above.

1999 _____ **17.** For OG tube insertion, you'll need:

    A. to measure the tube from the tip of the nose to the earlobe and down to the xiphoid process.

    B. an 8F feeding tube.

    C. a 20-mL syringe.

    D. all of the above.

1999 _____ **18.** What is the purpose of a 20-mL syringe during OG insertion?

    A. It's not used for OG insertion.

    B. To infuse a small amount of air and check for correct placement.

    C. To remove gastric contents.

    D. None of the above.

1999 _____ **19.** What method is used to choose the correct-sized ET tube for the newborn?

    A. Matching the diameter of the infant's little finger

    B. Based on the newborn's weight

    C. Based on the newborn's gestational age

    D. All of the above

1999 _____ **20.** Proper technique for intubating the newborn includes:

    A. preoxygenation.

    B. use of a pediatric-sized laryngoscope handle.

    C. an appropriate-sized ET tube.

    D. all of the above.

Vocabulary EMT-I

Define the following terms in the space provided.

1. Acrocyanosis:

_____

_____

_____

2. Meconium aspirator:

_____

_____

_____

3. Neonate:

_____

_____

_____

4. Peripheral cyanosis:

_____

_____

_____

5. Primary apnea:

_____

_____

_____

6. Secondary apnea:

_____

_____

_____

7. Umbilical vein catheterization:

_____

_____

_____

Fill-in

Read each item carefully, then complete the statement by filling in the missing word(s).

1. _____ of newborns will require some assistance to initiate adequate breathing after birth.

2. During the first _____ days of life, a baby is considered to be a neonate.

3. Prior to birth, most of the blood from the right side of the fetal heart bypasses the lungs through the

_____ _____.

4. When responding to a call for a possible delivery, ensure that the _____ in back of the

ambulance is _____ _____.

5. It may be necessary to place a _____ _____ in between the newborn's

shoulders to facilitate optimum head positioning.

6. Positive pressure ventilation is successful if you see _____ _____ of the

newborn's _____ _____ and hear breath sounds.

7. After _____ _____ of adequate ventilations, assess the heart rate.

1999 **8.** If prolonged ventilatory support or certain medications will be needed for the newborn, you should

_____ _____ _____.

9. For suspected hypovolemia in the newborn, administer _____ of an isotonic crystalloid

over _____ to _____ minutes.

10. If the pregnant woman describes a foul odor or dark liquid when her amniotic sac broke, you should

suspect _____ _____.

11. Because meconium is thick, a regular suction catheter will become easily occluded. Therefore, you

should use a _____ _____ to perform tracheal suctioning.

12. Grieving parents will be emotionally distraught and perhaps even _____ if the fetus has

died in the mother's uterus.

True/False

If you believe the statement to be more true than false, write the letter "T" in the space provided. If you believe
the statement to be more false than true, write the letter "F."

_____ **1.** Once the umbilical cord has been clamped, the fetus no longer receives prostaglandin-E2.

_____ **2.** If fetal distress occurs in utero, the problem is usually caused by compromised blood flow in
the placenta or umbilical cord.

_____ **3.** Fetal distress after delivery is usually the result of an airway or breathing problem.

_____ **4.** If a newborn remains depressed after drying, warming, and clearing the airway, you should
make several attempts at tactile stimulation.

_____ **5.** Newborn's bradycardia is usually the result of hypoxia, not primary cardiac disease.

_____ **6.** Assessment of the heart rate of a newborn can be accomplished by auscultation or by palpating
the base of the umbilical cord.

_____ **7.** If the heart rate is fewer than 60 beats/min, you should continue ventilation and begin chest
compressions.

_____ **8.** Free-flowing oxygen should be directed away from the newborn's eyes.

_____ **9.** Most problems can be corrected with oxygenation and ventilation.

_____ **10.** Venous access should only be gained for fluid delivery or for administration of essential medications.

_____ **11.** Shock is the last concern for the newborn if there has been a placental abruption or previa
blood loss from the umbilical cord.

_____ **12.** One should never give sodium bicarbonate via the ET tube and if adequate ventilation and
oxygenation have not been established.

Short Answer
Complete this section with short written answers in the space provided.

1. What are some clinical findings of fetal distress?

_____

_____

_____

2. When anticipating the need for newborn resuscitation, what four additional questions should you ask?

_____

_____

_____

3. List antepartum risk factors for neonatal resuscitation.

_____

_____

_____

4. List key elements of assessing the newborn.

_____

_____

_____

5. What is the danger of inserting an umbilical catheter too far?

_____

_____

_____

6. Why shouldn't naloxone (Narcan) be given to the newborn of a mother who is suspected of being addicted to narcotics?

_____

_____

_____

7. How is the meconium aspirator used?

_____

_____

_____

Word Fun EMT-I vocab explorer web

The following crossword puzzle is an activity provided to reinforce correct spelling and understanding of medical terminology associated with emergency care and the EMT-I. Use the clues in the column to complete the puzzle.

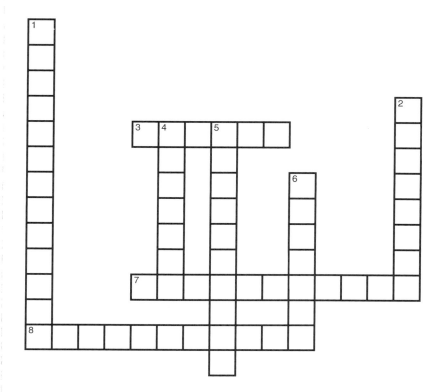

Across

3. A baby in the first 12 months of life

7. The phase that occurs during delivery

8. Auscultating the heart rate through the chest wall

Down

1. Slippery, cheesy-like substance that covers the newborn at birth

2. The newborn's first bowel movement

4. Phase from the first few minutes to the first few hours after birth

5. Phase before delivery of the newborn

6. Phase of life that occurs during the first 28 days

Ambulance Calls

The following real case scenarios provide an opportunity to explore the concerns associated with patient management. Read each scenario, then answer each question in detail.

1. On a hot 4th of July afternoon you're called for a "transient in labor" in a back alley. When you arrive, you find a 19-year-old woman who has delivered less than 30 seconds ago. Your partner heads straight to the mother, leaving you with the newborn.

How would you best manage this patient?

_____

_____

_____

_____

_____

_____

_____

_____

2. You're called to a home to assist a woman in labor. Upon arrival, you note a very foul odor and upon examination, you see an obviously dead newborn.

How would you best manage this patient?

_____

_____

_____

_____

_____

_____

_____

3. You've just delivered a premature newborn of 30 weeks' gestation.

How would you best manage this patient?

_____

_____

_____

_____

_____

_____

_____

Skill Drills

Skill Drill 30-1: Giving Chest Compressions to a Newborn

Test your knowledge of this skill drill by placing the photos below in the correct order. Number the first step with a "1," the second step with a "2," and so on.

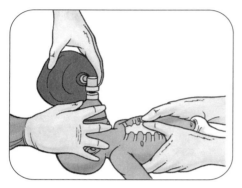

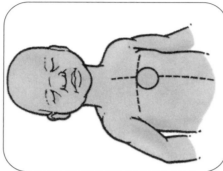

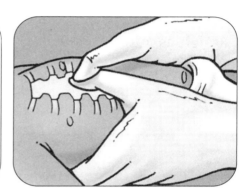

_____

_____

_____

Wrap your hands around the body, with your thumbs resting at that position.

Find the proper position: just below the nipple line, middle of the lower third of the sternum.

Press your thumbs gently against the sternum, compressing to a depth that is approximately one third the anteroposterior diameter of the chest. Deliver compressions and ventilations in a 3:1 ratio.

Skill Drill 30-2: Inserting an Orogastric Tube in the Newborn

Test your knowledge of this skill drill by filling the correct words in the photo captions.

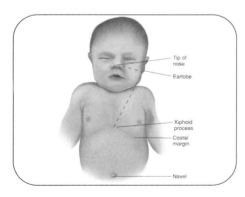

Tip of nose
Earlobe
Xiphoid process
Costal margin
Navel

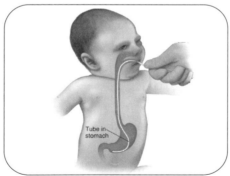

Tube in stomach

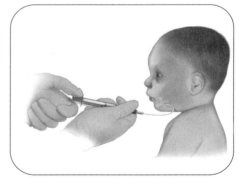

1. Measure for correct depth: from the _____ of the _____ to the _____ and from the _____ to the _____ _____.

2. Insert the _____ to the appropriate depth. Leave the _____ open to allow for _____.

3. Remove _____ contents with a _____ mL syringe. Remove the syringe and leave the tip of the _____ open to allow air to vent from the stomach. Tape the tube to the newborn's _____.

Workbook Activities

The following activities have been designed to help you. Your instructor may require you to complete some or all of these activities as a regular part of your EMT-I training program. You are encouraged to complete any activity that your instructor does not assign as a way to enhance your learning in the classroom.

Chapter Review

The following exercises provide an opportunity to refresh your knowledge of this chapter.

Matching

Match each of the terms in the left column to the appropriate definition in the right column.

_____ 1. Toddlerhood

_____ 2. Preschool age

_____ 3. Adolescence

_____ 4. Infancy

_____ 5. Neonate

_____ 6. Fontanelle

_____ 7. Croup

_____ 8. Epiglottitis

_____ 9. Asthma

_____ 10. Shock

_____ 11. Apical pulse

_____ 12. Greenstick

_____ 13. Meningitis

_____ 14. Febrile seizure

_____ 15. Osteomyelitis

_____ 16. Child abuse

_____ 17. Trauma

_____ 18. Child safety seats

_____ 19. Growth plate

_____ 20. Stridor

A. first year of life

B. infection of the soft tissue above the vocal cords

C. soft openings in the skull of an infant

D. bone and muscle inflammation

E. decreases severity of injury in MVC

F. incomplete fracture of a bone

G. ages 3 to 5 years

H. improper or excessive action that injures or otherwise harms a child

I. insufficient blood to body organs

J. inflammation of the meninges

K. infant in the first month after birth

L. weak spots in bones

M. infection of the soft tissue below the vocal cords

N. high-pitched inspiratory sound

O. age after infancy until about 3 years

P. number one killer of children in US

Q. acute bronchospasm and increased mucus

R. seizure relating to a fever

S. auscultating heart tones over the chest

T. ages 12 to 18 years

Pediatric Emergencies

Multiple Choice

Read each item carefully, then select the best response.

_____ 1. _____ is/are the number one killer of children in the United States.

    A. Heart problems

    B. Respiratory problems

    C. Trauma

    D. Dehydration

_____ 2. An effective injury or illness prevention program should focus on factors that can be changed or altered, such as:

    A. the appropriate use of car seats.

    B. the use of helmets.

    C. recognizing certain illnesses.

    D. all of the above.

_____ 3. Infants respond mainly to _____ stimuli.

    A. social

    B. mental

    C. physical

    D. all of the above

_____ 4. Injuries in the _____ age group are more frequent.

    A. infant

    B. toddler

    C. preschool

    D. school

_____ 5. At the _____ age, children are easily distracted with counting games and small toys.

    A. infant

    B. toddler

    C. preschool

    D. adolescent

_____ 6. A respiratory rate of _____ breaths/minute is normal for the newborn.

    A. 12 to 20

    B. 20 to 40

    C. 30 to 50

    D. 40 to 60

_____ 7. Breathing requires the use of the _____ and diaphragm.

    A. chest muscles

    B. neck muscles

    C. subclavian muscles

    D. abdominal muscles

_____ 8. Anything that puts pressure on the abdomen of a young child can block the movement of the _____ and cause respiratory distress.

    A. thorax

    B. air

    C. diaphragm

    D. lungs

_____ 9. The primary way the body compensates for decreased oxygenation is:

    A. increasing the respiratory rate.

    B. increasing the heart rate.

    C. increasing the blood pressure.

    D. increasing contractions of the diaphragm.

_____ 10. Anatomic differences between adults and children include all of the following EXCEPT:

    A. the heart is higher in the child's chest.

    B. the child's lungs are smaller.

    C. the adult's opening to the trachea is higher in the neck.

    D. the child's neck is shorter.

_____ 11. Because of the smaller diameter of the trachea in infants, which is about the same diameter as a drinking straw, their airway is easily obstructed by:

    A. secretions.

    B. blood.

    C. swelling.

    D. all of the above.

_____ 12. Because intercostal muscles are not well developed in children, movement of the _____ dictates the amount of air they inspire.

    A. diaphragm

    B. ribs

    C. abdomen

    D. lungs

_____ 13. Look for _____ when doing your initial assessment from across the room.

    A. work of breathing

    B. skin color and alertness

    C. level of activity

    D. all of the above

_____ 14. As the work of breathing increases, you may see:

    A. faster breathing.

    B. retractions along the chest wall.

    C. the child sitting in a position to allow for more chest expansion.

    D. all of the above.

_____ 15. Assessment of the _____ will give clues to the amount of oxygen reaching the end-organs of the body.

    A. heart rate

    B. respiratory rate

    C. level of responsiveness

    D. skin color

_____ **16.** Positioning the airway on a neutral sniffing position:

    A. keeps the trachea from kinking when the neck is hyperflexed.

    B. keeps the trachea from kinking when the neck is flexed.

    C. maintains the proper alignment if you have to immobilize the spine.

    D. all of the above.

_____ **17.** When evaluating the respiratory rate in children younger than 3 years and in infants you should count the number of times the:

    A. chest rises in 15 seconds.

    B. chest rises in 30 seconds.

    C. abdomen rises in 15 seconds.

    D. abdomen rises in 30 seconds.

_____ **18.** Signs of complete airway obstruction include:

    A. inability to speak or cry.

    B. increased respiratory difficulty with stridor.

    C. cyanosis.

    D. all of the above.

1999 _____ **19.** When suctioning the airway of the infant or child, you should do all of the following EXCEPT:

    A. apply the cardiac monitor.

    B. observe for tachycardia.

    C. stop suctioning and oxygenate if bradycardia occurs.

    D. limit suctioning time to 10 seconds in a child and 5 seconds in an infant.

_____ **20.** Benefits of using a nasopharyngeal airway include all of the following EXCEPT:

    A. it is usually well tolerated.

    B. it may be used in the presence of head trauma.

    C. it is not as likely as the oropharyngeal airway to cause vomiting.

    D. it is used for conscious patients or those with an altered level of consciousness.

_____ **21.** Indications for assisting ventilations in a child include:

    A. a respiratory rate that is too fast.

    B. a respiratory rate that is too slow.

    C. inadequate tidal volume.

    D. all of the above.

_____ **22.** Errors in technique when providing ventilations with a BVM device that may result in gastric distention include:

    A. providing too much volume.

    B. squeezing the bag too forcefully.

    C. ventilating too fast.

    D. all of the above.

1999 _____ **23.** Indications for endotracheal intubation for pediatric patients include:

    A. cardiopulmonary arrest.

    B. respiratory failure.

    C. inability to maintain a patent airway.

    D. all of the above.

1999 _____ **24.** Generally speaking, you should use a _____ blade to intubate a 2-year-old.

    A. size 1, straight blade

    B. size 1, curved blade

    C. size 2, straight blade

    D. size 2, curved blade

1999 _____ **25.** With regard to pediatric intubations, which of the following is NOT true?

    A. The child should be preoxygenated for 30 seconds.

    B. The head should be tilted back.

    C. The cardiac monitor and pulse oximeter should be placed on the patient.

    D. An airway adjunct can be inserted if needed.

1999 _____ **26.** _____ will decrease the risk of gastric distention and aspiration of vomitus by pushing the larynx back to compress and close off the esophagus.

    A. Using a BVM device

    B. The Sellick maneuver

    C. Abdominal compression

    D. None of the above

1999 _____ **27.** Indications for immediate ET tube removal include:

    A. no chest rise with ventilation.

    B. absence of breath sounds during auscultation.

    C. presence of epigastric gurgling sounds or vomitus in the ET tube.

    D. all of the above.

1999 _____ **28.** Gastric distention:

    A. increases tidal volume.

    B. slows downward movement of the diaphragm.

    C. decreases the risk of vomiting and aspiration.

    D. all of the above.

1999 _____ **29.** The way to measure the proper length of a NG tube is from the:

    A. tip of the earlobe to the xiphoid.

    B. earlobe to the xiphoid minus distance from the tip of nose to ear.

    C. tip of nose to earlobe plus distance from earlobe to xiphoid.

    D. lips to earlobe plus distance from earlobe to xiphoid.

1999 _____ **30.** Complications of NG or OG tube insertion include all of the following EXCEPT:

    A. placement of the tube in the trachea.

    B. gastric decompression.

    C. airway bleeding or obstruction.

    D. passage of tube into cranium.

_____ **31.** Chest compressions on the infant should be performed at a rate of:

    A. 100/min.

    B. 150/min.

    C. 80/min.

    D. 30/min.

_____ **32.** The ratio of compressions to breaths for infants should be:

    A. 100:1.

    B. 50:1.

    C. 30:2.

    D. 15:2.

1999 _____ **33.** Which is not considered a complication of IO therapy?

    A. Piercing the medullary canal

    B. Compartment syndrome

    C. Growth plate injury

    D. Osteomyelitis

_____ **34.** Fluid resuscitation for the infant or child in hypovolemic shock begins with an initial bolus of:

    A. 10 mL/kg.

    B. 20 mL/kg.

    C. 30 mL/kg.

    D. 40 mL/kg.

1999 _____ **35.** All of the following conditions can lead to V-fib or pulseless V-tach in the pediatric patient EXCEPT:

    A. respiratory arrest.

    B. electrocution.

    C. congenital heart defects.

    D. myocarditis.

1999 _____ **36.** The correct initial pediatric dose of adenosine is:

    A. 0.1 mg/kg up to 6.0 mg rapid IV or IO.

    B. 0.1 mg/kg up to 12.0 mg rapid IV or IO.

    C. 1.0 mg/kg up to 6.0 mg rapid IV or IO.

    D. 1.0 mg/kg up to 12.0 mg rapid IV or IO.

1999 _____ **37.** The maximum dose for lidocaine in the pediatric patient is:

    A. 400 mg

    B. 300 mg

    C. 200 mg

    D. 100 mg

_____ **38.** A way of providing emotional support and enhancing communication with pediatric patients is:

    A. positioning yourself on the same level as the child.

    B. using terminology appropriate for the child's age.

    C. allowing them to express their feelings.

    D. all of the above.

_____ **39.** Early signs of respiratory distress include all of the following EXCEPT:

    A. normal mentation.

    B. nasal flaring.

    C. bradycardia.

    D. grunting.

_____ **40.** When respiratory distress becomes respiratory failure, expect to see:

    A. decreased LOC.

    B. poor muscle tone.

    C. central cyanosis.

    D. all of the above.

1999 _____ **41.** If BVM ventilations do not improve a child's condition:

    A. squeeze the bag harder.

    B. squeeze the bag faster.

    C. perform endotracheal intubation.

    D. none of the above.

_____ **42.** _____ is an infection of the airway below the level of the vocal cords, usually caused by a virus.

    A. Croup

    B. Tonsillitis

    C. Epiglottitis

    D. Pharyngitis

1999 _____ **43.** Treatment for epiglottitis consists of all of the following EXCEPT:

    A. humidified oxygen.

    B. direct visualization of the epiglottitis.

    C. BVM ventilation if complete obstruction occurs.

    D. intubation if complete obstruction occurs.

1999 _____ **44.** Medical control may order subcutaneous _____ in children with severe respiratory distress or failure due to reactive airway disease.

    A. oxygen

    B. albuterol

    C. epinephrine 1:1000

    D. all of the above

1999 _____ **45.** Treatment for bronchiolitis includes all of the following EXCEPT:

    A. albuterol via nebulizer.

    B. possible BVM ventilations.

    C. cardiac monitoring.

    D. analgesics.

1999 _____ **46.** If BVM ventilations are ineffective or prolonged, ventilation support will be required in a patient with pneumonia. You should:

    A. perform ET intubation.

    B. apply a cardiac monitor.

    C. assess cardiac rhythms.

    D. all of the above.

_____ **47.** Severe coughing associated with _____ should lead you to suspect a foreign body lower airway obstruction.

    A. unilateral diminished breath sounds

    B. unilateral rales or rhonchi

    C. chest pain

    D. all of the above

_____ **48.** Common causes of shock in children include all of the following EXCEPT:

    A. heart attack.

    B. head trauma.

    C. dehydration.

    D. pneumothorax.

_____ **49.** Signs and symptoms of compensated shock include all of the following EXCEPT:

    A. tachycardia.

    B. tachypnea.

    C. weak peripheral pulses.

    D. increased urinary output.

_____ **51.** Signs and symptoms of decompensated shock include all of the following EXCEPT:

    A. lethargy or coma.

    B. slightly delayed capillary refill.

    C. mottled extremities.

    D. hypotension.

_____ **52.** _____ shock is the most common type of shock encountered in infants and children.

    A. Hypovolemic

    B. Distributive

    C. Anaphylactic

    D. Neurogenic

1999 _____ **53.** Treatment for neurogenic shock includes:

    A. spinal immobilization.

    B. 100% oxygen.

    C. vasopressors if IV fluids fail to increase perfusion.

    D. all of the above.

1999 _____ **54.** Treatment for anaphylaxis includes all of the following EXCEPT:

    A. epinephrine 1:1000 subcutaneously.

    B. epinephrine 1:10,000 IV or IO.

    C. Benadryl IV or IO.

    D. endotracheal intubation.

1999 _____ **55.** If tachydysrhythmia is the suspected cause of cardiogenic shock:

    A. consider adenosine 1.0 mg/kg.

    B. be prepared for ET intubation.

    C. consider adenosine 0.5 mg/kg.

    D. consider adenosine 0.2 mg/kg.

1999 _____ **56.** SVT is a narrow QRS complex tachycardia characterized by a heart rate greater than _____ beats/minute in the infant.

    A. 180

    B. 200

    C. 220

    D. 250

1999 _____ **57.** If your pediatric patient experiences unstable V-tach, you should do all of the following EXCEPT:

    A. transport immediately.

    B. apply 100% oxygen.

    C. syncronize cardiovert.

    D. be prepared to defibrillate if he or she becomes pulseless.

1999 _____ **58.** Bradycardia is defined as a heart rate less than _____ in the infant.

    A. 140

    B. 120

    C. 100

    D. 80

1999 _____ **59.** Atropine may be administered to patients with bradycardia, if needed, at a dose of:

    A. 0.01 mg/kg.

    B. 0.02 mg/kg.

    C. 0.1 mg/kg.

    D. 0.2 mg/kg.

1999 _____ **60.** Asystole:

    A. represents a total absence of electrical and mechanical activity.

    B. appears as a flat line on the cardiac monitor.

    C. has no electrical complexes.

    D. all of the above.

1999 _____ **61.** The "H" of asystole and PEA includes all of the following EXCEPT:

    A. hypoxemia.

    B. hypotension.

    C. hypovolemia.

    D. hypothermia.

1999 _____ **62.** The correct initial dose of electricity for defibrillation is:
   A. 1 J/kg.
   B. 2 J/kg.
   C. 3 J/kg.
   D. 4 J/kg.

_____ **62.** _____ is/are a continuous seizure or multiple seizures without a return to consciousness for 30 minutes or more.
   A. Status epilepticus
   B. Grand mal seizures
   C. Absence seizures
   D. Focal motor seizures

_____ **63.** During the postictal period, the patient may appear:
   A. sleepy.
   B. confused.
   C. unresponsive.
   D. all of the above.

_____ **64.** Most pediatric seizures caused by _____, which is why they are called febrile seizures.
   A. infection
   B. fever
   C. ingestion
   D. trauma

1999 _____ **65.** The maximum dose of diazepam for a 7-year-old child is:
   A. 2 mg.
   B. 4 mg.
   C. 5 mg.
   D. 10 mg.

_____ **66.** Nonverbal infants may demonstrate consciousness by:
   A. tracking.
   B. babbling and cooing.
   C. crying.
   D. all of the above.

_____ **67.** Signs and symptoms of poisoning vary widely, depending on:
   A. the substance.
   B. age.
   C. weight.
   D. all of the above.

_____ **68.** Common causes of high temperature in a child include all of the following EXCEPT:
   A. drug ingestion.
   B. infection.
   C. going from one temperature extreme to another.
   D. cancer.

_____ **69.** Meningitis is an infection caused by:
   A. bacteria.
   B. a virus.
   C. fungi.
   D. all of the above.

_____ **70.** Children with *N. meningitidis* are at serious risk of:
   A. sepsis.
   B. shock.
   C. death.
   D. all of the above.

_____ **71.** Life-threatening dehydration can overcome an infant in a matter of:

  A. minutes.

  B. hours.

  C. days.

  D. weeks.

_____ **72.** _____ is the leading cause of death in infants younger than 1 year.

  A. SIDS

  B. Congenital heart disease

  C. Respiratory arrest

  D. Foreign body airway obstruction

_____ **73.** When dealing with the death of an infant, your assessment of the scene should include:

  A. the site where the infant was discovered.

  B. the general condition of the house.

  C. family interaction.

  D. all of the above.

_____ **74.** A classic apparent life-threatening event is characterized by:

  A. a distinct change in muscle tone.

  B. choking or gagging.

  C. a child that may appear healthy after the event.

  D. all of the above.

_____ **75.** In dealing with the family after the death of a child, you should:

  A. use the child's name.

  B. acknowledge their feelings.

  C. keep any instructions short and simple.

  D. all of the above.

_____ **76.** Children differ from adults in that they:

  A. have less circulating blood volume.

  B. have a larger body surface area in relation to body mass.

  C. have more flexible and elastic bones.

  D. all of the above.

_____ **77.** When caring for children with sports-related injuries, you should remember to:

  A. elevate all the extremities.

  B. assist ventilations.

  C. immobilize the cervical spine.

  D. remove all helmets.

_____ **78.** _____ can occur as a result of head injuries in children.

  A. Cervical spine injuries

  B. Nausea and vomiting

  C. Respiratory arrest

  D. All of the above

_____ **79.** Children's bones bend more easily than adult's bones and, as a result, incomplete or _____ fractures can occur.

  A. spiral

  B. comminuted

  C. greenstick

  D. compound

_____ **80.** The most common cause(s) of burns in children is/are:

    A. exposure to hot substances.

    B. hot items on a stove.

    C. exposure to caustic substances.

    D. all of the above.

_____ **81.** In submersion situations, your first priority is to always take steps to:

    A. stay properly protected from body fluids.

    B. maintain the airway.

    C. ensure your own safety.

    D. retrieve the patient from the water.

_____ **82.** The principal injury from submersion is:

    A. lack of oxygen.

    B. neck and spinal cord injuries.

    C. drowning.

    D. hypothermia.

_____ **83.** Child abuse may include:

    A. physical abuse.

    B. neglect.

    C. emotional abuse.

    D. all of the above.

_____ **84.** The "H" in the CHILD ABUSE mnemonic stands for:

    A. history of present injury.

    B. history inconsistent with injury.

    C. history of previous injuries.

    D. history of sibling injuries.

_____ **85.** After difficult incidents involving children, _____ is helpful in working through the stress and trauma.

    A. having a drink

    B. talking with the family

    C. debriefing

    D. putting the incident out of your mind

Vocabulary EMT-I

Define the following terms in the space provided.

    1. Acrocyanosis:

_____

_____

_____

    2. Apical pulse:

_____

_____

_____

3. Apparent life-threatening event:

_____

_____

_____

4. Bronchiolitis:

_____

_____

_____

5. Child abuse:

_____

_____

_____

6. Croup:

_____

_____

_____

7. Epiglottitis:

_____

_____

_____

8. Epiphyseal plate:

_____

_____

_____

9. Fontanelles:

_____

_____

_____

10. Greenstick fracture:

_____

_____

_____

11. Grunting:

_____

_____

_____

12. Medullary canal:

_____

_____

_____

13. Nebulizer:

_____

_____

_____

14. Nuchal rigidity:

_____

_____

_____

15. Osteomyelitis:

_____

_____

_____

16. Pediatric assessment triangle:

_____

_____

_____

17. Reactive airway disease:

_____

_____

_____

18. Separation anxiety:

_____

_____

_____

19. Tenting:

_____

_____

_____

20. Volutrol:

_____

_____

_____

Fill-in

Read each item carefully, then complete the statement by filling in the missing word(s).

1. _____ is the number one killer of children in the United States.

2. Most _____ are able to think abstractly and can participate in decision making.

3. Infants have two soft openings within the skull called _____.

4. The _____ is longer and more rounded compared to the size of the mandible, or lower jaw, in younger children.

5. In a child, the _____ is softer and narrower.

6. A child's _____ are softer and more flexible than an adult's and may compress the heart and lungs, causing serious injury with no obvious external damage.

7. An infant's heart rate can become as high as _____ beats or more per minute if the body needs to compensate for injury or illness.

8. Injury to the _____ _____ of the bone during development or inadvertent puncture of the growth plate during intraosseous cannulation may result in abnormalities in normal bone growth and development.

9. The _____ _____ _____ is a structured assessment tool that allows you to form a general impression of the infant's or child's condition without touching him or her.

10. An _____ _____ is obtained by auscultating heart tones over the chest with a stethoscope.

11. _____ _____ is the amount of air that is delivered to the lungs in one inhalation.

12. A special kind of microdrip set called a _____ allows you to fill a large drip chamber with a specific amount of fluid and administer only this amount to avoid fluid overload.

1999 13. A commonly used IO catheter is the _____ needle.

1999 14. Because most cases of cardiopulmonary arrest in infants and children are related to respiratory failure, _____ is the most common medication you will administer to them in the prehospital setting.

15. _____ _____ indicates that the body has used up its available energy stores and cannot continue to support the extra work of breathing.

1999 16. Other than oxygen, the primary pharmacological agent used for an acute asthma attack is a beta-2 agonist called _____.

17. _____ _____ occurs when an invading organism, usually a bacterium, attacks the blood vessels, preventing them from constricting.

18. The term _____ _____ is used to describe a continuous seizure or multiple seizures without a return to consciousness for 30 minutes or more.

19. _____ is an increase in body temperature, usually in response to an infection.

20. _____ is an inflammation of the meninges that cover the brain and spinal cord.

21. The most common causes of dehydration in children are _____ and _____.

22. If you are unable to determine whether a child with an altered mental status has hypoglycemia or hyperglycemia, _____ _____.

23. Coping with the death of a child can be very _____ for health care professionals.

24. Although child safety seats are effective in decreasing the severity of injuries, children may still sustain

    _____ and lower spinal injuries as the result of trauma caused by improperly used

passenger restraints.

25. _____ is the second most common cause of unintentional death among children in the

    United States.

True/False

If you believe the statement to be more true than false, write the letter "T" in the space provided. If you believe the statement to be more false than true, write the letter "F."

_____ 1. Toddlers often resist separation and demonstrate stranger anxiety.

_____ 2. The skeletal system contains growth plates at the ends of long bones, which enable these bones to grow during childhood.

_____ 3. Adulthood begins at age 18.

_____ 4. Infants are usually afraid of strangers because they are the center of attention in most families.

_____ 5. Preschool aged children have a rich fantasy life, which can make them particularly fearful of pain and change involving their bodies.

_____ 6. Normal respirations are a common sign of illness or injury in children.

_____ 7. In infants, feel for a pulse over the brachial artery.

_____ 8. When checking capillary refill, color should return in less than 3 seconds after you let go.

_____ 9. Infants with inadequate breathing are in imminent danger of respiratory arrest.

_____ 10. Febrile seizures are self-limiting and do not need transport unless they recur.

_____ 11. Increasing irritability, especially with handling, may be a sign of meningitis in infants.

_____ 12. Children are simply little adults.

_____ 13. Children may experience significant internal injuries with little or no obvious outside signs.

_____ 14. Child safety seats are effective in decreasing the severity of injuries.

_____ 15. Head injuries are uncommon in children.

_____ 16. Children can lose a greater proportion of blood than adults before showing signs or symptoms of shock.

_____ 17. Children have soft and flexible ribs.

_____ 18. The intentional injury of a child is rare in our society.

_____ 19. EMT-Is must report all cases of suspected child abuse.

_____ 20. Child protection agencies are mandated to investigate all reported child abuse.

Short Answer

Complete this section with short written answers in the space provided.

1. List the three elements of the pediatric assessment triangle.

_____

_____

_____

1999 **2.** List the steps used to remove a foreign body obstruction with the Magill forceps.

_____

_____

_____

1999 **3.** List three methods for confirming ET tube placement in the pediatric patient.

_____

_____

_____

1999 **4.** List the steps of NG tube placement.

_____

_____

_____

5. List the steps of general shock management.

_____

_____

_____

6. List four identifiable risk factors for SIDS.

_____

_____

_____

7. Define the mnemonic CHILD ABUSE.

C: _____

H: _____

I: _____

L: _____

D: _____

A: _____

B: _____

U: _____

S: _____

E: _____

Word Fun EMT-I vocab explorer web

The following crossword puzzle is an activity provided to reinforce correct spelling and understanding of medical terminology associated with emergency care and the EMT-I. Use the clues in the column to complete the puzzle.

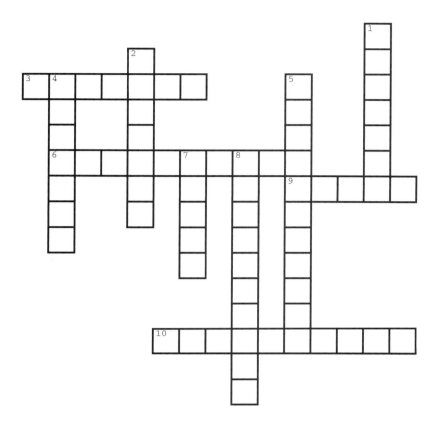

Across

3. Lower tip of sternum
6. 12 to 18 years of age
9. Absence of breathing
10. Incomplete fracture

Down

1. First month after birth
2. Terrible twos stage
4. First year of life
5. Two soft openings within the skulls of infants
7. Inadequate perfusion
8. Growth plate

Ambulance Calls

The following real case scenarios provide an opportunity to explore the concerns associated with patient management. Read each scenario, then answer each question in detail.

1. You are dispatched to a residence for an 8-year-old girl complaining of a possible tibia fracture. Her mother tells you that she tripped when she jumped out of a swing and twisted her leg when she landed. The child is lying on the ground and is fairly calm. You see obvious deformity to the lower left leg. How would you best manage this patient?

_____

_____

_____

_____

_____

_____

_____

_____

2. You are called to a child care center for a 3-year-old male with difficulty breathing. The patient is still alert but gasping for breath when you arrive. His respirations are 52 and shallow.

How would you best manage this patient?

_____

_____

_____

_____

_____

_____

_____

1999 **3.** You are called to the home of a 5-year-old asthmatic. His mother tells you the asthma attack started 10 minutes ago and that his inhaler is empty. You can hear wheezes from across the room, and the child appears tired and lethargic. His respiratory rate is 32 and his heart rate is 130.

How would you best manage this patient?

_____

_____

_____

_____

_____

_____

_____

Skill Drills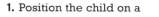

Skill Drill 31-1: Positioning the Airway in a Child
Test your knowledge by filling in the correct words in the photo captions.

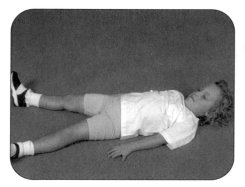

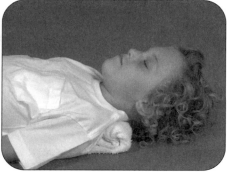

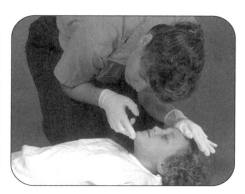

1. Position the child on a
_____ surface.

2. Place a _____ towel
about _____
inch(es) thick under the
_____ and
_____.

3. _____ the forehead
to limit _____.

Skill Drill 31-2: Removing a Foreign Body Airway Obstruction in an Unresponsive Child
Test your knowledge by filling in the correct words in the photo captions.

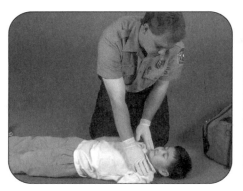

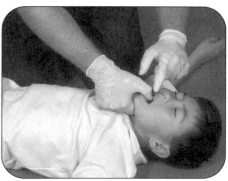

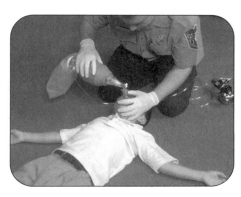

1. Place the child on a
_____,
_____ surface.

2. _____ the airway.
_____ any visible
foreign object.

3. Attempt _____
_____. If unsuc-
cessful, reposition the
_____ and try again.

Continued

Skill Drill 31-2: Removing a Foreign Body Airway Obstruction in an Unresponsive Child—cont'd

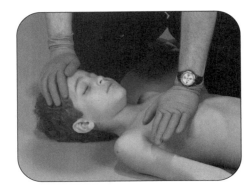

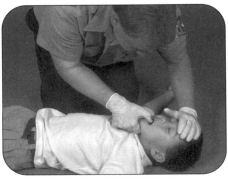

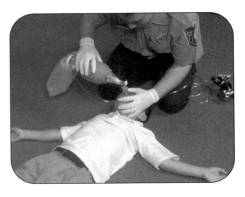

4. Provide _____ .

5. _____ the airway again to try to see the object. Try to remove the _____ only if you can see it.

6. Attempt _____ _____. If unsuccessful, _____ the head and try again. Repeat _____ _____ if obstruction persists.

Skill Drill 31-3: Inserting an Oropharyngeal Airway in a Child
Test your knowledge by placing the photos below in the correct order. Number the first step with a "1," the second step with a "2," etc.

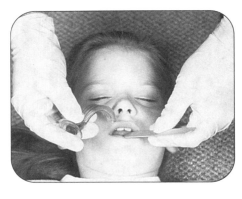

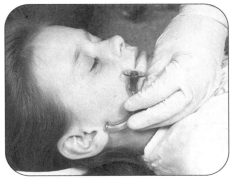

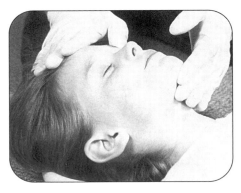

_____

Open the mouth.
Insert the airway until the flange rests against the lips.
Reassess the airway.

_____

Determine the appropriately sized airway by visualizing the device next to the patient's face.

_____

Position the child's airway with the appropriate method.

1999 **Skill Drill 31-6: Performing Pediatric Endotracheal Intubation**
Test your knowledge by filling in the correct words in the photo captions.

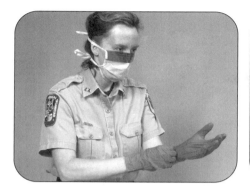

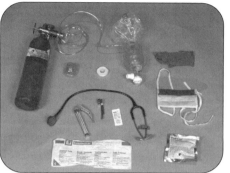

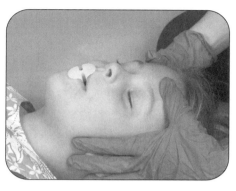

1. Take _____ precautions (gloves and face shield).

2. _____, _____, and _____ your equipment.

3. Manually open the patient's airway and insert an _____ if needed.

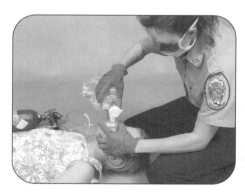

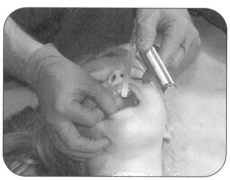

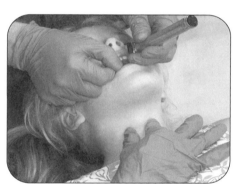

4. _____ the child with a BVM device and 100% oxygen for at least _____ seconds.

5. Insert the laryngoscope blade in the _____ side of the mouth and sweep the tongue to the _____. Lift the tongue with firm, gentle pressure. Avoid using the _____ or _____ as a _____.

6. Identify the _____ _____. If the cords are not visible, instruct your partner to apply _____ _____.

Continued

1999 Skill Drill 31-6: Performing Pediatric Endotracheal Intubation—cont'd

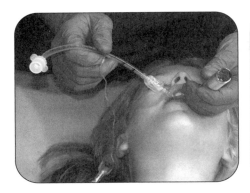

7. Introduce the ET tube in the
_____ corner of the
patient's mouth.

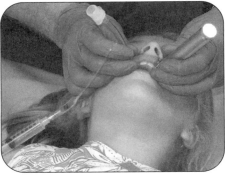

8. Pass the ET tube through the
_____
_____ to approxi-
mately 2 to 3 cm below the vocal
cords.

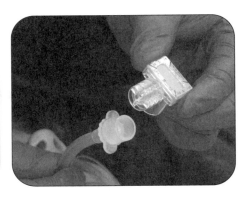

9. Attach a(n) _____
_____
_____
_____.

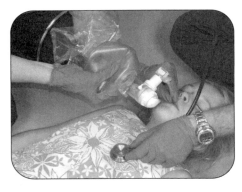

10. Attach the _____
device; ventilate and auscultate for
equal breath sounds over each lateral chest wall high in the .
_____. Ensure ab-
sence of breath sounds over the
_____.

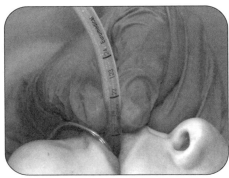

11. Secure the ET tube, noting the placement of the distance marker at the
patient's _____ or
_____, and recon-
firm tube placement.

Skill Drill 31-11: Immobilizing a Child

Test your knowledge by placing the photos below in the correct order. Number the first step with a "1," the second step with a "2," etc.

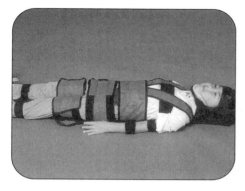

Ensure that the child is strapped in properly.

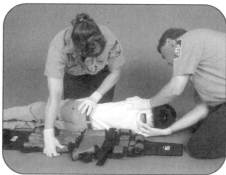

Log roll the child onto the immobilization device.

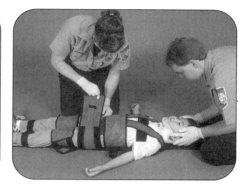

Secure the torso first.

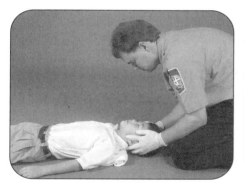

Use a towel under the shoulders to maintain the head in neutral position.

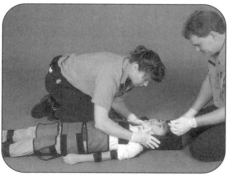

Secure the head.

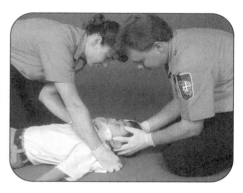

Apply an appropriately sized cervical collar.

Workbook Activities

The following activities have been designed to help you. Your instructor may require you to complete some or all of these activities as a regular part of your EMT-I training program. You are encouraged to complete any activity that your instructor does not assign as a way to enhance your learning in the classroom.

Chapter Review

The following exercises provide an opportunity to refresh your knowledge of this chapter.

Matching

Match each of the terms in the left column to the appropriate definition in the right column.

_____ **1.** Aneurysm

_____ **2.** Cataract

_____ **3.** Delirium

_____ **4.** Dementia

_____ **5.** Syncope

_____ **6.** Dyspnea

_____ **7.** Compensated shock

_____ **8.** Decompensated shock

_____ **9.** Collagen

_____ **10.** Vasodilation

_____ **11.** Vasoconstriction

A. a protein that is the chief component of connective tissue and bones

B. narrowing of a blood vessel

C. clouding of the lens of the eye

D. early shock

E. abnormal blood-filled dilation of a blood vessel

F. difficulty breathing

G. inability to focus, think logically, or maintain attention

H. late shock

I. slow onset of progressive disorientation

J. widening of a blood vessel

K. fainting

Multiple Choice

Read each item carefully, then select the best response.

_____ **1.** Leading causes of death in the elderly include all of the following, except:

   A. heart disease.

   B. AIDS.

   C. cancer.

   D. diabetes.

_____ **2.** Preventive intervention(s) for geriatric patients include:

   A. reviewing the home environment.

   B. providing information on preventing falls.

   C. making referrals to appropriate social services agencies.

   D. all of the above.

Geriatric Emergencies

_____ **3.** Simple preventive measures can help the elderly to avoid:

A. further injury.

B. costly medical treatment.

C. death.

D. all of the above.

_____ **4.** In elderly patients, acute illness and trauma are more likely to involve _____ beyond those initially involved.

A. organ systems

B. bones

C. fractures

D. vessels

_____ **5.** Risk factors that affect mortality in elderly patients include all of the following, except:

A. living alone.

B. unsound mind.

C. regular exercise.

D. recent hospitalization.

_____ **6.** Loss of collagen makes the skin:

A. wrinkled.

B. thinner.

C. more susceptible to injury.

D. all of the above.

_____ **7.** Driving and walking become more hazardous with age because the pupils of the eyes begin to lose the ability to:

A. dilate.

B. handle changes in light.

C. constrict.

D. detect color.

_____ **8.** Elderly patients' problems with balance are usually related to changes in the:

A. blood pressure.

B. vision.

C. inner eyes.

D. cardiovascular system.

_____ 9. Although the alveoli become enlarged with age, their elasticity decreases, resulting in a decreased ability to:

    A. cough, thereby increasing the chance of infection.

    B. exchange oxygen and carbon dioxide.

    C. monitor the changes in oxygen and carbon dioxide.

    D. force carbon dioxide out of the lungs.

_____ 10. Compensation for an increased demand on the cardiovascular system is accomplished by:

    A. increasing heart rate.

    B. increasing contraction of the heart.

    C. constricting the blood vessels to nonvital organs.

    D. all of the above.

_____ 11. Aging decreases a person's ability to _____ because of stiffer vessels.

    A. vasoconstrict

    B. vasodilate

    C. circulate blood

    D. exchange oxygen

_____ 12. An accumulation of fatty materials in the arteries is known as:

    A. myocardial infarction.

    B. stroke.

    C. atherosclerosis.

    D. aneurysm.

_____ 13. With a decrease in renal function, levels of _____ may rise, creating the impression of an overdose.

    A. medications

    B. toxins

    C. acid

    D. alkali

_____ 14. By age 85, a 10% reduction in brain weight can result in:

    A. increased risk of head trauma.

    B. short-term memory impairment.

    C. slower reflex times.

    D. all of the above.

_____ 15. As a person ages, fractures are more likely to occur because of a decrease in bone:

    A. cartilage.

    B. density.

    C. length.

    D. tissue.

_____ 16. Scene clues that can provide important information include:

    A. the general condition of the home.

    B. the number and type of pill bottles around.

    C. any hazards that could cause a fall.

    D. all of the above.

_____ 17. The best rule of thumb when assessing mental status is to always compare the patient's current level of consciousness or ability to function with the level or ability:

    A. of another adult in the household.

    B. before the problem began.

    C. of a person of the same age.

    D. none of the above.

_____ 18. The _____ is usually the key in helping to assess the elderly patient's problem.

    A. history

    B. medication

    C. environment

    D. all of the above

_____ **19.** An elderly patient's diminished _____ may hamper communication.
 A. sight
 B. hearing
 C. speaking ability
 D. all of the above

_____ **20.** The term applied to prescribing multiple medications is:
 A. hypermedicating.
 B. hyperpharmacy.
 C. polypharmacy.
 D. overmedicating.

_____ **21.** The sensation of pain may be _____ in an elderly patient, leading to "silent" heart attacks.
 A. enhanced
 B. diminished
 C. overstated
 D. false

_____ **22.** In order to understand a patient's baseline condition and how today's behavior differs from it, you should ask the nursing home staff questions concerning the patient's:
 A. mobility.
 B. activities of daily living.
 C. ability to speak.
 D. all of the above.

_____ **23.** You must consider the body's decreasing ability to _____ simple trauma when you are assessing and caring for an elderly patient.
 A. isolate
 B. separate
 C. heal
 D. recognize

_____ **24.** An isolated hip fracture in an 85-year-old patient can produce a systemic impact that results in:
 A. deterioration.
 B. shock.
 C. life-threatening conditions.
 D. all of the above.

_____ **25.** When assessing an elderly patient who has fallen, it is important to determine why the fall occurred, as it may have been the result of a medical problem such as:
 A. fainting.
 B. a cardiac rhythm disturbance.
 C. a medication interaction.
 D. all of the above.

_____ **26.** Your assessment of the patient's condition and stability must include past medical conditions, even if the patient('s condition) is not currently acute or:
 A. symptomatic.
 B. asymptomatic.
 C. complaining.
 D. on medication.

_____ **27.** A common complaint from the patient experiencing an abdominal aortic aneurysm (AAA) is pain in the:
 A. abdomen.
 B. back.
 C. leg, with decreased blood flow.
 D. all of the above.

_____ **28.** All of the following are true of delirium, except:
   A. It may have metabolic causes.
   B. The patient may be hypoglycemic.
   C. It develops slowly over a period of years.
   D. The memory remains mostly intact.

_____ **29.** For a DNR order to be valid, it must:
   A. be signed by the patient or legal guardian.
   B. be signed by one or more physicians.
   C. be dated within the preceding 12 months.
   D. all of the above.

_____ **30.** When in doubt about whether an advance directive is valid, or if one is in place, your best course of action is to:
   A. call medical control to see if an order is needed.
   B. take resuscitation action that is appropriate to the situation.
   C. wait for the family or caregivers to produce the appropriate document.
   D. none of the above.

_____ **31.** Signs and symptoms of possible abuse include all of the following, except:
   A. chronic pain.
   B. no history of repeated visits to the emergency department or clinic.
   C. depression or lack of energy.
   D. self-destructive behavior.

_____ **32.** Signs of neglect include:
   A. lack of hygiene.
   B. poor dental hygiene.
   C. lack of reasonable amenities in the home.
   D. all of the above.

_____ **33.** By the time we are in our 70s, we have approximately _____ fewer taste buds.
   A. 1/4
   B. 1/3
   C. 1/2
   D. 2/3

_____ **34.** If the patient has a history of _____, the cause may be cardiac related.
   A. pedal edema
   B. chest discomfort
   C. hypertension
   D. all of the above

_____ **35.** It is important to remember that an older person experiencing a myocardial infarction may only complain of _____.
   A. dyspnea.
   B. weakness.
   C. a syncopal episode.
   D. all of the above.

_____ **36.** Complaints of dizziness or weakness can be caused by _____.
   A. cardiac problems.
   B. inner-ear infections.
   C. hypo- or hypertension.
   D. all of the above.

_____ **37.** Geriatric patients are at risk for _____, also known as bacterial gastroenteritis, due to existing medical conditions such as dementia.

    A. food poisoning

    B. upset stomach

    C. diarrhea

    D. none of the above

Vocabulary EMT-I vocab explorer web

Define the following terms in the space provided.

1. Advance directives:

_____

_____

_____

2. Atherosclerosis:

_____

_____

_____

3. Arteriosclerosis:

_____

_____

_____

4. Elder abuse:

_____

_____

_____

5. Osteoporosis:

_____

_____

_____

6. Macular degeneration:

_____

_____

_____

Fill-in
Read each item carefully, then complete the statement by filling in the missing word(s).

1. Geriatric or elderly patients are individuals who are older than _____ years.

2. The aging body of the geriatric person may _____ serious medical conditions.

3. Common _____ about the elderly include the presence of mental confusion, illness, a sedentary lifestyle, and immobility.

4. Older skin feels dry because there are fewer _____.

5. _____ is a measure of the workload of the heart.

6. An _____ is an abnormal blood-filled dilation of the wall of a blood vessel.

7. Flexion at the neck and a forward curling of the shoulders produce a condition called

   _____.

8. _____ is the simultaneous use of many medications.

9. Deterioration of the central portion of the retina is known as _____

   _____.

10. _____ _____ _____ _____ include

    cooking and caring for oneself, bathing, housework, and personal hygiene, as well as toilet activities.

11. _____ _____ occurs when hypoperfusion follows a severe systemic

    infection.

12. A _____ is the body's immune response to combat an infection.

13. Consider the current _____ when assessing a patient's pain; many patients experience

    an exacerbation of pain when it changes.

14. Geriatric patients are at risk for _____ as a result of diarrhea.

15. Patients may ingest contaminated food without even being aware of it because of _____

    decline due to the aging process and improper hygiene.

True/False
If you believe the statement to be more true than false, write the letter "T" in the space provided. If you believe the statement to be more false than true, write the letter "F."

_____ 1. Vasodilation is a narrowing of a blood vessel.
_____ 2. Cardiovascular disease is one of the leading causes of death in the elderly.
_____ 3. Mental confusion and immobility are common stereotypes about the elderly.
_____ 4. Assessment of an elderly patient usually takes less time than assessment of a middle-aged person.
_____ 5. The sensation of pain in an elderly patient may be diminished.

_____ **6.** Elderly people are more prone to hypothermia than younger people.

_____ **7.** Falls are the leading cause of trauma, death, and disability in the elderly.

_____ **8.** 20% to 30% of elderly have "silent" heart attacks.

_____ **9.** Elderly abuse is on the decline in the United States.

_____ **10.** Dependent living is a type of care in which a person receives assistance based on family recommendations.

_____ **11.** Older people may not seek medical assistance because of concern over the cost.

_____ **12.** The sense of touch increases from loss of the end nerve fibers.

_____ **13.** The sense of smell is among the first to diminish.

_____ **14.** If the patient experiencing chest pain has a history of angina, you should determine if this episode is different from previous events.

_____ **15.** Nausea may be the older patient's complaint during a cardiac episode.

Short Answer

Complete this section with short written answers in the space provided.

1. List the three major categories of elder abuse.

_____

_____

_____

2. Briefly describe the three possible causes of syncope in an elderly patient.

_____

_____

_____

3. List at least five informational items that may be important in assessing possible elder abuse.

_____

_____

_____

4. Name three common signs and symptoms of a heart attack in an elderly patient.

_____

_____

_____

5. List the components of the "GEMS" diamond and what each represents.

_____

_____

_____

Word Fun EMT-I vocab explorer web

The following crossword puzzle is an activity provided to reinforce correct spelling and understanding of medical terminology associated with emergency care and the EMT-I. Use the clues in the column to complete the puzzle.

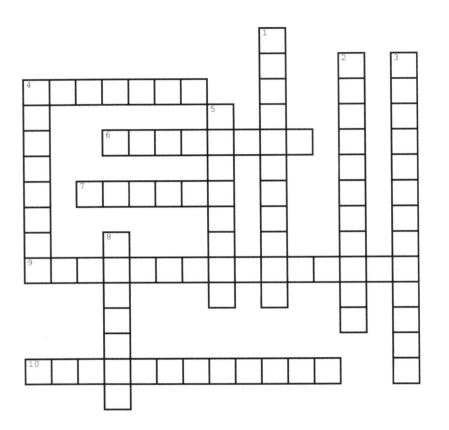

Across

4. Difficulty breathing
6. Chief component of connective tissue
7. Dark, tarry stool
9. Fatty materials deposited
10. Generalized bone disease

Down

1. Early shock
2. Vomiting blood
3. Late shock
4. Slow onset of progressive disorientation
5. Clouding of the lens
8. Ear wax

Ambulance Calls

The following real case scenarios provide an opportunity to explore the concerns associated with patient management. Read each scenario, then answer each question in detail.

1. You are called to the residence of an 87-year-old woman who is "not acting right." Family members tell you they think she may have taken her medication twice this morning. She is lethargic, confused, and hypotensive.

How would you best manage this patient?

_____

_____

_____

_____

_____

_____

_____

2. You are dispatched to a single vehicle motor vehicle crash with minor damage to the front where the car rolled into a culvert at a low speed. Bystanders tell you that the driver, an 82-year-old man, slumped over the steering wheel before the vehicle veered off the road. The patient is now alert and says he does not remember what happened. He has a 2-inch laceration above his right eye with moderate bleeding.

How would you best manage this patient?

_____

_____

_____

_____

_____

_____

_____

3. You are dispatched to a residence for a fall. Upon arrival, you find an 87-year-old woman complaining of severe pain in her left hip. Her daughter tells you that she falls a lot. You notice that the patient appears malnourished and lethargic. In the process of immobilizing the patient on a long spine board, you see what appear to be small circular burns to the backs of her thighs. Her daughter tells you she has a history of dementia and accidentally sat on a heater grate. The pattern is incompatible with such an injury.

How would you best manage this patient?

_____

_____

_____

_____

_____

_____

_____

Workbook Activities

The following activities have been designed to help you. Your instructor may require you to complete some or all of these activities as a regular part of your EMT-I training program. You are encouraged to complete any activity that your instructor does not assign as a way to enhance your learning in the classroom.

Chapter Review

The following exercises provide an opportunity to refresh your knowledge of this chapter.

Matching

Match each of the terms in the left column to the appropriate definition in the right column.

_____ **1.** Footprint	**A.** the process of increasing speed
_____ **2.** Chassis	**B.** area of contact between tire and road surface
_____ **3.** Friction	**C.** the killing of pathogenic agents by direct application of chemicals
_____ **4.** Sterilization	**D.** the process of removing dirt, dust, blood, or other visible contaminants
_____ **5.** Acceleration	
_____ **6.** Ambulance	**E.** vehicle frame
_____ **7.** Cleaning	**F.** the process of slowing down
_____ **8.** Deceleration	**G.** resistance to motion
_____ **9.** Disinfection	**H.** specialized vehicle for treating and transporting sick and injured patients
	I. removes microbial contamination

Multiple Choice

Read each item carefully, then select the best response.

_____ **1.** Ambulances today are designed according to strict government regulations based on _____ standards.
   A. local
   B. state
   C. national
   D. individual

_____ **2.** Features of the modern ambulance include all of the following EXCEPT:
   A. self-contained breathing apparatus.
   B. a patient compartment.
   C. two-way radio communication.
   D. a driver's compartment.

Ambulance Operations

_____ **3.** During the _____ phase, make sure that equipment and supplies are in their proper place.

A. preparation

B. dispatch

C. arrival at scene

D. transport

_____ **4.** The type _____ ambulance is a standard van with forward-control integral cab-body.

A. I

B. II

C. III

D. IV

_____ **5.** Items needed to care for life-threatening conditions include:

A. equipment for airway management.

B. equipment for artificial ventilation.

C. oxygen delivery devices.

D. all of the above.

_____ **6.** Oropharyngeal airways can be used for:

A. adults.

B. children.

C. infants.

D. all of the above.

_____ **7.** A BVM device, when attached to oxygen supply with the oxygen reservoir in place, is able to supply almost _____ oxygen.

A. 100%

B. 95%

C. 90%

D. 85%

_____ **8.** Masks on BVM devices should be transparent so that you can:

A. monitor the patient's respirations.

B. notice any color changes in the patient.

C. detect vomiting.

D. all of the above.

_____ **9.** Oxygen masks, with and without nonrebreathing bags, should be transparent and disposable and in sizes for:

    A. adults.

    B. children.

    C. infants.

    D. all of the above.

_____ **10.** Basic wound care supplies include all of the following EXCEPT:

    A. sterile sheets.

    B. an OB kit.

    C. an assortment of bandages.

    D. large safety pins.

_____ **11.** Think of the jump kit as containing anything you might need in the first _____ minutes with the patient except for the semiautomated external defibrillator and/or cardiac monitor and possibly the oxygen cylinder and portable suctioning unit.

    A. 2

    B. 3

    C. 4

    D. 5

_____ **12.** Stretchers must be easy to move, store, clean, and:

    A. fold.

    B. disinfect.

    C. lift.

    D. wash.

_____ **13.** Deceleration straps over the shoulders prevent the patient from continuing to move _____ in case the ambulance suddenly slows or stops.

    A. forward

    B. backward

    C. laterally

    D. down

_____ **14.** The ambulance inspection should include checks of:

    A. fuel levels.

    B. brake fluid.

    C. wheels and tires.

    D. all of the above.

_____ **15.** All medical equipment and supplies should be checked at least:

    A. after every call.

    B. after every emergency transport.

    C. every 12 hours.

    D. every day.

_____ **16.** For every emergency request, the dispatcher should gather and record all of the following EXCEPT:

    A. the nature of the call.

    B. the location of the patient(s).

    C. medications that the patient is currently taking.

    D. the number of patients and possible severity of their condition.

_____ **17.** During the _____ phase, the team should review dispatch information and assign specific initial duties and scene management tasks to each team member.

    A. preparation

    B. dispatch

    C. en route

    D. transport

_____ **18.** Basic requirements for the driver to safely operate an ambulance include:

    A. physical fitness.

    B. emotional fitness.

    C. proper attitude.

    D. all of the above.

_____ **19.** The _____ phase may be the most dangerous part of the call.

    A. preparation

    B. en route

    C. transport

    D. on-scene

_____ **20.** In order to operate an emergency vehicle safely, you must know how it responds to _____ under various conditions.

    A. steering

    B. braking

    C. acceleration

    D. all of the above.

_____ **21.** You must always drive:

    A. offensively.

    B. defensively.

    C. under the speed limit.

    D. all of the above.

_____ **22.** When driving with lights and siren, you are _____ drivers to yield the right of way.

    A. requesting

    B. demanding

    C. all of the above

    D. none of the above

_____ **23.** The _____ is a measure of the tire's grip on the road.

    A. coefficient of friction

    B. friction

    C. footprint

    D. centrifugal force

_____ **24.** Steering technique includes:

    A. the way you hold the steering wheel.

    B. the way it moves.

    C. the timing of the movements.

    D. all of the above.

_____ **25.** _____ is the transfer of weight to different points on the chassis.

    A. Chassis set

    B. Acceleration

    C. Deceleration

    D. Sliding

_____ **26.** Vehicle size and _____ greatly influence braking and stopping distances.

A. length

B. height

C. weight

D. width

_____ **27.** When on an emergency call, before proceeding past a stopped school bus with its lights flashing, you should stop before reaching the bus and wait for the driver to:

A. make sure the children are safe.

B. close the bus door.

C. turn off the warning lights.

D. all of the above.

_____ **28.** The _____ is probably the most overused piece of equipment on an ambulance.

A. stethoscope

B. siren

C. cardiac monitor

D. stretcher

_____ **29.** The _____ is the most visible and effective warning device for clearing traffic in front of the vehicle.

A. front light bar

B. rear light bar

C. high-beam flasher unit

D. standard headlight

_____ **30.** If you are involved in a motor vehicle crash while operating an emergency vehicle and are found to be at fault, you may be charged:

A. civilly.

B. criminally.

C. both civilly and criminally.

D. neither civilly nor criminally.

_____ **31.** _____ crashes are the most common and usually the most serious type of collision in which ambulances are involved.

A. T-bone

B. Intersection

C. Lateral

D. Rollover

_____ **32.** Guidelines for sizing up the scene include:

A. looking for safety hazards.

B. evaluating the need for additional units or other assistance.

C. evaluating the need to stabilize the spine.

D. all of the above.

_____ **33.** The main objectives in directing traffic include:

A. warning other drivers.

B. preventing additional crashes.

C. keeping vehicles moving in an orderly fashion.

D. all of the above.

_____ **34.** Transferring the patient to receiving staff member occurs during the _____ phase.

A. arrival

B. transport

C. delivery

D. postrun

_____ **35.** Cleaning the vehicle inside and out, refueling, disposing of contaminated waste, and replacing equipment and supplies all are accomplished during the _____ phase.

   A. preparation

   B. transport

   C. delivery

   D. postrun

_____ **36.** Air medical unit crews may include:

   A. EMTs.

   B. paramedics.

   C. physicians.

   D. all of the above.

_____ **37.** The proper approach area for a helicopter is between the _____ o'clock and _____ o'clock positions as the pilot faces forward.

   A. 2 and 10

   B. 11 and 5

   C. 1 and 11

   D. 3 and 9

_____ **38.** When clearing a landing site for an approaching helicopter, look for:

   A. loose debris.

   B. electric or telephone wires.

   C. poles.

   D. all of the above.

Vocabulary EMT-I vocab explorer web

Define the following terms in the space provided.

1. Air ambulances:

_____

_____

_____

2. Coefficient of friction:

_____

_____

_____

3. Decontaminate:

_____

_____

_____

4. Hydroplaning:

_____

_____

_____

5. High-level disinfection:

_____

_____

_____

Fill-in
Read each item carefully, then complete the statement by filling in the missing word.

1. A _____ is a portable kit containing items that are used in the initial care of the patient.

2. The six-pointed star that identifies vehicles that meet federal specifications as licensed or certified ambulances is known as the _____.

3. For many decades after 1906, a _____ was the vehicle that was most often used as an ambulance.

4. _____ respond initially to the scene with personnel and equipment to treat the sick and injured until an ambulance can arrive.

5. An ambulance call has _____ phases.

6. Devices should be either disposable or easy to clean and _____, which means to remove radiation, chemicals, or other hazardous materials.

7. Suction tubing must reach the patient's _____, regardless of the patient's position.

8. A _____ provides a firm surface under the patient's torso so that you can give effective chest compressions.

9. _____ is resistance to the motion of one body against another.

10. Vehicle _____ and _____ are critical factors in maneuvering, driving, and parking an emergency vehicle.

True/False

If you believe the statement to be more true than false, write the letter "T" in the space provided. If you believe the answer to be more false than true, write the letter "F."

_____ **1.** Equipment and supplies should be placed in the unit according to their relative importance and frequency of use.

_____ **2.** A CPR board is a pocket-sized reminder that the EMT-I carries to help recall CPR procedures.

_____ **3.** Having the ability to exchange equipment between units or between your unit and the emergency department decreases the time that you and your unit must stay at the hospital.

_____ **4.** In most instances, if the patient is properly assessed and stabilized at the scene, speeding during transport is unnecessary, undesirable, and dangerous.

_____ **5.** The en route or response phase of the emergency call is the least dangerous for the EMT-I.

_____ **6.** Controlled acceleration is the use of acceleration to control the vehicle.

_____ **7.** When the siren is on, you can speed up and assume that you have the right-of-way.

_____ **8.** You should use the "4-second rule" to help you maintain a safe following distance.

_____ **9.** Always approach a helicopter from the front.

_____ **10.** Fixed-wing air ambulances are generally used for short-haul patient transfers.

_____ **11.** A clear landing zone of 50' by 50' is recommended for EMS helicopters.

_____ **12.** The ambulance chassis and engine components are subjected to no more stress than the typical automobile or truck.

Short Answer

Complete this section with short written answers in the space provided.

1. Describe the three basic ambulance designs.

_____

_____

_____

2. Describe "right of way" privileges.

_____

_____

_____

3. List the five factors that contribute to the use of excessive speed.

_____

_____

_____

4. Describe the three basic principles that govern the use of warning lights and sirens.

_____

_____

_____

5. List four guidelines for safe ambulance driving.

_____

_____

_____

6. Describe the correct technique for approaching a helicopter that is "hot" (rotors turning).

_____

_____

_____

7. List the general considerations used for selecting a helicopter landing site.

_____

_____

_____

8. Explain what is meant by "siren syndrome."

_____

_____

_____

9. Explain why the use of escorts is a dangerous practice.

_____

_____

_____

Word Fun EMT-I vocab explorer web

The following crossword puzzle is an activity provided to reinforce correct spelling and understanding of medical terminology associated with emergency care and the EMT-I. Use the clues in the column to complete the puzzle.

Across

1. Vehicle used for transporting patients
5. Emblem identifying vehicles that meet ambulance specifications
7. Using a police _____ is an extremely dangerous practice
9. The proper _____ is very important for the driver of an ambulance
10. Lifting the tire off the road as water "piles up" under it

Down

2. Vehicle frame
3. Resistance to the motion of one body against another
4. Process of removing visible contaminants from a surface
5. Removes all microbial contamination
6. Area of contact between the tire and the surface of the road
8. 5-minute kit

Ambulance Calls

The following real case scenarios provide an opportunity to explore the concerns associated with patient management. Read each scenario, then answer each question in detail.

1. You are dispatched to a call on the opposite side of town. The dispatcher tells you that the bridge over Second Street is still blocked from an earlier crash. This was the shortest, most direct route to your destination. You do not know of another route.

   How would you best manage this situation?

   _____

   _____

   _____

   _____

   _____

   _____

   _____

2. You are called to the scene of a motor vehicle crash. En route to the scene, in heavy rain, your ambulance begins to hydroplane. You are on a straightaway and no one is in the oncoming lane.

   How would you best manage this situation?

   _____

   _____

   _____

   _____

   _____

   _____

   _____

3. You are called to the scene of a motor vehicle crash. The car is situated on a curve and traffic is heavy. Police are not on the scene. Your patient is alert and looking around, but stuck in the vehicle because of traffic. You see blood smeared across her face, but it appears to be minimal.

How would you best manage this situation?

_____

_____

_____

_____

_____

_____

_____

_____

Workbook Activities

The following activities have been designed to help you. Your instructor may require you to complete some or all of these activities as a regular part of your EMT-I training program. You are encouraged to complete any activity that your instructor does not assign as a way to enhance your learning in the classroom.

Chapter Review

The following exercises provide an opportunity to refresh your knowledge of this chapter.

Matching

Match each of the terms in the left column to the appropriate definition in the right column.

_____ **1.** Extremity lift	**A.** separates into two or four pieces
_____ **2.** Flexible stretcher	**B.** tubular framed stretcher with rigid fabric stretched across it
_____ **3.** Stair chair	**C.** used for patients without a spinal injury who are supine or sitting on the ground
_____ **4.** Basket stretcher	
_____ **5.** Scoop stretcher	**D.** specifically designed stretcher that can be rolled along the ground
_____ **6.** Backboard	**E.** used to carry patients across uneven terrain
_____ **7.** Direct ground lift	**F.** used for patients who are found lying supine with no suspected spinal injury
_____ **8.** Portable stretcher	
_____ **9.** Wheeled ambulance stretcher	**G.** can be folded or rolled up
	H. used to carry patients up and down stairs
	I. spine board or longboard

Multiple Choice

Read each item carefully, then select the best response.

_____ **1.** _____ safety depends on the use of proper lifting techniques and maintaining a proper hold when lifting or carrying a patient.

    A. Your

    B. Your team's

    C. The patient's

    D. All of the above

_____ **2.** You should perform an urgent move:

    A. if a patient has an altered level of consciousness.

    B. if a patient has inadequate ventilation or shock.

    C. in extreme weather conditions.

    D. all of the above.

Lifting and Moving

_____ **3.** The _____ is the mechanical weight-bearing base of the spinal column and the fused central posterior section of the pelvic girdle.

A. coccyx

B. sacrum

C. lumbar region

D. thorax

_____ **4.** You may injure your back if you lift:

A. with your back curved.

B. with your back straight but bent significantly forward at the hips.

C. with the shoulder girdle anterior to the pelvis.

D. all of the above.

_____ **5.** When lifting you should:

A. spread your legs shoulder width apart.

B. never lift a patient while reaching any significant distance in front of your torso.

C. keep the weight that you are lifting as close to your body as possible.

D. all of the above.

_____ **6.** When carrying a patient on a cot, be sure:

A. to flex at the hips.

B. to bend at the knees.

C. that you do not hyperextend your back.

D. all of the above.

_____ **7.** In lifting with the palm down, the weight is supported by the _____ rather than the palm.

A. fingers

B. forearm

C. lower back

D. wrist

_____ **8.** When you must carry a patient up or down a flight of stairs or other significant incline, use a _____ if possible.

A. backboard

B. stair chair

C. stretcher

D. short spine board

_____ **9.** If you need to lean to either side to compensate for a weight imbalance, you have probably _____ your weight limitation.

   A. met

   B. exceeded

   C. increased

   D. countered

_____ **10.** A backboard is a device that provides support to patients who you suspect have:

   A. hip injuries.

   B. pelvic injuries.

   C. spinal injuries.

   D. all of the above.

_____ **11.** The team leader should do all of the following, except _____, before any lifting is initiated.

   A. give a command of execution

   B. indicate where each team member is to be located

   C. rapidly describe the sequence of steps that will be performed

   D. give a detailed overview of the stages

_____ **12.** Special _____ are usually required to move any patient who weighs more than 300 lb to an ambulance.

   A. techniques

   B. equipment

   C. resources

   D. all of the above

_____ **13.** When carrying a patient in a stair chair, always remember to:

   A. keep your back in a locked-in position.

   B. flex at the hips, not at the waist.

   C. keep the patient's weight and your arms as close to your body as possible.

   D. all of the above.

_____ **14.** When you use a body drag to move a patient:

   A. your back should always be locked and straight.

   B. you should avoid any twisting so that the vertebrae remain in normal alignment.

   C. avoid hyperextending.

   D. all of the above.

_____ **15.** When pulling a patient, you should do all of the following EXCEPT:

   A. extend your arms no more than about 15 to 20 inches.

   B. reposition your feet so that the force of pull will be balanced equally.

   C. when you can pull no further, lean forward another 15 to 20 inches.

   D. pull the patient by slowly flexing your arms.

_____ **16.** When log rolling a patient:

   A. kneel as close to the patient's side as possible.

   B. lean solely from the hips.

   C. use your shoulder muscles to help with the roll.

   D. all of the above.

_____ **17.** If the weight you are pushing is lower than your waist, you should push from:

   A. the waist.

   B. a kneeling position.

   C. the shoulder.

   D. a squatting position.

_____ **18.** To protect your _____ from injury, never push an object with your arms fully extended in a straight line and with your elbows locked.

    A. elbows

    B. shoulders

    C. neck

    D. arms

_____ **19.** If you are alone and must remove an unconscious patient from a car, you should first move the patient's:

    A. legs.

    B. head.

    C. torso.

    D. pelvis.

_____ **20.** Situations in which you should use an emergency move include those where:

    A. fire, explosives, or hazardous materials are present.

    B. you are unable to protect the patient from other hazards.

    C. you are unable to gain access to others in a vehicle who need lifesaving care.

    D. all of the above.

_____ **21.** You should use a one-person technique to move a patient only:

    A. if a potentially life-threatening danger exists and you are alone.

    B. because of the pressing nature of the danger.

    C. if your partner is moving a second patient.

    D. all of the above.

_____ **22.** You can move a patient on his or her back along the floor or ground by using all of the following methods EXCEPT:

    A. pulling on the patient's clothing in the neck and shoulder area.

    B. placing the patient on a blanket, coat, or other item that can be pulled.

    C. pulling the patient by the legs if they are the most accessible part.

    D. placing your arms under the patient's shoulders and through the armpits while grasping the patient's arms, dragging the patient backward.

_____ **23.** An urgent move may be necessary for moving a patient with:

    A. an altered level of consciousness.

    B. inadequate ventilation.

    C. shock.

    D. all of the above.

_____ **24.** Use the rapid extrication technique in the following situation(s):

    A. The vehicle on the scene is unsafe.

    B. The patient's condition cannot be properly assessed before being removed from the car.

    C. The patient blocks access to another seriously injured patient.

    D. All of the above.

_____ **25.** Before you attempt any move, the team leader must be sure:

    A. that there are enough personnel and that the proper equipment is available.

    B. that any obstacles have been identified or removed.

    C. that the procedure and path to be followed have been clearly identified and discussed.

    D. all of the above.

_____ **26.** To avoid the strain of unnecessary lifting and carrying, you should use _____ or assist an able patient to the cot whenever possible.

    A. the direct ground lift

    B. the extremity lift

    C. the draw sheet method

    D. a scoop stretcher

_____ **27.** To move a patient from the ground or the floor onto the cot, you should:

    A. lift and carry the patient to the nearby prepared cot with a direct body carry.

    B. use a scoop stretcher.

    C. use a log roll or long-axis drag to place the patient onto a backboard and then lift and carry the backboard to the cot.

    D. all of the above.

_____ **28.** The _____ is the most uncomfortable of all the various devices; however, it provides excellent support and immobilization.

    A. portable stretcher

    B. flexible stretcher

    C. wooden backboard

    D. scoop stretcher

_____ **29.** If _____ are used, you must follow infection control procedures before you can reuse the backboards.

    A. plastic backboards

    B. wooden backboards

    C. metal backboards

    D. all of the above

_____ **30.** You should use a rigid _____, often called a Stokes litter, to carry a patient across uneven terrain from a remote location that is inaccessible by ambulance or other vehicle.

    A. basket stretcher

    B. scoop stretcher

    C. molded backboard

    D. flotation device

_____ **31.** Basket stretchers can be used:

    A. for technical rope rescues and some water rescues.

    B. to carry a patient across fields on an all-terrain vehicle.

    C. to carry a patient on a toboggan.

    D. all of the above.

_____ **32.** Every time you have to move a patient, you must take special care that _____ are/is not injured.

    A. you

    B. your team

    C. the patient

    D. all of the above

_____ **33.** Certain patient conditions, such as _____, call for special lifting and moving techniques.

    A. head or spinal injury

    B. shock

    C. pregnancy

    D. all of the above

Vocabulary EMT-I vocab explorer web

Define the following terms in the space provided.

1. Diamond carry:

_____

_____

_____

2. Rapid extrication technique:

_____

_____

_____

3. Power grip:

_____

_____

_____

4. Power lift:

_____

_____

_____

5. Emergency move:

_____

_____

_____

Fill-in

Read each item carefully, then complete the statement by filling in the missing word(s).

1. To avoid injury to you, the patient, or your partners, you will have to learn how to lift and carry the
patient properly, using proper _____ _____ and a power grip.

2. The key rule of lifting is to always keep the back in a straight, _____ position and to lift
without twisting.

3. The safest and most powerful way to lift, lifting by extending the properly placed flexed legs, is called a

_____ _____.

4. The arm and hand have their greatest lifting strength when facing _____ up.

5. Be sure to pick up and carry the backboard with your back in the _____ position.

6. You should not attempt to lift a patient who weighs more than _____ pounds with
fewer than four rescuers, regardless of individual strength.

7. During a body drag where you and your partner are on each side of the patient, you will have to alter the
usual pulling technique to prevent pulling _____ and producing adverse lateral leverage
against your lower back.

8. When you are rolling the wheeled ambulance stretcher, your back should be _____, straight, and untwisted.

9. Be careful that you do not push or pull from a(n) _____ position.

10. Remember to always consider whether there is an option that will cause _____ _____ to you and the other EMT-Is.

11. The manual support and immobilization that you provide when using the rapid extrication technique produce a greater risk of _____ _____.

12. The _____ _____ _____ is used for patients with no suspected spinal injury who are found lying supine on the ground.

13. The _____ _____ may be especially helpful when the patient is in a very narrow space or when there is not enough room for the patient and a team of EMTs to stand side by side.

14. The mattress on a stretcher must be _____ _____ so that it does not absorb any type of potentially infectious material, including water, blood, or other body fluid.

15. A _____ _____ may be used for patients who have been struck by a motor vehicle.

True/False

If you believe the statement to be more true than false, write the letter "T" in the space provided. If you believe the statement to be more false than true, write the letter "F."

_____ **1.** Patient packaging and handling are technical skills you will learn and perfect through practice and training.

_____ **2.** A portable stretcher is typically a lightweight folding device that does not have the undercarriage and wheels of a true ambulance stretcher.

_____ **3.** The term "power lift" refers to a posture that is safe and helpful for EMT-Is when they are lifting.

_____ **4.** If you find that lifting a patient is a strain, try to move to the patient as quickly as possible to minimize the possibility of back injury.

_____ **5.** The use of adjunct devices and equipment, such as sheets and blankets, may make the job of lifting and moving a patient more difficult.

_____ **6.** One-person techniques for moving patients should only be used when immediate patient movement is necessary because of a life-threatening hazard and only one EMT-I is available.

_____ **7.** A scoop stretcher may be used alone for standard immobilization of a patient with a spinal injury.

_____ **8.** When carrying a patient down stairs or on an incline, make sure the stretcher is carried head end first.

_____ **9.** The rapid extrication technique is the preferred technique to use on all sitting patients with possible spinal injuries.

_____ **10.** It is unprofessional for you to discuss and plan a lift at the scene in front of the patient.

Short Answer

Complete this section with short written answers in the space provided.

1. List the one-rescuer drags, carries, and lifts.

_____

_____

_____

2. List the situations in which the rapid extrication technique is used.

_____

_____

_____

3. List the three guidelines for loading the cot into the ambulance.

_____

_____

_____

4. List the five guidelines for carrying a patient on a cot.

_____

_____

_____

5. Describe the key rule of lifting.

_____

_____

_____

Word Fun ![EMT-I vocab explorer web]

The following crossword puzzle is an activity provided to reinforce correct spelling and understanding of medical terminology associated with emergency care and the EMT-I. Use the clues in the column to complete the puzzle.

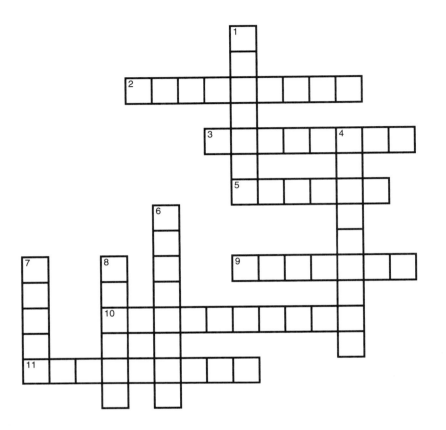

Across

2. Using the patient's limbs to lift
3. Stretcher that becomes rigid when secured around patient
5. A ground lift used with no suspected spinal injury
9. Four-rescuer carry with one at the head, one at the foot, and one on each side
10. Folding device for moving seated patients up or down floors
11. Safest way to lift

Down

1. Stretcher designed to roll along the ground
4. Used to support patient with hip, pelvic, or spine injury
6. Tubular framed stretcher with fabric across
7. Stretcher that can be split into two or four sections
8. Stretcher used with technical rescues, particularly when water is involved

Ambulance Calls

The following real case scenarios provide an opportunity to explore the concerns associated with patient management. Read each scenario, then answer each question in detail.

1. You are dispatched to a construction site for a 26-year-old male who fell into a ravine. He is approximately 35 feet down a rocky ledge. He is alert, with an unstable pelvis and weak radial pulses. You have all the help you need from the construction crew and the volunteer fire department.

   How would you best manage this patient?

   _____

   _____

   _____

   _____

   _____

   _____

   _____

   _____

2. You are working a head-on motor vehicle crash where you have the two drivers in critical condition. As your partner works with the driver of one vehicle, you assess the driver of the second car. He is a 58-year-old male with weak radial pulses and a respiratory rate of 4 breaths/min. No other help has arrived on the scene, and your partner's patient is equally critical. You cannot effectively ventilate the patient where he is seated. The fire department is en route to your location.

How would you best manage this patient?

_____

_____

_____

_____

_____

_____

_____

3. You are working a motor vehicle crash and note that the patient, a 34-year-old female, responds to pain and has absent radial pulses. She is breathing shallowly at a rate of 10 breaths/min.

How would you best manage this patient?

_____

_____

_____

_____

_____

_____

_____

Skill Drills EMT-I video clips web

Skill Drill 34-1: Performing the Power Lift

Test your knowledge by filling in the correct words in the photo captions.

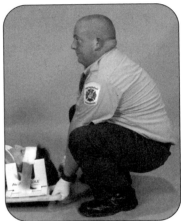 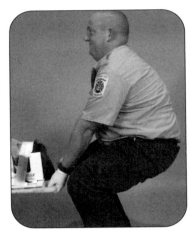 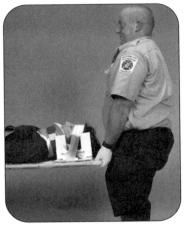

1. Lock your back into a(n) _____, inward curve. _____ and bend your legs. Grasp the backboard, palms up and just in front of you. _____ and _____ the weight between your arms.

2. Position your feet, _____ the object, and _____ weight.

3. _____ your legs and lift, keeping your back locked in.

Skill Drill 34-2: Performing the Diamond Carry

Test your knowledge by placing the photos below in the correct order. Number the first step with a "1," the second step with a "2," etc.

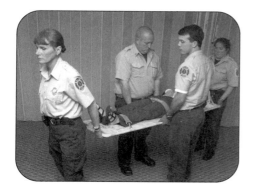

_____

After the patient has been lifted, the EMT-I at the foot turns to face forward.

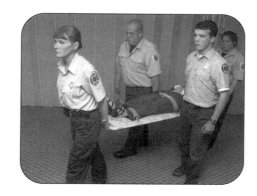

_____

EMT-Is at the side turn toward the foot end.

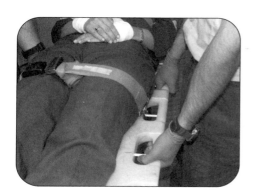

_____

EMT-Is at the side each turn the head-end hand palm down and release the other hand.

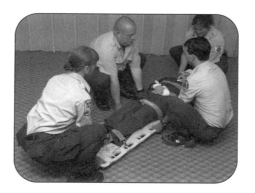

_____

Position yourselves facing the patient.

Skill Drill 34-3: Performing the One-Handed Carrying Technique
Test your knowledge by filling in the correct words in the photo captions.

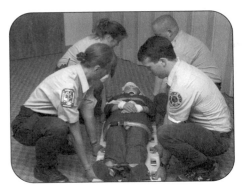

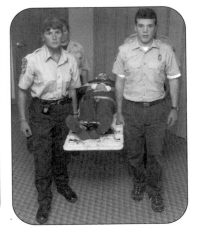

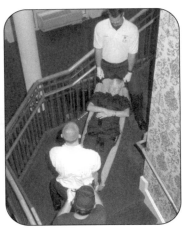

1. _____ each other and use both _____.

2. Lift the backboard to _____ _____.

3. _____ in the direction you will walk and _____ to using one hand.

Skill Drill 34-4: Carrying a Patient on Stairs
Test your knowledge by filling in the correct words in the photo captions.

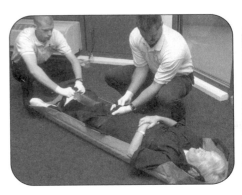

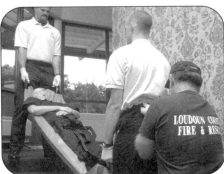

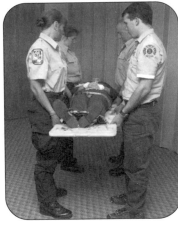

1. _____ the patient securely.

2. Carry a patient down stairs with the _____ end first, _____ elevated.

3. Carry the _____ end first going up stairs.

Skill Drill 34-5: Using a Stair Chair
Test your knowledge by filling in the correct words in the photo captions.

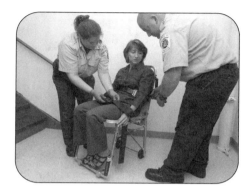

1. Position and secure the patient on the
   _____.

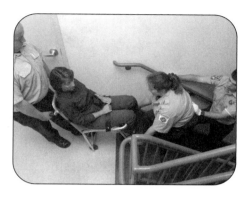

2. Take your places at the
   _____ and
   _____ of the chair.

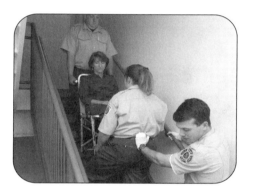

3. A third _____ pre-
   cedes and "backs up" the rescuer
   carrying the _____.

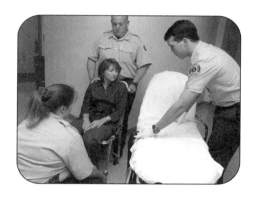

4. _____ the chair to
   roll on landings, or for transfer to the
   cot.

Skill Drill 34-6: Performing Rapid Extrication Technique

Test your knowledge by placing the photos below in the correct order. Number the first step with a "1," the second step with a "2," etc.

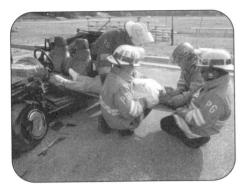 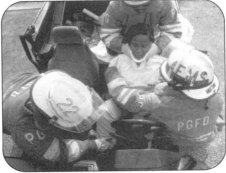 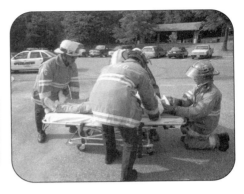

_____

_____

_____

Third EMT-I exits the vehicle, moves to the backboard opposite Second EMT-I, and they continue to slide the patient until patient is fully on the board.

Second EMT-I supports the torso. Third EMT-I frees the patient's legs from the pedals and moves the legs together, without moving the pelvis or spine.

First (or Fourth) EMT-I continues to stabilize the head and neck while Second and Third carry the patient away from the vehicle.

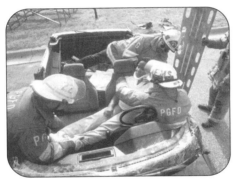 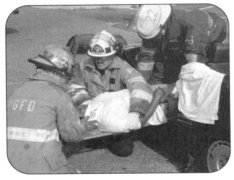 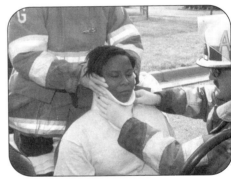

_____

_____

_____

Second and Third EMT-Is rotate the patient as a unit in several short, coordinated moves. First EMT-I (relieved by Fourth EMT-I or bystander as needed) supports the head and neck during rotation (and later steps).

Third EMT-I moves to an effective position for sliding the patient.

Second and Third EMT-Is slide the patient along the backboard in coordinated, 8" to 12" moves until the hips rest on the backboard.

Second EMT-I gives commands, applies a cervical collar, and performs the initial assessment.

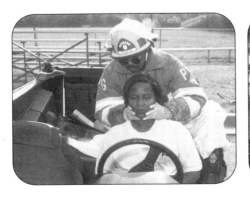 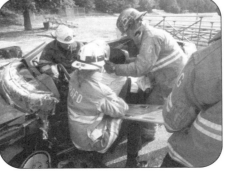

_____

_____

First EMT-I provides in-line manual support of the head and cervical spine.

First (or Fourth) EMT-I places the backboard on the seat against the patient's buttocks.

Skill Drill 34-7: Extremity Lift

Test your knowledge by filling in the correct words in the photo captions.

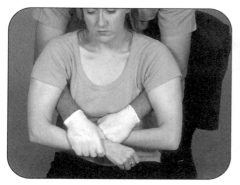

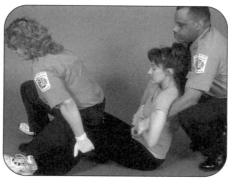

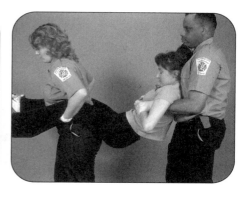

1. Patient's hands are

_____ over the

chest. The First EMT-I grasps the pa-

tient's wrists or

_____ and pulls

patient to a _____

position.

2. When the patient is sitting, First

EMT-I passes his or her arms through

patient's _____ and

grasps the patient's opposite (or his

or her own) _____

or _____. Second

EMT-I kneels between the

_____, facing the

feet, and places his or her hands un-

der the _____.

3. Both EMT-Is rise to a

_____ position. On

_____, both lift and

begin to move.

Skill Drill 34-8: Using a Scoop Stretcher

Test your knowledge by filling in the correct words in the photo captions.

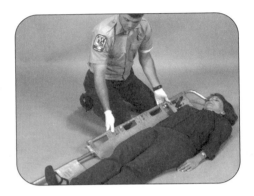

1. Adjust stretcher

   _____.

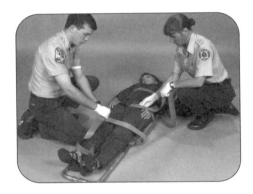

2. _____ patient
   slightly and _____
   stretcher into place, one side at a
   time.

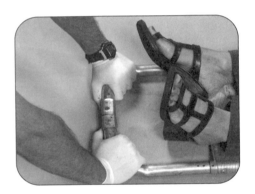

3. _____ the stretcher
   ends together, avoiding
   _____.

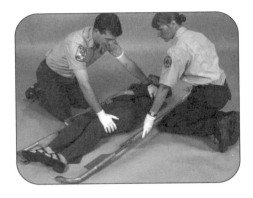

4. _____ the patient
   and _____ to the
   cot.

Skill Drill 34-9: Loading a Cot into an Ambulance

Test your knowledge by placing the photos below in the correct order. Number the first step with a "1," the second step with a "2," etc.

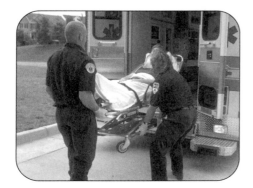

_____

Second rescuer on the side of the cot releases the undercarriage lock and lifts the undercarriage.

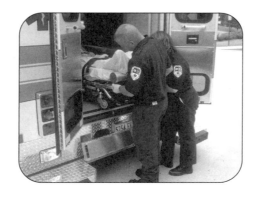

_____

Roll the cot into the back of the ambulance.

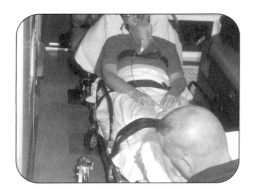

_____

Secure the cot to the brackets mounted in the ambulance.

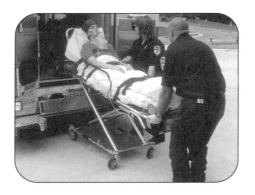

_____

Tilt the head of the cot upward, and place it into the patient compartment with the wheels on the floor.

Workbook Activities

The following activities have been designed to help you. Your instructor may require you to complete some or all of these activities as a regular part of your EMT-I training program. You are encouraged to complete any activity that your instructor does not assign as a way to enhance your learning in the classroom.

Chapter Review

The following exercises provide an opportunity to refresh your knowledge of this chapter.

Matching

Match each of the terms in the left column to the appropriate definition in the right column.

_____ **1.** Extrication	**A.** access requiring no special tools and training
_____ **2.** Simple access	**B.** individual who has overall command of the scene in the field
_____ **3.** Complex access	**C.** a substance that causes injury or death with exposure
_____ **4.** Access	**D.** access requiring special tools and training
_____ **5.** Incident commander	**E.** removal from entrapment or a dangerous situation or position
_____ **6.** Structure fire	**F.** gaining entry to an enclosed area to reach a patient
_____ **7.** Hazardous material	**G.** fire in a house, apartment building, or other building

Multiple Choice

Read each item carefully, then select the best response.

_____ **1.** Aside from EMS personnel, other rescuers at a crash scene include:

  A. fire fighters.

  B. law enforcement.

  C. a rescue group.

  D. all of the above.

_____ **2.** Of the four teams at a crash scene, the _____ team is responsible for investigating the crash or crime scene.

  A. fire fighter

  B. law enforcement

  C. rescue group

  D. EMS personnel

CHAPTER 35

Gaining Access

_____ **3.** Of the four teams at a crash scene, the _____ team is responsible for properly securing and stabilizing the vehicle.

A. fire fighter

B. law enforcement

C. rescue group

D. EMS personnel

_____ **4.** Of the four teams at a crash scene, the _____ team is responsible for washing down any spilled fuel.

A. fire fighter

B. law enforcement

C. rescue group

D. EMS personnel

_____ **5.** Before proceeding with an extrication you should:

A. position your unit in a safe location.

B. make sure the scene is properly marked.

C. determine if any additional resources will be needed.

D. all of the above.

_____ **6.** While you are gaining access to the patient and during extrication, you must make sure that the patient:

A. remains safe.

B. stays conscious.

C. holds his/her head completely still.

D. all of the above.

_____ **7.** When dealing with multiple patients, you should locate and rapidly _____ each patient.

A. treat

B. triage

C. transport

D. extricate

_____ **8.** When preparing for patient removal, you should determine:

A. how urgently the patient needs to be extricated.

B. where you should be positioned during extrication.

C. how you will best move the patient from the vehicle.

D. all of the above.

_____ **9.** Once the patient has been extricated, additional assessment should be completed:

    A. once the patient has been placed on the stretcher.

    B. inside the ambulance inclement weather.

    C. en route if the patient's condition requires rapid transport.

    D. all of the above.

_____ **10.** Even when a technical rescue group includes a paramedic or physician, generally nothing but essential _____ is provided until the rescuers can bring the patient to the nearest point where a safe, stable setting exists.

    A. bandaging

    B. triage

    C. simple care

    D. splinting

_____ **11.** When called to a person lost outdoors, your role involves:

    A. standing by at the search base until the lost person is found.

    B. preparing necessary equipment.

    C. obtaining any medical history from relatives on scene.

    D. all of the above.

_____ **12.** Tactical situations involve all of the following EXCEPT:

    A. an armed hostage situation.

    B. a structure fire.

    C. the presence of a sniper.

    D. an exchange of shots.

Vocabulary EMT-I vocab explorer web

Define the following terms in the space provided.

1. Entrapment:

_____

_____

_____

2. Technical rescue situation:

_____

_____

_____

3. Danger zone:

_____

_____

_____

4. Tactical situation:

_____

_____

_____

5. Technical rescue group:

_____

_____

_____

Fill-in
Read each item carefully, then complete the statement by filling in the missing word(s).

1. _____ is the final phase of extrication, and this usually results in the patient being

placed on the ambulance stretcher.

2. During all phases of rescue, your primary concern is _____.

3. Good _____ among team members and clear leadership are essential to safe, efficient

provision of proper emergency care.

4. You should not attempt to gain access to the patient or enter the vehicle until you are sure that the

vehicle is _____.

5. When gaining access, it is up to you to identify the _____, most efficient way to gain

access.

6. Moving the patient in one fast continuous step increases the risk of _____ and

confusion.

7. Search and rescue is performed by teams of fire fighters wearing full turnout gear and

_____ _____ _____ _____ (SCBA)

and carrying tools and fully charged hose lines.

True/False
If you believe the statement to be more true than false, write the letter "T" in the space provided. If you believe the statement to be more false than true, write the letter "F."

_____ **1.** There should be no talking throughout the extrication process.

_____ **2.** A team leader must be identified and agreed on before you arrive at the scene.

_____ **3.** If you will be involved with extrication, you should wear leather gloves over your disposable gloves.

_____ **4.** Once a physician arrives at an emergency scene and is properly identified, all care should be turned over to him or her.

_____ **5.** The first step in simple access is to try to get to the patient as quickly as possible using tools or other forcible entry methods.

_____ **6.** You should not try to access the patient until you are sure that the vehicle is stable and that hazards have been identified and rendered safe.

Short Answer

Complete this section with short written answers in the space provided.

1. Explain the four different basic functions that must be addressed at any crash scene.

_____

_____

_____

2. To determine the exact location and position of the patient, what questions should you and your team consider?

_____

_____

_____

3. List the steps for assessing and caring for a patient who is entrapped once access has been gained.

_____

_____

_____

4. When examining the exposed area of the limb or other part of the patient that is trapped, explain what you are assessing.

_____

_____

_____

5. Explain the proper technique for patient removal once the patient is disentangled.

_____

_____

_____

Word Fun EMT-I vocab explorer web

The following crossword puzzle is an activity provided to reinforce correct spelling and understanding of medical terminology associated with emergency care and the EMT-I. Use the clues in the column to complete the puzzle.

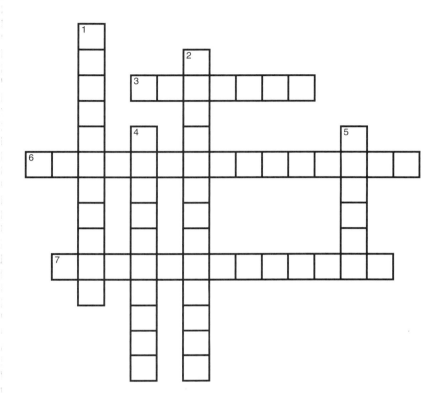

Across

3. Danger zone

6. Cave rescue, dive rescue, etc.

7. Requires tools and special training

Down

1. Removal from trapped area

2. Fire in a house, office, or other building

4. To be caught with no way out

5. Gaining entry to an enclosed area

Ambulance Calls

The following real case scenarios provide an opportunity to explore the concerns associated with patient management. Read each scenario, then answer each question in detail.

1. You are dispatched to the scene of a personal care home where an elderly resident has wandered off into nearby woods. The staff searched for half an hour before calling for assistance. You are in the staging area with the daughter and son-in-law. Staff members told you earlier that the patient has a history of Alzheimer's and some other details they could not remember.

How would you best manage this situation?

_____

_____

_____

_____

_____

_____

_____

_____

2. You are called to the scene of a motor vehicle crash with a 24-year-old male who is pinned underneath the dashboard. Firefighters are setting up the equipment for extrication. The patient is alert but confused, and his breathing is slightly shallow at 24 breaths/min. He has weak radial pulses.

How would you best manage this patient?

_____

_____

_____

_____

_____

_____

_____

_____

3. You are dispatched to a chemical spill where a train car derailed. The patient is the engineer who went back to look at the damage. He is lying beside the tracks and appears to be breathing from your vantage point at the staging area. HazMat team members are suiting up to go in and retrieve the patient. They will decontaminate him before bringing him to the staging area.

How will you best manage this situation and patient?

_____

_____

_____

_____

_____

_____

_____

_____

Workbook Activities

The following activities have been designed to help you. Your instructor may require you to complete some or all of these activities as a regular part of your EMT-I training program. You are encouraged to complete any activity that your instructor does not assign as a way to enhance your learning in the classroom.

Chapter Review

The following exercises provide an opportunity to refresh your knowledge of this chapter.

Matching

Match each of the terms in the left column to the appropriate definition in the right column.

_____ **1.** Mass-casualty incident

_____ **2.** Incident command

_____ **3.** Toxicity level

_____ **4.** Triage

_____ **5.** Chemical transportation

_____ **6.** Protection level

_____ **7.** Casualty collection area

_____ **8.** Disaster

_____ **9.** Hazardous materials

_____ **10.** Rehabilitation area

_____ **11.** Transportation area

_____ **12.** Treatment officer

A. incident in which a hazardous material is no longer properly contained and isolated

B. area where patients can receive further system triage and medical care

C. individual who is in charge of and directs EMS personnel at the treatment area

D. the process of sorting patients based on the severity of injury and medical need, to establish treatment and transportation priorities

E. a measure of the amount and type of protective equipment that an individual needs to avoid injury during contact with a hazardous material

F. provides protection and treatment to firefighters and other personnel working at an emergency

G. area where ambulances and crews are organized

H. an agency that assists emergency personnel in identifying and handling hazardous materials transport incidents

I. widespread event that disrupts community incident resources and functions

J. an emergency situation involving more than one patient, and which can place such demand on equipment or personnel that the system is stretched to its limit or beyond

K. an organizational system to help control, direct, and coordinate emergency responders and resources; known more generally as an incident management system (IMS)

L. a measure of the risk that a hazardous material poses to the health of an individual who comes in contact with it

CHAPTER 36

Special Operations

Multiple Choice

Read each item carefully, then select the best response.

_____ 1. Functions normally centered at the command post include:

   A. information.

   B. safety.

   C. liaison with other agencies and groups that are responding.

   D. all of the above.

_____ 2. In extended operations, the typical incident command structure may have multiple sectors, including:

   A. operations.

   B. planning.

   C. logistics.

   D. all of the above.

_____ 3. With a major airplane crash, the leading agency is typically the:

   A. EMS department.

   B. law enforcement.

   C. fire department.

   D. HazMat team.

_____ 4. The _____ is a holding area for arriving ambulances and crews until they can be assigned a particular task.

   A. staging area

   B. treatment area

   C. transportation area

   D. rehabilitation area

_____ 5. The _____ provides protection and treatment to firefighters and other personnel working at the emergency scene.

   A. staging area

   B. treatment area

   C. transportation area

   D. rehabilitation area

_____ **6.** The _____ is where ambulances and crews are organized to transport patients from the treatment area to local hospitals.

A. staging area

B. treatment area

C. transportation area

D. rehabilitation area

_____ **7.** As patients are loaded into the ambulance, the transport officer logs:

A. each patient's mass-casualty tag number.

B. each patient's overall condition.

C. the hospital to which they will be taken.

D. all of the above.

_____ **8.** The _____ is where a more thorough assessment is made and on-scene treatment is begun while transport is being arranged.

A. staging area

B. treatment area

C. transportation area

D. rehabilitation area

_____ **9.** Examples of mass-casualty incidents include:

A. airplane crashes.

B. earthquakes.

C. railroad crashes.

D. all of the above.

_____ **10.** To make decontaminating the ambulance easier after a HazMat incident:

A. tape the cabinet doors shut.

B. place any equipment that will not be used en route in the front of the truck.

C. turn on the power vent ceiling fan and patient compartment air-conditioning unit fan.

D. all of the above.

_____ **11.** If you are treating and transporting a patient who has not been fully and properly decontaminated, you should do all of the following, except:

A. wear two pairs of gloves.

B. remove goggles.

C. wear a protective coat.

D. wear respiratory protection.

_____ **12.** EMT-Is providing care in the treatment area should assess and treat the patient:

A. as contaminated.

B. with respect.

C. from the point where the previous caregiver left off.

D. in the same way as a patient who has not previously been assessed or treated.

_____ **13.** To avoid entrapment and communication of contaminants, only _____ are applied, until the "clean" patient has been moved to the treatment area.

A. pressure dressings that are needed to control bleeding

B. bandages

C. splints

D. cervical collars

_____ **14.** When a material is hazardous because of its flammability or potential for explosion rather than its toxicity, you will need to be at an even greater distance and behind a windowless wall or other strong barrier that will shield you and others from:

A. heat.

B. the blast force.

C. flying debris.

D. all of the above.

_____ **15.** When toxic gas, fumes, or airborne droplets or particles are involved, the safe area is upwind and at least _____ from the site of any visible cloud or other discharge.

    A. 50'

    B. 100'

    C. 150'

    D. 200'

_____ **16.** If you can see and read the placard or other warning sign, note _____, and, if included, the four-digit number that appears on it or on any orange panel near it.

    A. its color

    B. its wording

    C. any symbols that it contains

    D. all of the above

_____ **17.** Once you have reached a safe place, try to rapidly assess the situation and provide as much information as possible when calling for the HazMat team, including:

    A. your specific location.

    B. the size and shape of the containers of the hazardous material.

    C. what you have observed and been told has occurred.

    D. all of the above.

_____ **18.** In the event of a leak or spill, a hazardous materials incident is often indicated by presence of:

    A. a visible cloud or strange-looking smoke resulting from the escaping substance.

    B. a leak or spill from a tank, etc., with or without HazMat placards or labels.

    C. an unusual, strong, noxious, acrid odor in the area.

    D. all of the above.

_____ **19.** Safety of _____ must be your most important concern.

    A. you and your team

    B. the other responders

    C. the public

    D. all of the above

_____ **20.** In some incidents, a large number of people are _____ and may be injured or killed before the presence of a hazardous materials incident is identified.

    A. transported

    B. exposed

    C. injected

    D. decontaminated

_____ **21.** Often, the presence of hazardous materials is easily recognized from warning signs, placards, or labels found:

    A. on buildings or areas where hazardous materials are produced, used, or stored.

    B. on trucks and railroad cars that carry any amount of hazardous material.

    C. on barrels or boxes that contain hazardous material.

    D. all of the above.

_____ **22.** To provide for interoperability and compatibility among federal, state, and local capabilities, the NIMS will include a core set of concepts, principles, terminology, and technologies covering:

    A. training.

    B. qualifications and certifications.

    C. the incident command system.

    D. all of the above.

_____ **23.** The odors produced during the drug production process in a P-2-P lab can be mistaken for the smell of:

    A. dried cat urine.

    B. cat litter.

    C. rotten garbage.

    D. all of the above.

_____ **24.** Many of the chemicals used in clandestine drug labs are _____ if the proper air-to-product ratio is attained.

    A. inert

    B. gelatinous

    C. explosive

    D. soluble

_____ **25.** Chemicals used in labs can be absorbed into the walls and floors of the building. This can create a potential health hazard that lasts _____ after a lab is dismantled and all chemicals and equipment are removed from the site.

    A. minutes to hours

    B. hours to days

    C. days to weeks

    D. weeks to months

For the remainder of the multiple-choice section, apply the following answers:

    A. First priority (red)

    B. Second priority (yellow)

    C. Third priority (green)

    D. Fourth priority (black)

Classify the following emergencies according to triage priority:

_____ **26.** Shock

_____ **27.** Major or multiple bone or joint injuries

_____ **28.** Cardiac arrest

_____ **29.** Minor fractures

_____ **30.** Decreased level of consciousness

_____ **31.** Obvious death

_____ **32.** Airway and breathing difficulties

_____ **33.** Burns without airway problems

_____ **34.** Major open brain trauma

_____ **35.** Minor soft-tissue injuries

Vocabulary EMT-I vocab explorer web

Define the following terms in the space provided.

1. Command post:

_____

_____

_____

2. Danger zone:

_____

_____

_____

3. Hazardous material:

_____

_____

_____

4. Incident commander:

_____

_____

_____

5. Sector commander:

_____

_____

_____

Fill-in

Read each item carefully, then complete the statement by filling in the missing word(s).

1. The _____ _____ _____ is more effective when used to organize large numbers of personnel at complex incidents such as hazardous materials spills and mass-casualty incidents.

2. The incident commander usually remains at a _____ _____, the designated field command center.

3. The _____ _____ is responsible for protecting all personnel and any victims of the incident.

4. When you arrive at the scene of a possible _____ _____ _____, you must first step back and assess the situation.

5. If patients are entrapped, _____ is required.

6. A _____ is a widespread event that disrupts functions and resources of a community and threatens lives and property.

7. _____ is the sorting of patients based on the severity of their conditions to establish priorities for care based on available resources.

8. The _____ _____ is a sorting point, run by a _____

_____, where each patient is assessed and tagged according to their injuries.

9. Transporting a _____ patient merely increases the size of the event.

10. Most serious injuries and deaths from hazardous materials result from _____ and

_____ problems.

11. _____ is the process of removing or neutralizing and properly disposing of hazardous

materials from equipment, patients, and rescue personnel.

12. When dealing with a HazMat situation, be sure to check the wind direction periodically, and

_____ if a change in wind direction dictates.

13. The _____ _____ manages the transportation area and assigns patients

to waiting ambulances.

14. Some substances are not hazardous; however, when mixed with another substance, they may become

_____ or volatile.

15. When you enter a building or vehicle to treat an overdose victim, look for glassware and other

fundamental items that you might find in a _____ _____ laboratory.

16. In most cases, the package or tank must contain a certain amount of a hazardous material before a

_____ is required.

17. All personnel and equipment used at the scene of an illegal drug lab will be _____.

18. The incident command post is located in the _____ zone.

19. Everyone and everything must be _____ before leaving the hot zone.

20. When a fire or chemical spill is involved, consider evacuating people _____ from the

incident.

21. An ALS unit should be assigned to all clandestine drug lab operations to monitor everyone working in

the _____ _____.

22. _____ is a powerful CNS stimulant that can be injected, snorted, smoked, or swallowed.

True/False

If you believe the statement to be more true than false, write the letter "T" in the space provided. If you believe
the statement to be more false than true, write the letter "F."

_____ 1. When you are responding to a hazardous materials incident, you must first take time to
accurately assess the scene.

_____ 2. Moving patients from the contaminated area is your main responsibility in a hazardous
materials situation.

_____ **3.** Toxicity level 1 is more dangerous than level 4.

_____ **4.** Protective clothing level A is the least level of protection.

_____ **5.** Patients with major or multiple bone or joint injuries should be assigned to the second priority triage category.

_____ **6.** Patients with severe burns should be assigned to the black triage category.

_____ **7.** A large number of hazardous gases and fluids are essentially odorless.

_____ **8.** Only the original patients who leave the hazard zone must pass through the decontamination area.

_____ **9.** Most hazardous materials have specific antidotes or treatments for exposure.

_____ **10.** The volatile nature and toxic effects of the chemicals involved decreases the physical danger for emergency services personnel who may not realize the incident involves an illicit drug operation.

_____ **11.** The success of any incident command system depends on all personnel performing their assigned tasks and working within the system.

_____ **12.** All of the necessary ingredients for producing methamphetamine can be purchased at any discount department store, and recipes are available over the Internet.

_____ **13.** When material is hazardous because of its flammability or potential for explosion rather than its toxicity, the damage or hazard zone is smaller.

_____ **14.** A portable radio transmission may activate an explosive device.

_____ **15.** The runoff of contaminated water produced by suppression efforts will not cause any ecological damage.

_____ **16.** Higher doses and chronic use of methamphetamines will produce irritability and paranoia.

Short Answer

Complete this section with short written answers in the space provided.

1. Define the five levels of toxicity as classified by the NFPA.

_____

_____

_____

2. Describe the four levels of protection and the type of protective gear required for each level.

_____

_____

_____

3. List the eight major EMS-related positions within an incident command system.

_____

_____

_____

4. List and define the four triage priorities.

_____

_____

_____

5. For each of the following hazardous materials classifications, list the general category of hazard.

Class	Type
Class 1	
Class 2	
Class 3	
Class 4	
Class 5	
Class 6	
Class 7	
Class 8	
Class 9	

6. Define and describe the process of decontamination and the decontamination area.

_____

_____

_____

7. List the components of the NIMS that work together as a system to provide a national framework for preparing for, preventing, responding to, and recovering from domestic incidents.

_____

_____

_____

8. To protect the operation, operators of clandestine drug labs set booby traps. List three outside mechanisms and three inside traps.

_____

_____

_____

9. List five symptoms associated with exposure to toxic chemicals.

_____

_____

_____

Word Fun EMT-I vocab explorer web

The following crossword puzzle is an activity provided to reinforce correct spelling and understanding of medical terminology associated with emergency care and the EMT-I. Use the clues in the column to complete the puzzle.

Across

1. Measures of health risk of a substance
4. Determines amount of gear to be worn around a given hazard
6. Area of least safety, exposure to harm possible
7. Where patients are reassessed, treated, and monitored until transport

Down

2. Responsible for sorting of patients
3. Designated field command center
5. Sorting by priority

Ambulance Calls

The following real case scenarios will give you an opportunity to explore the concerns associated with patient management. Read each scenario, then answer each question in detail.

1. You are dispatched to a multi-vehicle crash where you encounter three patients: a 4-year-old man with bilateral femur fractures and absent radial pulse, a 27-year-old woman with a laceration to the head and a humerus fracture, and a 42-year-old man who is apneic and pulseless with an open skull fracture. How should you triage these patients?

_____

_____

_____

_____

_____

_____

_____

2. You respond to an overturned vehicle to find a tanker truck lying on its side with a white liquid pooling underneath. The driver is still restrained and is not moving. You see blood on the side of his head that faces you. There are no placards visible on the vehicle.

How would you best manage this situation?

_____

_____

_____

_____

_____

_____

_____

3. You are called to transport patients from a hazardous materials spill at a local chemical plant. The patients have gone through a partial decontamination, but are not "clean."

How would you best manage this situation?

_____

_____

_____

_____

_____

_____

_____

4. You are called to a person down on the front porch of a residence found by law enforcement officers who were on scene to serve a warrant for the arrest of a known drug dealer. There is a strong odor of ammonia, similar to strong cat urine, emanating from the residence. You notice that the windows of the residence are covered with cardboard, and the officers tell you that the kitchen looks like a chemical laboratory.

What steps should you take, and which agencies should be notified?

_____

_____

_____

_____

_____

_____

_____

_____

Workbook Activities

The following activities have been designed to help you. Your instructor may require you to complete some or all of these activities as a regular part of your EMT-I training program. You are encouraged to complete any activity that your instructor does not assign as a way to enhance your learning in the classroom.

Chapter Review

The following exercises provide an opportunity to refresh your knowledge of this chapter.

Matching

Match each of the terms in the left column to the appropriate definition in the right column.

_____ **1.** Domestic terrorists

_____ **2.** Persistency

_____ **3.** Mutagen

_____ **4.** Covert

_____ **5.** Pulmonary agents

_____ **6.** Contamination

_____ **7.** Vapor hazard

_____ **8.** Nerve agents

_____ **9.** Chemical agents

_____ **10.** Incubation

_____ **11.** Secondary device

_____ **12.** Volatility

_____ **13.** Contact hazard

_____ **14.** Bacteria

_____ **15.** Biologic agents

_____ **16.** Anthrax

_____ **17.** Smallpox

_____ **18.** Cross contamination

_____ **19.** Viruses

_____ **20.** Viral hemorrhagic fevers

A. organisms that cause disease

B. do not require a host to live

C. enters the body through the skin

D. deadly bacterium that lays dormant in a spore

E. man-made substance that can have devastating effects on living organisms

F. Ebola, Rift Valley and Yellow fever

G. direct contact with WMD or exposure to it

H. native citizens that carry out terrorism against their own country

I. remains on a surface for a long period of time

J. germs that require a living host to multiply

K. public safety community has no prior knowledge of time, location, or nature of attack

L. evaporates relatively quickly

M. contact with contaminated persons

N. immediate harm when exposed to them

O. enters the body through the respiratory tract

P. set to explode after the initial bomb

Q. mutates, damages, or destroys structure of the cells

R. the most deadly chemicals developed

S. period between exposure and symptoms

T. lesions are identical in size and shape

CHAPTER 37

Response to Terrorism and Weapons of Mass Destruction

_____ **1.** Examples of groups that turn toward terrorism as a means of achieving their goals are:

    A. violent religious groups.

    B. extremists political groups.

    C. technology terrorists.

    D. all of the above.

_____ **2.** The primary route of exposure to vesicants is:

    A. oral.

    B. respiratory.

    C. skin contact.

    D. all of the above.

_____ **3.** The military designation for phosgene is:

    A. H.

    B. CX.

    C. L.

    D. CL.

_____ **4.** Signs of vesicant exposure include all of the following EXCEPT:

    A. swollen, closed eyes.

    B. gray discoloration of the skin.

    C. painless blistering.

    D. reddening of the skin.

_____ **5.** If vesicant vapors are inhaled, the patient may experience:

    A. hoarseness.

    B. severe cough.

    C. hemoptysis.

    D. all of the above.

_____ **6.** Absorption of sulfur mustard through the skin or mucous membranes occurs within seconds, and the damage to cells takes place within:

    A. 1 to 2 minutes.

    B. 1 to 2 hours.

    C. 1 to 2 days.

    D. 1 to 2 weeks.

_____ **7.** On the surface, the patient will generally not produce any signs and symptoms from mustard exposure for:

A. 4 to 6 minutes.

B. 4 to 6 hours.

C. 4 to 6 days.

D. 4 to 6 weeks.

1999 _____ **8.** Treatment for a patient exposed to a vesicant includes all of the following EXCEPT:

A. decontamination before ABCs.

B. ABCs then decontamination.

C. early intubation and cardiac monitoring.

D. analgesics.

_____ **9.** The first chemical used in warfare was _____.

A. mustard.

B. phosgene.

C. Lewisite.

D. chlorine.

_____ **10.** Phosgene is:

A. a chemical produced for warfare.

B. a product of combustion that might be produced in a house fire.

C. produced by burning freon refrigerant..

D. all of the above.

1999 _____ **11.** Treatment for exposure to pulmonary agents includes all of the following EXCEPT:

A. performing ABCs and gaining IV access.

B. placing the patient in a comfortable position with the head elevated.

C. analgesics.

D. early intubation and ECG monitoring.

_____ **12.** Sarin is primarily a:

A. vapor hazard.

B. contact hazard.

C. blistering hazard.

D. none of the above.

_____ **13.** Soman is twice as persistent as sarin and _____ as lethal.

A. 2 times.

B. 5 times.

C. 50 tmes.

D. 200 times.

_____ **14.** Under the proper conditions, VX will remain relatively unchanged for:

A. minutes to hours.

B. hours to days.

C. days to weeks.

D. weeks to months.

_____ **15.** The medical mnemonic DUMBELS is used to describe the symptoms of nerve agent exposure. The "S" refers to:

A. seizures.

B. sweating.

C. salivation.

D. all of the above.

_____ **16.** _____ is derived from the mash that is left from the castor bean.
   A. Botulinum
   B. VX
   C. Ricin
   D. Anthrax

_____ **17.** _____ rays cannot travel fast or through most objects.
   A. Alpha
   B. Beta
   C. Gamma
   D. Neutron

_____ **18.** _____ rays require a layer of clothing to stop them.
   A. Alpha
   B. Beta
   C. Gamma
   D. Neutron

_____ **19.** _____ rays penetrate the human body.
   A. Alpha
   B. Beta
   C. Gamma
   D. Neutron

_____ **20.** Radioactive wastes can be found at:
   A. hospitals.
   B. colleges and universities.
   C. chemical and industrial sites.
   D. all of the above.

_____ **21.** The best way to protect yourself from the effects of radiation is to use:
   A. time.
   B. distance.
   C. shielding.
   D. all of the above.

Vocabulary EMT-I vocab explorer web

Define the following terms in the space provided.

1. Weapons of mass destruction:

_____

_____

_____

2. Weaponization:

_____

_____

_____

3. Off-gassing:

_____

_____

_____

4. Dissemination:

_____

_____

_____

5. Syndromic surveillance:

_____

_____

_____

6. Points of distribution:

_____

_____

_____

7. Special atomic demolition munitions:

_____

_____

_____

Fill-in

Read each item carefully, then complete the statement by filling in the missing word(s).

1. The EMT-I must be _____ and _____ prepared for the possibility of a

terrorist attack.

2. The best location for staging at a WMD scene is _____ and _____ from

the incident.

3. As with burns, the primary complication associated with vesicant blisters is _____

_____.

4. The components used to manufacture _____ are easy to acquire, and the agent is easy

to manufacture.

5. The seizures associated with nerve agent exposure are unlike those found in patients with a history of seizures. The patient will continue to seize until _____.

6. The MARK 1 kit contains _____ and _____, which are antidotes for nerve agent exposure.

7. _____ is a gas that smells like almonds.

8. _____ _____ infects the lymphatic system while _____ _____ is a lung infection.

9. _____ is the most potent neurotoxin.

10. The destructive capabilities of a dirty bomb is limited to the _____ that are attached to it.

True/False

If you believe the statement to be more true than false, write the letter "T" in the space provided. If you believe the statement to be more false than true, write the letter "F."

_____ **1.** When dealing with a WMD scene, it is safe to assume that you will not be able to enter where the event has occurred.

_____ **2.** There may be more than one type of device or agent present at a WMD scene.

_____ **3.** Sulfur mustard is not very persistent.

_____ **4.** The fluid from blisters of a patient exposed to sulfur mustard contains small amounts of the chemical.

_____ **5.** Phosgene and Lewisite are highly volatile and have a rapid onset of symptoms.

_____ **6.** There are no known antidotes to counteract the pulmonary agents.

_____ **7.** Miosis is the most common symptom of nerve agent exposure and can remain for days to weeks.

_____ **8.** Atropine eliminates nerve agents from the body and 2-PAM chloride blocks the effects of nerve agents.

`1999` _____ **9.** When treating the patient exposed to cyanide, place the patient on the cardiac monitor and consider early intubation.

_____ **10.** The sense of smell is a poor tool to use to determine whether there is a chemical agent present.

_____ **11.** Nuclear energy is artificially made by altering radioactive atoms.

_____ **12.** Being exposed to a radiation source makes a patient contaminated and radioactive.

Short Answer

Complete this section with short written answers in the space provided.

1. List four forms of chemical agents.

_____

_____

_____

2. List three types of biologic agents.

_____

_____

_____

3. In determining the potential for a terrorist attack, on every call you should observe:

_____

_____

_____

4. List the common signs of acute radiation sickness.

Low exposure:

_____

Moderate exposure:

_____

Severe exposure:

_____

Word Fun EMT-I vocab explorer web

The following crossword puzzle is an activity provided to reinforce correct spelling and understanding of medical terminology associated with emergency care and the EMT-I. Use the clues in the column to complete the puzzle.

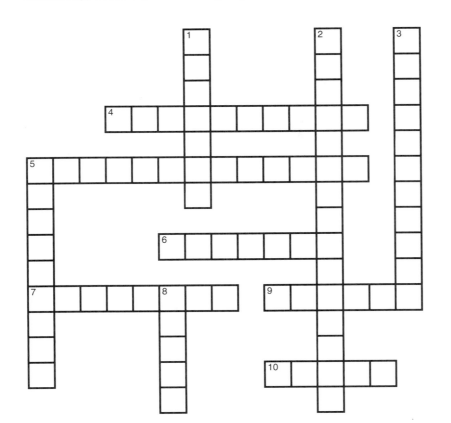

Across

4. How long a chemical will stay on a surface

5. Animal that spreads a disease to other animals

6. Lays dormant in spores

7. Does not require a living host to survive

9. Bilateral pinpoint pupils

10. Requires a living host to multiply

Down

1. Damages and changes the structures of DNA

2. Manner by which a toxic substance enters the body

3. Organophosphates

5. Used as a radiological dispersal device

8. Derived from the castor bean

Ambulance Calls

The following real case scenarios provide an opportunity to explore the concerns associated with patient management. Read each scenario, then answer each question in detail.

1. You are called to the local shopping mall for a man down in the food court. As you enter the mall, you are told there are now five patients that are unresponsive.

   What is the best way to manage this situation?

   _____

   _____

   _____

   _____

   _____

   _____

   _____

2. You are working for a hospital based ambulance service where you are frequently called to assist in the emergency room. Over the last hour, three patients have needed x-rays. The nurse on duty asks you to assist in holding a patient but does not have a spare apron for you to wear.

   How would you best manage this situation?

   _____

   _____

   _____

   _____

   _____

   _____

   _____

Workbook Activities

The following activities have been designed to help you. Your instructor may require you to complete some or all of these activities as a regular part of your EMT-I training program. You are encouraged to complete any activity that your instructor does not assign as a way to enhance your learning in the classroom.

Chapter Review

The following exercises provide an opportunity to refresh your knowledge of this chapter.

Matching

Match each of the terms in the left column to the appropriate definition in the right column.

_____ **1.** Field impression	**A.** expected findings that are absent
_____ **2.** Assessment	**B.** carrying the right equipment to the patient
_____ **3.** Dynamic	**C.** working diagnosis
_____ **4.** Pertinent negatives	**D.** foundation of patient care
_____ **5.** "Right stuff"	**E.** continuously changing

Multiple Choice

Read each item carefully, then select the best response.

_____ **1.** Regardless of the type of call, you must:
- **A.** evaluate the scene.
- **B.** evaluate the patient's condition.
- **C.** make the appropriate choices for patient care and transportation.
- **D.** all of the above.

_____ **2.** Oftentimes, _____ of the diagnosis is attributed to the patient's history.
- **A.** 50%
- **B.** 60%
- **C.** 70%
- **D.** 80%

_____ **3.** You should gather information from:
- **A.** the environment.
- **B.** history.
- **C.** patient status.
- **D.** all of the above.

Assessment-Based Management

_____ **4.** In a mass-casualty situation the _____ acts as the triage group leader.

    A. patient care person

    B. transportation officer

    C. team leader

    D. safety officer

_____ **5.** Even though the patient may have an extensive _____, make sure you are focused toward the systems associated with the current complaint and any associated problems.

    A. medicine collection

    B. knowledge

    C. history

    D. family present

_____ **6.** In order to be effective in gathering information, you must have a good understanding of _____ disease processes.

    A. various

    B. infectious

    C. communicable

    D. minor

_____ **7.** On calls that involve ACLS intervention, the team leader:

    A. reads the ECG.

    B. relays information on the radio.

    C. controls the drug box.

    D. all of the above.

_____ **8.** During the _____ phase of the initial assessment, the team leader also designates who will perform critical interventions and actively participates in patient care.

    A. scene survey

    B. resuscitative

    C. vital signs

    D. restorative

_____ **9.** "Labels" applied by responders sometimes:

    A. set an inappropriate tone.

    B. are distracting.

    C. cause biased assessment.

    D. all of the above.

_____ **10.** The _____ assessment sets the tone for the patient encounter.

    A. secondary

    B. initial

    C. tertiary

    D. focused

_____ **11.** Immediate evacuation to the ambulance may be required if:

    A. the patient needs lifesaving interventions that cannot be provided by the EMT-I.

    B. the scene is unsafe.

    C. the scene is too unstable or chaotic to allow for an effective and accurate assessment.

    D. all of the above.

_____ **12.** It is impossible to get an accurate history by:

    A. proxy.

    B. audience participation.

    C. committee.

    D. family interviews.

_____ **13.** _____ is not necessarily in direct proportion to the life-threat potential.

    A. Pain severity

    B. Blood loss

    C. Angulation

    D. Vocal ability

_____ **14.** The key to developing _____ is repetition and understanding the format.

    A. confidence

    B. proficiency

    C. integrity

    D. security

Vocabulary EMT-I vocab explorer web

Define the following terms in the space provided.

    1. Multitasking:

_____

_____

_____

    2. ABCDEs:

_____

_____

_____

Fill-in

Read each item carefully, then complete the statement by filling in the missing word(s).

1. Your assessment and _____ _____ may be all that is standing between

 the patient and morbidity or mortality.

2. You must be able to accurately assess not only the patient but the _____ as well.

3. _____ is the foundation of patient care.

4. You must work in the capacity of a _____ _____ and put together the

 clues that you find.

5. _____ is the key to expanding your knowledge base.

6. When you are assessing a patient, look for _____.

7. Members of the EMS team need to have a _____ for determining roles.

8. The _____ _____ generally manages patient care throughout the call.

9. Use the initial scene size-up to gather clues and help formulate an _____.

10. The patient may not be able to rate your medical performance, but he or she can rate your

 _____ skills.

11. As _____ of the physician's authority, EMT-Is must contact their supervising physician

 for orders at one time or another.

True/False

If you believe the statement to be more true than false, write the letter "T" in the space provided. If you believe the statement to be more false than true, write the letter "F."

_____ 1. The goal of practice sessions should be to choreograph the EMS response team.

_____ 2. Medical conditions or the medication taken for those conditions will not interfere with or mask signs and symptoms of the current problem.

_____ 3. The number of responders on scene often makes effective assessment challenging.

_____ 4. You must learn how to adapt your treatment for the problem presented.

_____ 5. By designating roles, confusion on scene is maximized.

_____ 6. As an EMT-I you must assure that your attitude is nonjudgmental.

_____ 7. The most obvious problems are often the most life threatening.

_____ 8. The patient will lose confidence if you have to run back and forth to the ambulance to obtain necessary equipment.

Short Answer

Complete this section with short written answers in the space provided.

1. Explain what is meant by "tunnel vision."

_____

_____

_____

2. List the roles of the team leader.

_____

_____

_____

3. List the roles of the patient care person(s).

_____

_____

_____

4. In all uncooperative, restless, belligerent patients, what possible causes should you consider?

_____

_____

_____

5. Immediate intervention is required for any patient with a life-threatening problem such as:

_____

_____

_____

Word Fun EMT-I vocab explorer web

The following crossword puzzle is an activity provided to reinforce correct spelling and understanding of medical terminology associated with emergency care and the EMT-I. Use the clues in the column to complete the puzzle.

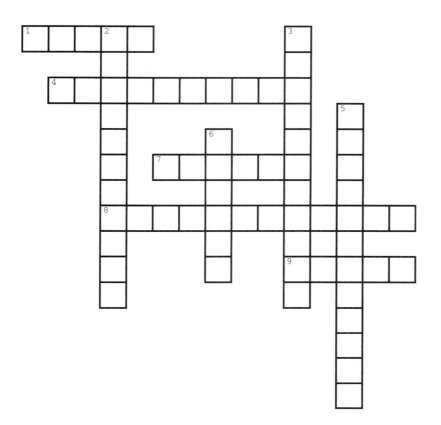

Across

1. Mnemonic for initial survey
4. Foundation of patient care
7. Slang for National Registry or state-approved test
8. Causes distraction
9. Provides for an organized and concise report

Down

2. Obvious injuries that may look bad
3. Causes a rush to judgment too early
5. Doing multiple things simultaneously
6. Set inappropriate tone; cause biased assessment

Ambulance Calls

The following real case scenarios will give you an opportunity to explore the concerns associated with patient management. Read each scenario, then answer each question in detail.

1. You are called to the scene of a "person down" in an office. According to bystanders, there was a crash that came from "Mary's" cubicle and they found her on the floor. No one knows her medical history. Your general impression is of a woman in her late 30s who appears to be incontinent and is lying on her side with dried blood around her mouth. The objects on the top of her desk are overturned. She is diaphoretic and breathing heavily.

Based on the patterns presented, what is your field impression of this patient and how should she be managed?

_____

_____

_____

_____

_____

_____

_____

_____

2. You are called to the local playground for an unresponsive teenage boy with a possible leg fracture. Upon arrival you find a 16-year-old boy with obvious angulation and deformity of the right thigh with minimal bleeding.

How will you proceed with your assessment and treatment?

_____

_____

_____

_____

_____

_____

_____

_____

3. You are called to the scene of a busy restaurant at rush hour for a 72-year-old woman in cardiac arrest. As you and your partner work with the patient, bystanders question what you are doing and why. Several children have gathered around and are looking through your jump kit.

How can you best manage this situation?

_____

_____

_____

_____

_____

_____

_____

_____

Workbook Activities

The following activities have been designed to help you. Your instructor may require you to complete some or all of these activities as a regular part of your EMT-I training program. You are encouraged to complete any activity that your instructor does not assign as a way to enhance your learning in the classroom.

Chapter Review

The following exercises provide an opportunity to refresh your knowledge of this chapter.

Matching

Match each of the terms in the left column to the appropriate definition in the right column.

_____ **1.** Artificial ventilation

_____ **2.** Abdominal-thrust maneuver

_____ **3.** Basic life support (BLS)

_____ **4.** Advanced life support

_____ **5.** Cardiopulmonary resuscitation

A. steps used to establish artificial ventilation and circulation in a patient who is not breathing and has no pulse

B. noninvasive emergency lifesaving care used maneuver for patients in respiratory or cardiac arrest

C. procedures such as cardiac monitoring, starting IV fluids, and using advanced airway adjuncts

D. a method of dislodging food or other material from the throat of a choking victim

E. use of CPR to open the airway and restore breathing by mouth-to-mask ventilation and/or the use of mechanical devices

Multiple Choice

Read each item carefully, then select the best response.

_____ **1.** Basic life support is noninvasive emergency lifesaving care that is used to treat:

    A. airway obstruction.

    B. respiratory arrest.

    C. cardiac arrest.

    D. all of the above.

_____ **2.** Exhaled gas from you to the patient contains _____ oxygen.

    A. 8%

    B. 12%

    C. 16%

    D. 21%

BLS Review

_____ **3.** BLS differs from advanced life support, involving advanced lifesaving procedures that include all of the following EXCEPT:

 A. cardiac monitoring.

 B. mouth-to-mouth.

 C. administration of IV fluids and medications.

 D. use of advanced airway adjuncts.

_____ **4.** In some instances such as _____, early BLS measures may be all that a patient needs to be resuscitated.

 A. choking

 B. near drowning

 C. lightning injuries

 D. all of the above

_____ **5.** In addition to checking level of consciousness, it is also important to protect the _____ from further injury while assessing the patient and performing CPR.

 A. spinal cord

 B. ribs

 C. internal organs

 D. facial structures

_____ **6.** In most cases, cardiac arrest in children younger than 9 years results from:

 A. choking.

 B. aspiration.

 C. congenital heart disease.

 D. respiratory arrest.

_____ **7.** Causes of respiratory arrest in infants and children include:

 A. aspiration of foreign bodies.

 B. airway infections.

 C. sudden infant death syndrome (SIDS).

 D. all of the above.

_____ **8.** Signs of irreversible or biological death include clinical death, along with:

 A. rigor mortis.

 B. dependent lividity.

 C. decapitation.

 D. all of the above.

_____ **9.** Once you begin CPR in the field, you must continue until:

    A. the fire department arrives.

    B. the funeral home arrives.

    C. a physician arrives who assumes responsibility.

    D. law enforcement arrives and assumes responsibility.

_____ **10.** Once the patient is properly positioned, you can easily assess:

    A. the airway.

    B. breathing.

    C. disability.

    D. all of the above.

_____ **11.** The chin lift has the added advantage of holding _____ in place, making obstruction by the lips less likely.

    A. loose dentures

    B. the tongue

    C. the mandible

    D. the maxilla

_____ **12.** To perform a _____, place your fingers behind the angles of the patient's lower jaw and then move the jaw forward.

    A. head tilt–chin lift maneuver

    B. jaw-thrust maneuver

    C. tongue–jaw lift maneuver

    D. all of the above

_____ **13.** Providing slow, deliberate ventilations prevents:

    A. overexpansion of the lungs.

    B. rupture of the bronchial tree.

    C. gastric distention.

    D. rupture of the alveoli.

_____ **14.** A _____ is an opening that connects the trachea directly to the skin.

    A. tracheostomy

    B. stoma

    C. laryngectomy

    D. none of the above

_____ **15.** The _____ position helps to maintain a clear airway in a patient with a decreased level of consciousness who has not had traumatic injuries and is breathing on his or her own.

    A. recovery

    B. lithotomy

    C. Trendelenburg's

    D. Fowler's

_____ **16.** Excessive pressure applied to the carotid artery can:

    A. obstruct the carotid circulation.

    B. dislodge blood clots.

    C. produce marked reflex slowing of heart rate.

    D. all of the above.

_____ **17.** The lower tip of the breastbone is the:

    A. xiphoid process.

    B. sternum.

    C. manubrium.

    D. intercostal space.

_____ **18.** Complications from chest compressions can include:

    A. fractured ribs.

    B. a lacerated liver.

    C. a fractured sternum.

    D. all of the above.

_____ **19.** When checking for a pulse in an infant, you should palpate the _____ artery.

    A. radial

    B. brachial

    C. carotid

    D. femoral

_____ **20.** The technique for chest compressions in infants and children differs because of a number of anatomic differences, including:

    A. the position of the heart.

    B. the size of the chest.

    C. the fragile organs.

    D. all of the above.

_____ **21.** The rate of compressions for an infant is about _____ compressions per minute.

    A. 70

    B. 80

    C. 90

    D. 100

_____ **22.** The rate of compression to ventilation for infants and children is _____ for two-rescuer CPR.

    A. 1:5

    B. 5:1

    C. 15:2

    D. 2:15

_____ **23.** Sudden airway obstruction is usually easy to recognize in someone who is eating or has just finished eating because they suddenly:

    A. are unable to speak or cough.

    B. turn cyanotic.

    C. make exaggerated efforts to breathe.

    D. all of the above.

_____ **24.** You should suspect an airway obstruction in the unresponsive patient if:

    A. the standard maneuvers to open the airway and ventilate the lungs are not effective.

    B. you feel resistance to blowing into the patient's lungs.

    C. pressure builds up in your mouth.

    D. all of the above.

_____ **25.** You should use _____ for women in advanced stages of pregnancy, patients who are very obese, and children younger than 1 year.

    A. the Heimlich maneuver

    B. chest thrusts

    C. the abdominal-thrust maneuver

    D. any of the above

_____ **26.** For a patient with a mild (partial) airway obstruction, you should:

    A. perform the Heimlich maneuver.

    B. attempt a finger sweep to remove the foreign body.

    C. not interfere with the patient's attempt to expel the foreign body.

    D. all of the above.

_____ **27.** Most out-of-hospital cardiac arrests occur as the result of a sudden cardiac rhythm disturbance (dysrhythmia) such as:

   A. sinus tachycardia.

   B. ventricular fibrillation.

   C. atrial fibrillation.

   D. asystole.

Vocabulary EMT-I vocab explorer web

Define the following terms in the space provided.

1. Gastric distention:

_____

_____

_____

2. Head tilt–chin lift maneuver:

_____

_____

_____

3. Jaw-thrust maneuver:

_____

_____

_____

4. Recovery position:

_____

_____

_____

5. Asynchronous CPR:

_____

_____

_____

Fill-in

Read each item carefully, then complete the statement by filling in the missing word(s).

1. Permanent brain damage may occur if the brain is without oxygen for _____ to

_____ minutes.

2. CPR does not require any equipment; however, you should use a _____ device to

perform rescue breathing.

3. Because of the urgent need to start CPR in a pulseless, nonbreathing patient, you must complete an

initial assessment as soon as possible, evaluating the patient's _____.

4. Infants and children have smaller _____ than adults.

5. Although _____ arrest in adults usually occurs before _____ arrest, the

reverse is true in infants and children.

6. _____ _____, such as living wills, may express the patient's wishes, but

these documents are not binding for all health care providers.

7. For CPR to be effective, the patient must be lying supine on a _____ surface.

8. Without an open _____, rescue breathing will not be effective.

9. Early _____ is the link in the chain of survival that is most likely to improve survival

rates.

True/False

If you believe the statement to be more true than false, write the letter "T" in the space provided. If you believe
the statement to be more false than true, write the letter "F."

_____ **1.** During the initial assessment, you need to quickly evaluate the patient's airway, breathing,
circulation, and level of consciousness.

_____ **2.** All unresponsive patients need all elements of BLS.

_____ **3.** A patient who is not fully conscious often needs some degree of BLS.

_____ **4.** The recovery position should be used to maintain an open airway in a patient with a head or
spinal injury.

_____ **5.** You should always remove a patient's dentures before initiating artificial ventilation.

_____ **6.** You should not start CPR if the patient has obvious signs of irreversible death.

_____ **7.** After you apply pressure to depress the sternum, you must follow with an equal period of
relaxation so that the chest returns to normal position.

_____ **8.** The ratio of compressions to ventilations for one-person CPR on an adult is 2:1.

_____ **9.** When performed correctly, external chest compressions provide 50% of the blood normally
pumped by the heart.

_____ **10.** For infants, the preferred technique of artificial ventilation is mouth-to-nose-and-mouth
ventilation with a mask or other barrier device.

_____ **11.** You need to use less ventilatory pressure to inflate a child's lungs because the airway is smaller
than that of an adult.

_____ **12.** For each minute the patient remains in V-fib or pulseless V-tach, there is a 7% to 10% smaller chance of survival.

_____ **13.** The AED should not be applied to the patient with traumatic cardiac arrest.

Short Answer

Complete this section with short written answers in the space provided.

1. List the four obvious signs of death, in addition to absence of pulse and breathing, that are used as a general rule to not start CPR.

_____

_____

_____

2. Complete the following table regarding pediatric BLS by listing the procedure parameters or guidelines for each age group as they relate to the action noted on the left.

Procedure	Infants (younger than 1 y)	Children (1 y to onset of puberty)
Airway		
Breathing		
Initial breaths		
Subsequent breaths		
Circulation		
Pulse check		
Compression area		
Compression width		
Compression depth		
Compression rate		
Ratio of compressions to ventilations		
Foreign body obstruction		

3. List the four acceptable reasons for stopping CPR.

_____

_____

_____

4. Describe how to perform a head tilt–chin lift maneuver.

_____

_____

_____

5. Describe how to perform a jaw-thrust maneuver.

_____

_____

_____

6. Describe the "two thumb–encircling hands technique" for performing two-rescuer infant CPR.

_____

_____

_____

7. Describe the process of chest compressions during one-rescuer adult CPR.

_____

_____

_____

8. List and describe the method for "switching positions" during two-rescuer adult CPR.

_____

_____

_____

9. Describe the process of abdominal thrusts for a standing patient and a supine patient.

_____

_____

_____

10. Describe the process for chest thrusts on a standing and a supine patient.

_____

_____

_____

11. Describe the process for removing a foreign body airway obstruction in an infant.

_____

_____

_____

Word Fun EMT-I

The following crossword puzzle is an activity provided to reinforce correct spelling and understanding of medical terminology associated with emergency care and the EMT-I. Use the clues in the column to complete the puzzle.

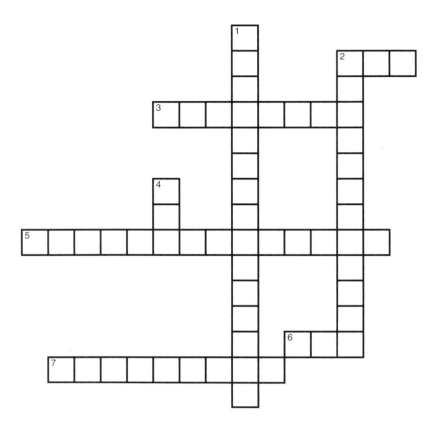

Across

2. High level of care, beyond basic

3. Position after patient regains consciousness

5. Link most likely to improve survival rates

6. First level of care

7. Opening airway by moving lower bone forcibly forward

Down

1. Preferred method to remove airway obstruction

2. CPR without a pause in compressions for ventilation

4. Chest compression and artificial ventilation

Ambulance Calls

The following real case scenarios provide an opportunity to explore the concerns associated with patient management. Read each scenario, then answer each question in detail.

1. You are dispatched to a "person down." The dispatcher informs you that the caller said the patient is not breathing. On arrival, you find a 78-year-old female in bed, apneic and pulseless. In the process of moving the patient to place a CPR board underneath her, you note the discoloration of her back and hips known as dependent lividity.

How would you best manage this patient?

_____

_____

_____

_____

_____

_____

_____

2. You are called to a business office downtown where CPR is in progress. On arrival, you immediately attach the pads of the AED to the patient while your partner checks the airway. He advises you that the patient is now breathing and palpation reveals a faint radial pulse.

How would you best manage this patient?

_____

_____

_____

_____

_____

_____

_____

3. You arrive on the scene of a possible cardiac arrest to find a 48-year-old male with no related medical history, apneic and pulseless. Bystanders tell you he was breathing up until about 3 minutes ago.

How would you best manage this patient?

_____

_____

_____

_____

_____

_____

_____

Skill Drills EMT-I video clips web

Skill Drill 39-1: Positioning the Patient

Test your by placing the photos below in the correct order. Number the first step with a "1," the second step with a "2," etc.

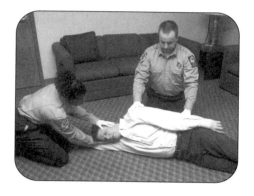

_____

Move the head and neck as a unit with the torso as your partner pulls on the distant shoulder and hip.

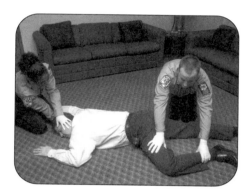

_____

Kneel beside the patient, leaving room to roll the patient toward you.

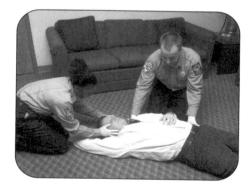

_____

Move the patient to a supine position with legs straight and arms at the sides.

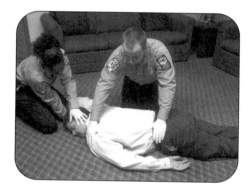

_____

Grasp the patient, stabilizing the cervical spine if needed.

Skill Drill 39-2: Performing Chest Compressions

Test your knowledge by filling in the correct words in the photo captions.

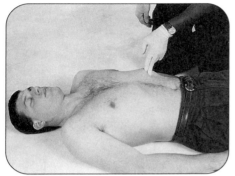

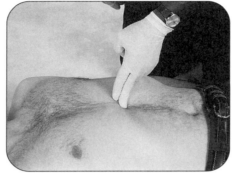

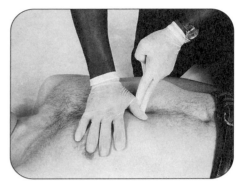

1. Slide your _____ and _____ fingers along the rib cage to the _____ in the center of the chest.

2. Push the middle finger high into the notch, and lay the index finger on the _____ _____ of the sternum.

3. Place the _____ of the second hand on the lower half of the sternum, touching the _____ _____ of your first hand.

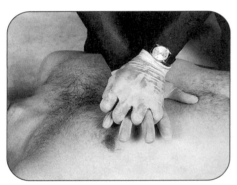

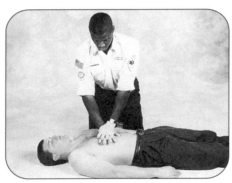

4. Remove your first hand from the notch, and place it over the _____ on the sternum.

5. With your arms straight, _____ your elbows, and position your shoulders directly _____ your hands. Depress the sternum _____ inch(es) to _____ inch(es) using a rhythmic motion.

Skill Drill 39-3: Performing One-Rescuer Adult CPR

Test your knowledge by placing the photos below in the correct order. Number the first step with a "1," the second step with a "2," etc.

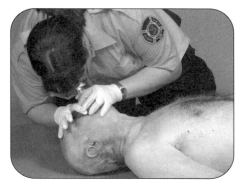

_____

If not breathing, give two breaths of 1 second each.

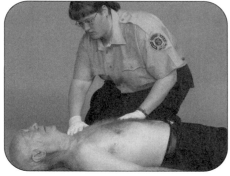

_____

Establish unresponsiveness, and call for help.

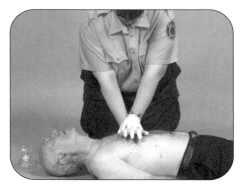

_____

If no pulse is found, apply your AED.

If there is no AED, place your hands in the proper position for chest compressions.

Give 30 compressions at about 100/min.

Open the airway, and give two ventilations of 1 second each.

Perform five cycles of compressions.

Stop CPR, and check for return of the carotid pulse.

Depending on the patient's condition, continue CPR, continue rescue breathing only, or place the patient in the recovery position and monitor breathing and pulse.

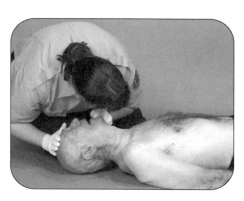

_____

Look, listen, and feel for breathing. If the patient is breathing adequately, place in the recovery position and monitor.

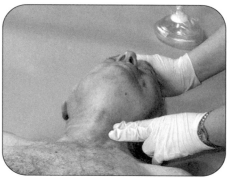

_____

Check for carotid pulse.

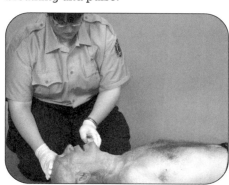

_____

Open the airway.

Skill Drill 39-4: Performing Two-Rescuer Adult CPR
Test your knowledge by filling in the correct words in the photo captions.

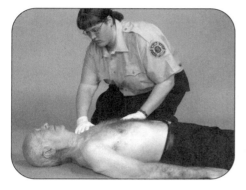

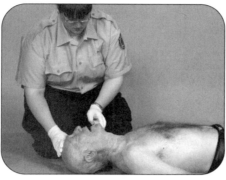

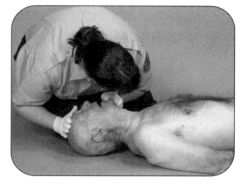

1. Establish _____ and take positions.

2. _____ the airway.

3. Look, listen, and feel for breathing. If breathing, place in the _____ position and _____.

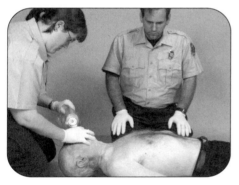

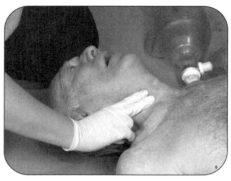

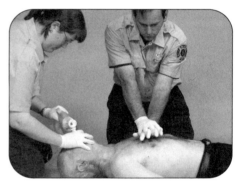

4. If the patient is not breathing, give _____ breaths of _____ second each.

5. Check for _____ pulse. If no pulse is felt in 10 seconds, begin CPR.

6. If there is no pulse but an AED is available, apply it now. If no _____ is available, begin _____ _____ at about _____/min. After every _____ cycles, switch rescuer positions in order to minimize fatigue. Keep switch time to 5 to 10 seconds. Depending on patient _____, continue CPR, continue rescue breathing only, or place in the recovery position and monitor.

Chapter 1: Preparing to Be an EMT-I

Matching

1. H	(page 10)		**8.** C	(page 6)
2. F	(page 10)		**9.** L	(page 19)
3. M	(page 6)		**10.** E	(page 14)
4. G	(page 6)		**11.** I	(page 13)
5. A	(page 6)		**12.** D	(page 13)
6. K	(page 14)		**13.** J	(page 9)
7. B	(page 14)			

Multiple Choice

1. B – These are among the training or "scope of practice" of the EMT-Basic. Other levels of EMT (A, C, D) include advanced procedures in their practice. (page 6)

2. D – EMS is regulated entirely by the state in which you are certified. NHTSA, which is part of the DOT, created funding sources and programs to develop improved systems of prehospital emergency care. US DOT published the first National Standard Curriculum. NREMT was established to certify and register EMS professionals. (page 11)

3. A (page 14)

4. C (page 14)

5. A – Medical control may be online over radio or telephone or off-line as protocols or standing orders, which describe the care authorized by the medical director. Dispatchers are not authorized to guide patient care by the EMS team. (page 14)

6. D – (A), (B), and (C) are among the circular system of CQI. The public is not a part of CQI. However, a complaint may lead to a CQI investigation. (page 14)

7. C – Quality control ensures that all staff members involved in caring for patients meet appropriate standards on each call. Periodic audits or reviews may be employed; these may be yearly, quarterly, or more frequently (A). EMT training in skills is a component of regulation and certification (B). Billing information (D) is an important aspect of documentation but not a matter for the medical director in quality control. (page 14)

8. A – Ensuring your safety and that of your fellow EMTs is a primary responsibility. (B), (C), and (D) are among the concerns upon arrival at the scene during scene size-up. (page 18)

9. B – The emergency care of patients occurs in three phases. The first phase consists of assessment, packaging, and transport; the second phase continues care in the emergency department (C); and in the third phase the patient receives the necessary definitive care. Public recognition (A) and accurate dispatching (D) are components of access to the EMS system. (page 17)

10. B – EMT-I training is divided into three main categories: life-threatening conditions, non–life-threatening conditions, and important nonmedical issues as listed in the textbook. (pages 7 to 8)

11. C – EMT-B training is divided into three main categories: life-threatening conditions, non–life-threatening conditions, and important nonmedical issues as listed in the textbook. (pages 7 to 8)

12. B – The material and skills taught in the EMT-I training program were developed in the US Department of Transportation EMT-Basic National Standard Curriculum. (A) The AAOS assists the development of EMS through research, quality standards, and publications. (C) The AHA conducts research, provides training standards, and certification in CPR. (D) The NAEMT represents EMS on the national, regional, and state levels. (page 10)

13. B – AEDs are designed to be used by the "untrained" layperson. (A), (C), and (D) are correct statements about the AED. (page 11)

Vocabulary

1. Emergency medical services: A multidisciplinary system that represents the combined efforts of several professionals and agencies to provide prehospital emergency care to the sick and injured. (page 6)

2. First responder: The first trained individual, such as police officer, fire fighter, or other rescuer, to arrive at the scene to provide initial medical assistance. (page 11)

3. Primary service area: The designated area in which the EMS agency is responsible for the provision of prehospital emergency care and transportation to the hospital. (page 13)

4. Emergency medical technician: An EMS professional who is trained and licensed by the state to provide emergency medical care in the field. (page 6)

Fill-in

1. Reciprocity (page 8)

2. GPS (page 13)

3. EMD (page 13)

4. state (page 10)

5. 9-1-1 (page 12)

6. medical control (page 14)

True/False

1. F   (page 6)

2. T   (page 14)

3. T   (page 14)

4. F   (page 14)

5. T   (page 18)

6. T   (page 18)

7. F   (page 16)

Short Answer

1. The EMT-I is one of the five levels of prehospital care. The EMT-I provides some advanced care such as IV therapy, advanced airway management, and cardiac monitoring. (page 12)

2. The Department of Transportation (DOT) has developed a series of guidelines, curricula, funding ources, and assessment tools, all designed to develop and improve EMS in the United States. (page 10)

3. -Ensuring your own safety and the safety of your fellow EMTs, the patient, and others at the scene

-Locating and safely driving to the scene

-Sizing up the scene and situation

-Rapidly assessing the patient's gross neurologic, respiratory, and circulatory status

-Providing any essential immediate intervention

-Performing a thorough, accurate patient assessment

-Obtaining an expanded SAMPLE history

-Reaching a clinical impression and providing prompt, efficient, prioritized patient care based on your assessment

-Communicating effectively with and advising the patient of any procedures you will perform

-Properly interacting and communicating with fire, rescue, and law enforcement responders at the scene

-Identifying patients who require rapid packaging and initiating transport without delay

-Identifying patients who do not need emergency care and will benefit from further detailed assessment and care before they are moved and transported

-Properly packaging the patients

-Safely lifting and moving the patient to the ambulance and loading the patient into it

-Providing safe appropriate transport to the hospital emergency department or other ordered facility

-Giving the necessary radio report to the medical control center or receiving hospital emergency department

-Providing any additional assessment or treatment while en route

-Monitoring the patient and checking vital signs while en route

-Documenting all findings and care on the run report

-Unloading the patient safely and, after giving a proper verbal report, transferring the patient's care to the emergency department staff

-Safeguarding the patient's rights (page 18)

4. Online medical direction is provided through radio or telephone connections between the EMT-I and the medical control facility. Off-line medical direction is provided through written protocols, procedures, and standing orders. (page 14)

Word Fun

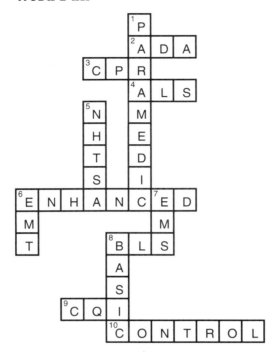

Ambulance Calls

1. Most services would require that you continue on the original call in order not to commit an act of negligence. The only exception would be if the route were blocked by the crash and another unit could reach the original call quicker from another direction. The crash should be reported to the dispatcher so that a unit could be dispatched and then proceed according to local protocols.

2. Call the dispatcher to send police if the environment appears hostile. Wait for them to arrive and then proceed to care for the patient. It would also be appropriate for the boy to come to you. Ask someone close by to bring the boy to the ambulance so that you can examine his injury. If in any doubt, wait for law enforcement.

3. The paramedics cannot transfer care of the patient to you in any area of the country. This would constitute abandonment by turning care over to someone with less training. You should tell the paramedics that you cannot accept transfer of this patient and notify your dispatcher to send a paramedic unit for the transport. It is only acceptable to transport a patient with an intermediate unit from one facility to another under a doctor's orders, not from the scene.

4. Treat the patient first: oxygen, oral glucose. Educate the patient and her family: explain how to eat properly, explain how to take the appropriate amount of medication

Chapter 2: The Well-Being of the EMT-I

Matching

1. D (page 66)	**9.** M (page 56)
2. A (page 38)	**10.** J (page 55)
3. C (page 45)	**11.** K (page 46)
4. F (page 35)	**12.** O (page 58)
5. B (page 47)	**13.** I (page 56)
6. E (page 45)	**14.** G (page 45)
7. N (page 45)	**15.** L (page 55)
8. H (page 56)	

Multiple Choice

1. B (page 26)

2. C (page 26)

3. D (page 27)

4. A – This is a presumptive sign. (page 27)

5. D – Cases for the medical examiner also include those in which the patient is dead on arrival; death without previous medical care or when the physician is unable to state the cause of death; poisoning, known or suspected; and death resulting from accidents. (page 28)

6. D (page 28)

7. C (page 28)

8. A (page 28)

9. D (page 28)

10. B (page 29)

11. A (page 29)

12. D (page 29)

13. C (page 30)

14. B (page 30)

15. D – Fear may also be expressed as withdrawal, tension, "butterflies" in the stomach, or nervousness. (page 30)

16. D (page 30)

17. B – Loss of contact with reality, regression, and diminished control of basic impulses and desires are other common characteristics of mental health problems. (page 31)

18. D (page 31)

19. D (page 33)

20. A – Other factors that influence how a patient reacts to the stress of an EMS incident include alcohol or substance abuse, history of chronic disease, mental disorders, reaction to medications, nutritional status, and feelings of guilt. (page 34)

21. B – This is a form of positive stress. (page 35)

22. D (page 35)

23. C – This is a sign, not a symptom. (page 35)

24. D – Prolonged or excessive stress has also been proven to be a strong contributor to alcoholism and depression. (page 35)

25. B (page 35)

26. D (page 35)

27. A (page 36)

28. B (page 36)

29. D – Stress management strategies also include changing or eliminating stressors; cutting back on overtime; stopping complaining and worrying about things you cannot change; adopting a more relaxed, philosophical outlook; expanding your social support system; sustaining friends and interests outside EMS; and minimizing the physical response to stress. (page 38)

30. D   (page 38)

31. B   (page 38)

32. C   (page 40)

33. D   (page 40)

34. D – Other components of the CISM system are on-scene peer support, one-on-one support, disaster support services, CISD, follow-up services, community outreach programs, and other health and welfare programs, such as wellness. (page 41)

35. D   (page 42)

36. B – Drug and alcohol use in the workplace can lead to poor treatment decisions, not enhanced treatment decisions. (page 43)

37. C – Personal safety begins with mentally preparing yourself and wearing seat belts, etc. (page 44)

38. C   (page 45)

39. B   (page 46)

40. D – Modes of transmission also include oral contamination due to lack of or improper handwashing. (page 47)

41. A   (page 50)

42. C   (page 50)

43. B   (page 52)

44. D – The tetanus-diphtheria booster is also recommended every 10 years. (page 53)

45. B   (page 55)

46. D   (page 56)

47. B   (page 57)

48. B   (page 58)

49. C   (page 50)

50. B   (page 52)

51. D – Factors to take into consideration for potential violence also include the behavior triad of truancy, fighting, and uncontrollable temper; instability of family structure; tattoos; and functional disorder. (page 57)

52. D   (page 59)

Vocabulary

1. Critical incident stress management (CISM): A process that confronts the responses to critical incidents and diffuses them, directing the emergency services personnel toward physical and emotional equilibrium. (page 35)

2. Posttraumatic stress disorder (PTSD): A delayed stress reaction to a prior incident. This delayed reaction is the result of one or more unresolved issues concerning the incident that might have been alleviated with the use of CISM. (page 35)

3. Critical incident stress debriefing (CISD): A confidential group discussion of a severely stressful incident that usually occurs within 24 to 72 hours of the incident. (page 40)

4. Concealment: The use of objects such as shrubs or bushes to limit a person's visibility of you. (page 66)

Fill-in

1. well-being (page 26)

2. emotional stress (page 26)

3. heart disease (page 26)

4. physician (page 27)

5. warm (page 27)

6. medical examiner (page 28)

7. Fear (page 30)

8. minor (page 34)

9. high-stress (page 34)

10. SARS (page 57)

11. Stress, stressors (page 35)

True/False

1. T (page 26)
2. F (page 27)
3. F (page 27)
4. T (page 28)
5. T (page 28)
6. F (page 47)
7. F (page 36)
8. T (pages 38 to 39)

Short Answer

1. An infection control practice that assumes all body fluids are potentially infectious. (page 47)

2. -Unresponsiveness to painful stimuli

-Lack of a pulse or heartbeat

-Absence of breath sounds

-No deep tendon or corneal reflexes

-Absence of eye movement; no systolic blood pressure

-Profound cyanosis

-Lowered or decreased body temperature (page 27)

3. 1. Obvious mortal damage (decapitation)

2. Dependent lividity

3. Rigor mortis

4. Putrefaction (pages 27 to 28)

4. 1. Denial

2. Anger/hostility

3. Bargaining

4. Depression

5. Acceptance (pages 28 to 29)

5. -Irritability toward coworkers, family, and friends

-Inability to concentrate

-Difficulty sleeping, increased sleeping, or nightmares

-Anxiety, indecisiveness, guilt

-Loss of appetite (gastrointestinal disturbances)

-Loss of interest in sexual activities

-Isolation

-Loss of interest in work

-Increased use of alcohol

-Recreational drug use (page 35)

6. -Change or eliminate stressors

-Change partners to avoid a negative or hostile personality

-Change work hours

-Cut back on overtime

-Change your attitude about the stressor

-Stop wasting your energy complaining or worrying about things you cannot change

-Try to adopt a more relaxed, philosophical outlook

-Expand your social support system apart from your coworkers

-Sustain friends and interests outside emergency services

-Minimize the physical response to stress by employing various techniques (page 38)

7. 1. Use soap and water

2. Rub hands together for at least 10 to 15 seconds to work up a lather

3. Rinse hands and dry with a paper towel

4. Use paper towel to turn off faucet (page 47)

8.

Level	Hazard	Protection Needed
0	Little to no hazard	None
1	Slightly hazardous	SCBA only (level C suit)
2	Slightly hazardous	SCBA only (level C suit)
3	Extremely hazardous	Full protection, with no exposed skin (level A or B suit)
4	Minimal exposure causes death	Special HazMat gear (level A suit) (page 61)

9. 1. Thin inner layer

2. Thermal middle layer

3. Outer layer (page 63)

10. 1. Past history

2. Posture

3. Vocal activity

4. Physical activity (page 67)

12. -Duty to act: having a duty to respond

-Breech of duty: failure to respond

-Injury: an injury has occurred

-Proximate cause: injury was caused by your action or inaction

Word Fun

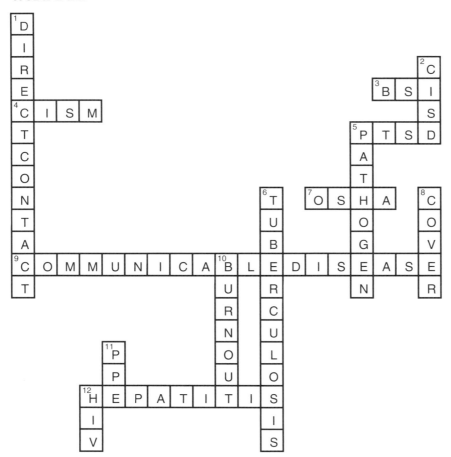

Ambulance Calls

1. -Say "I'm sorry."

-Explain why CPR will be ineffective.

-Say "If you want to cry, it's okay."

-Offer to call a relative or religious advisor.

-Notify your supervisor, dispatcher, or coroner as protocol dictates.

-Offer a hug and just listen.

2. -Your attention must focus on the mother-clearing her airway, assisting ventilations.

-Have a fire fighter or bystander talk to the child and try to comfort him.

-Advise them NOT to remove him from his seat.

-Have the child brought to the ambulance in the seat and strapped into the Captain's chair; he should be immobilized in his seat.

-Continue your care of the mother and have help ride with you to care for the child.

2. -Continue to treat your patient appropriately, including c-spine stabilization and transport.

-Allow your cut to bleed as long as it is minimal; it will help to wash/clean it out.

-Clean your wound with an alcohol gel if available.

-Once patient care has been transferred at the receiving facility, immediately wash thoroughly with soap and water and report to your supervisor.

-Follow up with prompt medical attention.

Skill Drills

Skill Drill 2-1: Proper Glove Removal Technique

1. Partially remove the first glove by pinching at the wrist. Be careful to touch only the outside of the glove.

2. Remove the second glove by pinching the exterior with the partially gloved hand.

3. Pull the second glove inside out toward the fingertips.

4. Grasp both gloves with your free hand, touching only the clean interior surfaces. (page 48)

Chapter 3: Medical, Legal, and Ethical Issues

Matching

1. H (page 84)

2. I (page 82)

3. G (page 86)

4. E (page 84)

5. L (page 80)

6. A (page 86)

7. D (page 82)

8. F (page 81)

9. B (page 83)

10. C (page 84)

11. M (page 83)

12. N (page 83)

13. J (page 81)

14. K (page 78)

Multiple Choice

1. C – The scope of practice outlines the care the EMT-I is able to provide. (A) Duty to act is the responsibility to provide care. (B) Competency is the ability to make qualified decisions. (D) Certification is the process whereby an individual or agency is recognized for meeting a set of standards. (page 78)

2. A – The standard of care is a certain, definable way the EMT-I is required to act, regardless of the activity involved. Generally, a standard of care is how a reasonably prudent individual with similar training would act with similar equipment and situation. (page 78)

3. D – Certification obliges the EMT to conform to predetermined standards. (page 80)

4. D (page 81)

5. B (page 81)

6. A (page 81)

7. D (page 82)

8. D – Negligence is proven when all four elements—duty, breach, cause, and damages—are met, regardless of whether consent was expressed (A) or implied, care was terminated or not (B), or how the patient was transported (C). (pages 68 to 81)

9. A – Consent for emergency treatment of a mentally incompetent individual should be obtained from the person's legal guardian. In cases where this is not possible, many states have provisions to take the individual into protective custody. (B, C) Expressed or informed consent requires that the patient or guardian fully understand the condition and consequences of accepting or refusing treatment. Implied consent (D) is limited to true emergency situations where the individual is unconscious or delusional. (page 84)

10. C – If you leave patients alone, you risk being accused of negligence or abandonment. (page 82)

11. B – Good Samaritan laws protect individuals who provide care within their scope of practice and in good faith. Proper performance of CPR (A), improvising BLS materials (C), and supportive care given to a patient with an advance directive or DNR (D) are each appropriate to the scope of practice of the EMT-I. (page 85)

12. D – Confidential information includes history, assessment, treatments, diagnosis, and mental or physical conditions (A, B, and C) and cannot be disclosed without authorization of the patient. The location of an emergency call is generally not considered confidential. (page 88)

13. C (page 88)

14. A (page 88)

15. B (page 88)

16. D – Most experts agree that a complete and accurate record of an emergency incident is an important safeguard against legal complications. Not every call requires use of emergency lights and siren (A) or transport to an emergency department (C). Ambulance equipment and supplies should be checked (B) and restocked with every shift or after each run, but this is not necessarily related to legal issues. (page 89)

Vocabulary

1. Abandonment: Unilateral termination of care by the EMT-I without the patient's consent and without making provisions for transferring care to another medical professional with skills of at least the same level. (page 82)

2. Advance directive: Written documentation that specifies medical treatment for a competent patient should the patient become unable to make decisions. (page 86)

3. Assault: Unlawfully placing a patient in fear of bodily harm. (page 84)

4. Battery: Touching a patient or providing emergency care without consent. (page 84)

5. DNR order: Written documentation giving permission to medical personnel not to attempt resuscitation in the event of cardiac arrest. (page 86)

6. Certification: A process in which a person, an institution, or a program is evaluated and recognized as meeting certain predetermined standards to provide safe and ethical care. (page 80)

7. Duty to act: A medicolegal term relating to certain personnel who either by statute or by function have a responsibility to provide care. (page 81)

8. Expressed consent: A type of consent in which a patient gives express authorization for provision of care or transport. (page 83)

9. Good Samaritan laws: Statutory provisions enacted by many states to protect citizens from liability for errors and omissions in giving good faith emergency medical care, unless there is wanton, gross, or willful negligence. (page 85)

10. Implied consent: Type of consent in which a patient who is unable to give consent is given treatment under the legal assumption that he or she would want treatment. (page 83)

11. Negligence: Failure to provide the same care that a person with similar training would provide. (page 81)

12. Standard of care: Written, accepted levels of emergency care expected by reason of training and profession; written by legal or professional organizations so that patients are not exposed to unreasonable risk or harm. (page 78)

13. Criminal law: An area of law in which the federal, state, or local government prosecutes individuals on behalf of society for violating laws designed to safeguard society. (page 81)

14. Civil law: An area of law dealing with private complaints brought by a plaintiff against a defendant for an illegal act or wrongdoing. (page 81)

15. Ethics: Principles that identify conduct deemed morally desirable. (page 87)

16. Licensure: The process by which a governmental agency, such as a state medical board, grants permission to an individual who meets established qualifications to engage in a profession or occupation. (page 80)

17. Protocols: Precise and detailed plans for a regimen of therapy. (page 78)

18. Standing orders: Localized protocols, usually pertaining to a particular service or area. (page 78)

Fill-in

1. scope, practice (page 78)

2. diagnosis, treatment (page 80)

3. standard, care (page 78)

4. duty, act (page 81)

5. negligence (page 81)

6. termination (page 82)

7. Expressed, implied (page 83)

8. assault, battery (page 84)

9. advance directive, DNR order (page 86)

10. moral obligation (page 87)

11. protected (page 88)

12. refuse treatment (page 85)

13. special reporting (page 89)

True/False

1. T   (page 80)

2. T   (page 81)

3. F   (page 83)

4. T   (page 83)

5. T   (page 84)

6. F   (page 86)

7. T   (page 84)

8. T   (pages 87 to 88)

Short Answer

1. If the minor is emancipated, married, or pregnant. (page 83)

2. You must continue to care for the patient until the patient is transferred to another medical professional of equal or higher skill level or to another medical facility. (page 82)

3. 1. Obtain the refusing party's signature on an official medical release form that acknowledges refusal.

   2. Obtain a signature from a witness of the refusal.

   3. Keep the refusal form with the incident report.

4. Note the refusal on the incident report.

5. Keep a department copy of the records for future reference. (page 85)

4. 1. If it was not documented, it did not happen.

2. Incomplete or disorderly records equate to incomplete or inexpert medical care. (page 89)

5. 1. Inform medical control.

2. Treat the patient as you would any patient.

3. Take any steps necessary to preserve life.

4. If saving the patient is not possible, take steps to make sure the organs remain viable. (pages 90 to 91)

Word Fun

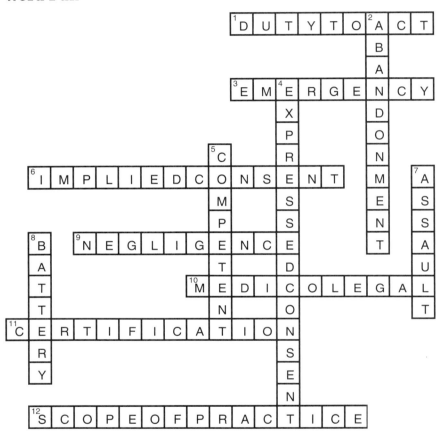

Ambulance Calls

1. You should not enter the scene until law enforcement arrives. The ambulance should "stage" several blocks from the residence and wait for police. Once the scene is safe, the EMTs will be summoned to enter the scene and provide care for the patient.

2. The child should be treated based on implied consent. A loss of function constitutes an emergency, and the child can be treated and transported without consent from the parent since not treating him could result in a loss of the extremity. The hospital will try to reach the child's mother once you arrive. You might also tell the other children to try to contact her and tell her to come to the hospital.

3. Assess the patient's mental status. If he is intoxicated, or has an altered mental status, he is treated under implied consent. If he is alert and oriented, you may attempt to talk him into being treated by explaining what you feel is necessary and what may happen if he does not receive care. If he has an altered mental status, you can obtain orders from medical control to restrain the patient with the help of law enforcement and transport him to the hospital.

Chapter 4: Medical Terminology

Matching

Prefixes

1. G (page 99)
2. H (page 100)
3. D (page 99)
4. A (page 99)
5. B (page 100)

6. I (page 99)
7. E (page 99)
8. C (page 99)
9. F (page 100)

Suffixes

1. D (page 101)
2. E (page 101)
3. G (page 101)
4. B (page 101)

5. H (page 101)
6. C (page 101)
7. A (page 101)
8. F (page 101)

Root Words

1. F (page 102)
2. H (page 102)
3. E (page 102)
4. B (page 103)
5. A (page 102)

6. I (page 104)
7. C (page 103)
8. D (page 103)
9. G (page 103)

Abbreviations

1. F (page 105)
2. E (page 105)
3. K (page 106)
4. G (page 108)
5. A (page 105)
6. D (page 107)

7. C (page 105)
8. B (page 105)
9. J (page 109)
10. L (page 108)
11. H (page 106)
12. I (page 106)

Multiple Choice

1. B (page 101)
2. C (page 101)
3. D (page 99)
4. C (page 99)
5. B (page 99)
6. B (page 99)
7. A (page 100)
8. A (page 100)
9. C (page 100)
10. C (page 101)

11. B (page 100)
12. D (page 101)
13. B (page 101)
14. A (page 101)
15. B (page 101)
16. D (page 102)
17. A (page 103)
18. A (page 103)
19. C (page 101)
20. C (page 102)

21. A (page 102)
22. C (page 103)
23. D (page 103)
24. D (page 104)
25. B (page 105)
26. C (page 105)
27. A (page 107)
28. C (page 107)
29. B (page 105)
30. C (page 108)

Vocabulary

1. Prefix: Appears at the beginning of a word and generally describes location and intensity.

2. Suffix: Placed at the end of a word to change the meaning and usually indicates a procedure, condition, disease, or part of speech.

3. Root word: The main part or stem of a word that conveys the essential meaning of the word and frequently indicates a body part.

Fill-in

1. Greek, Latin (page 98)
2. prefix (page 98)
3. suffix (page 101)
4. root word (page 101)
5. infra-, inter-, intra- (page 99)
6. -ectomy, -ostomy (page 101)
7. bid (page 105)
8. OS, OD, OU (page 108)
9. Cervic(o) (page 99)
10. Hypo (page 99)
11. Tachy (page 100)
12. -cyte (page 101)
13. Serum (page 104)

True/False

1. T   (page 99)
2. F   (page 99)
3. T   (page 100)
4. T   (page 100)
5. T   (page 101)

Short Answer

1. It is necessary for communicating with other medical personnel. (page 98)
2. Using incorrect terminology can relay the wrong information to other medical personnel, leading to confusion and detrimental patient care. (page 98)

Word Fun

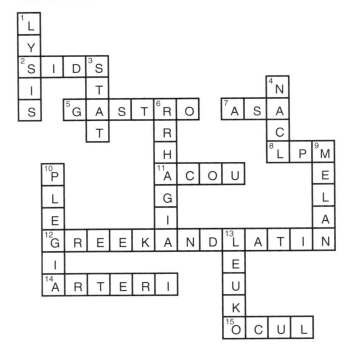

Ambulance Calls

1. Pt with hx NIDDM c/o N/V x 4d. VS WNL.
2. 64-year-old patient with history of acute myocardial infarction. Presented to emergency room complaining of chest pain for 2 hours, dyspnea on exertion, and nausea and vomiting. Was given aspirin by mouth and nitroglycerin sublingual. Intravenous access, sodium chloride, at to-keep-open rate. Electrocardiogram and chest x-ray normal.
3. Responded to a MVC. Pt was 20 y/o male. AVPU= P. Multiple lacs and abrasions to forehead. + spider web fx to windshield. Removed from veh on LSB. Pt placed on O2 at 15 lpm via NRB. IV NS KVO with 18g cath to R forearm. ECG-ST.

Chapter 5: The Human Body

Matching

1. O	(page 120)	**14.** Y	(page 127)
2. M	(page 118)	**15.** C	(page 118)
3. J	(page 114)	**16.** Z	(page 121)
4. Q	(page 129)	**17.** H	(page 118)
5. V	(page 129)	**18.** I	(page 128)
6. R	(page 122)	**19.** F	(page 126)
7. L	(page 120)	**20.** D	(page 121)
8. B	(page 118)	**21.** U	(page 121)
9. P	(page 126)	**22.** N	(page 127)
10. K	(page 127)	**23.** W	(page 128)
11. A	(page 120)	**24.** E	(page 118)
12. G	(page 122)	**25.** T	(page 128)
13. S	(page 128)	**26.** X	(page 120)

Multiple Choice

1. A (page 126)

2. B (page 129)

3. D (page 129)

4. B (page 130)

5. B (page 131)

6. C (page 135)

7. B (page 137)

8. C (page 138)

9. C (page 141)

10. A (page 144)

11. C (page 144)

12. D – The hip joint is a ball-and-socket joint; the thumb is a saddle joint; the vertebrae make up slightly moveable joints. (page 147)

13. D – The ileum is part of the small intestine. (page 148)

14. B (page 152)

15. D (page 154)

16. C (page 169)

17. C (page 174)

18. A (page 184)

19. B (page 198)

20. D (page 200)

21. A (page 204)

Labeling

Directional Terms (page 119)

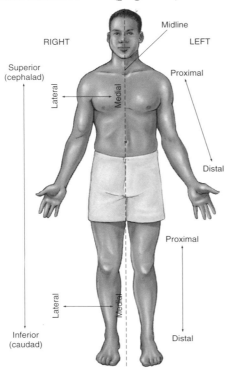

Abdominal Quadrants (page 123)

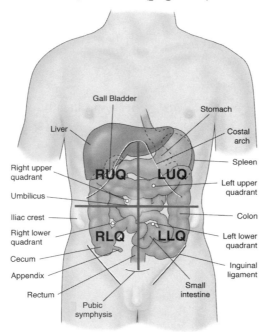

Anatomic Positions (page 124)

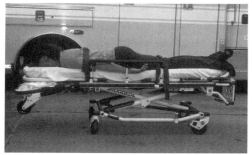

A. Prone.

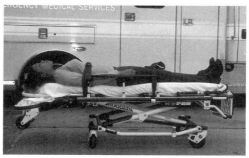

B. Supine.

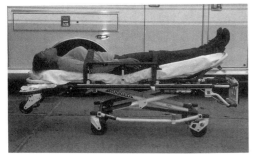

C. Trendelenburg's.

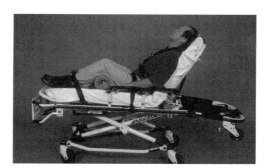

D. Semi-Fowler's.

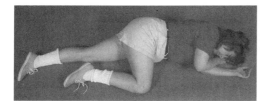

E. Lateral recumbent.

The Neuron (page 131)

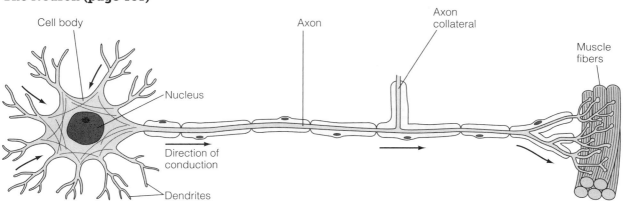

Cell body

Nucleus

Direction of conduction

Dendrites

Axon

Axon collateral

Muscle fibers

The Skin (page 133)

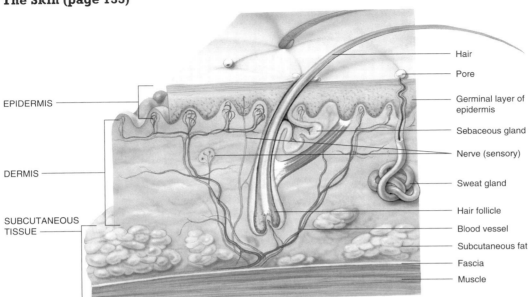

EPIDERMIS

DERMIS

SUBCUTANEOUS
TISSUE

Hair

Pore

Germinal layer of
epidermis

Sebaceous gland

Nerve (sensory)

Sweat gland

Hair follicle

Blood vessel

Subcutaneous fat

Fascia

Muscle

Skeletal System (page 134)

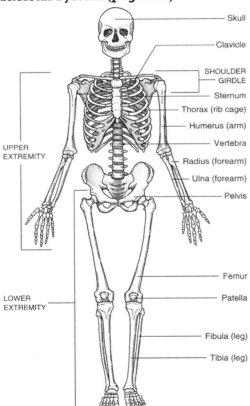

Skull

Clavicle

SHOULDER
GIRDLE

Sternum

Thorax (rib cage)

Humerus (arm)

Vertebra

Radius (forearm)

Ulna (forearm)

Pelvis

UPPER
EXTREMITY

LOWER
EXTREMITY

Femur

Patella

Fibula (leg)

Tibia (leg)

The Skull (page 136)

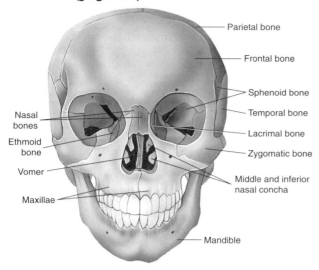

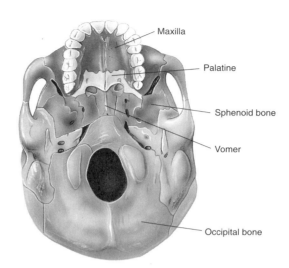

Parietal bone
Frontal bone
Sphenoid bone
Temporal bone
Lacrimal bone
Zygomatic bone
Middle and inferior nasal concha
Mandible
Nasal bones
Ethmoid bone
Vomer
Maxillae

Maxilla
Palatine
Sphenoid bone
Vomer
Occipital bone

The Thorax (page 141)

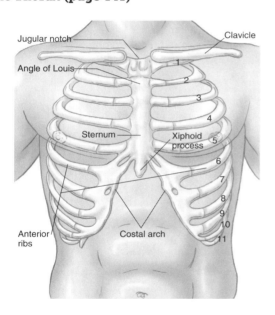

Jugular notch
Angle of Louis
Sternum
Xiphoid process
Anterior ribs
Costal arch
Clavicle
1 2 3 4 5 6 7 8 9 10 11

Shoulder Girdle (page 145)

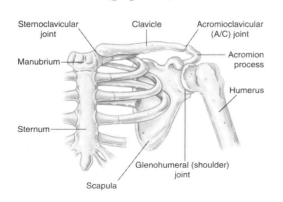

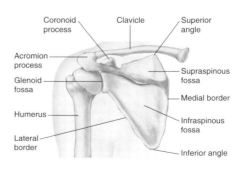

Sternoclavicular joint
Clavicle
Acromioclavicular (A/C) joint
Acromion process
Humerus
Glenohumeral (shoulder) joint
Manubrium
Sternum
Scapula

Coronoid process
Clavicle
Superior angle
Acromion process
Supraspinous fossa
Glenoid fossa
Medial border
Humerus
Infraspinous fossa
Lateral border
Inferior angle

Upper Extremity (page 148)

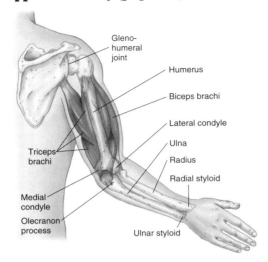

Gleno-humeral joint
Humerus
Biceps brachi
Lateral condyle
Ulna
Radius
Radial styloid
Triceps brachi
Medial condyle
Olecranon process
Ulnar styloid

Wrist and Hand (page 148)

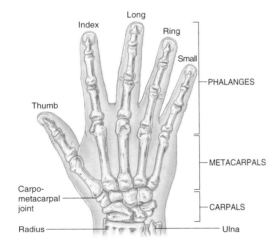

Long
Index
Ring
Small
Thumb
PHALANGES
METACARPALS
Carpo-metacarpal joint
CARPALS
Radius
Ulna

Pelvic Girdle (page 149)

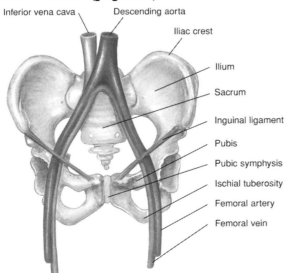

Inferior vena cava
Descending aorta
Iliac crest
Ilium
Sacrum
Inguinal ligament
Pubis
Pubic symphysis
Ischial tuberosity
Femoral artery
Femoral vein

Hip Joint (page 149)

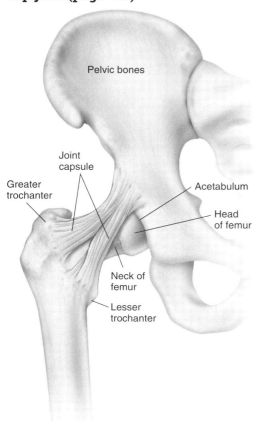

Pelvic bones

Joint
capsule

Greater
trochanter

Acetabulum

Head
of femur

Neck of
femur

Lesser
trochanter

Lower Extremity (page 152)

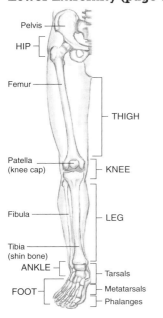

Pelvis

HIP

Femur

THIGH

Patella
(knee cap)

KNEE

Fibula

LEG

Tibia
(shin bone)

ANKLE

Tarsals

FOOT

Metatarsals

Phalanges

The Knee (page 157)

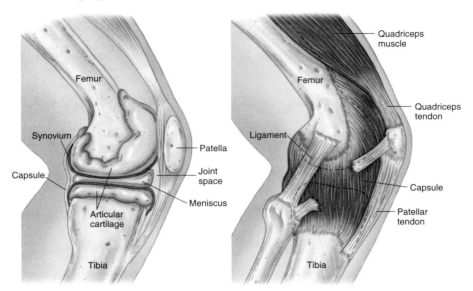

The Brain (page 162)

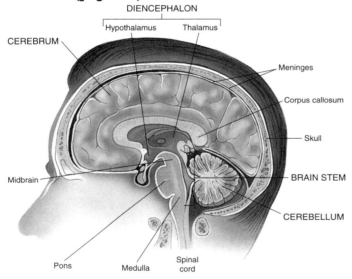

Spinal Cord (page 166)

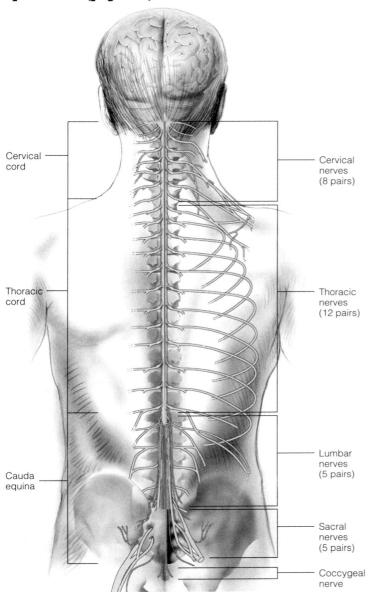

Cervical cord

Thoracic cord

Cauda equina

Cervical nerves (8 pairs)

Thoracic nerves (12 pairs)

Lumbar nerves (5 pairs)

Sacral nerves (5 pairs)

Coccygeal nerve

Cardiac Conduction System (page 185)

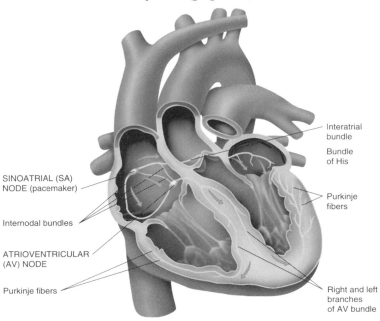

Interatrial bundle

Bundle of His

SINOATRIAL (SA) NODE (pacemaker)

Purkinje fibers

Internodal bundles

ATRIOVENTRICULAR (AV) NODE

Purkinje fibers

Right and left branches of AV bundle

Coronary Arteries (page 190)

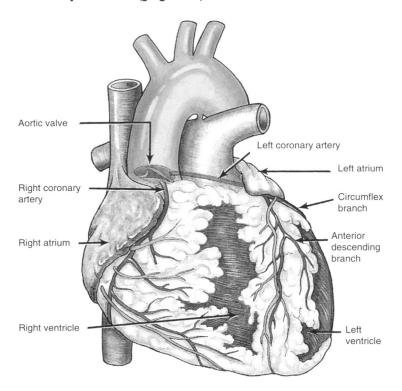

Aortic valve

Left coronary artery

Left atrium

Right coronary artery

Circumflex branch

Right atrium

Anterior descending branch

Right ventricle

Left ventricle

Cardiovascular System (page 190)

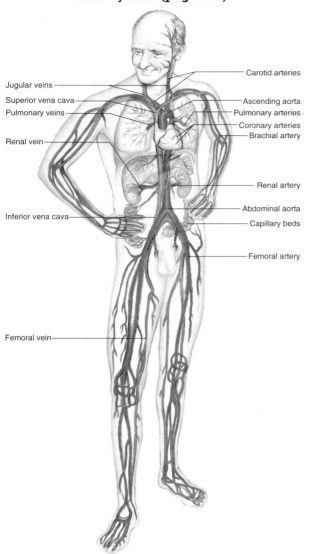

Jugular veins

Superior vena cava

Pulmonary veins

Renal vein

Inferior vena cava

Femoral vein

Carotid arteries

Ascending aorta

Pulmonary arteries

Coronary arteries

Brachial artery

Renal artery

Abdominal aorta

Capillary beds

Femoral artery

Veins of the Head and Neck (page 195)

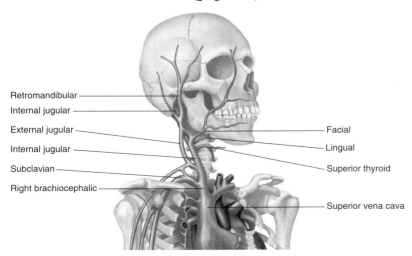

Retromandibular

Internal jugular

External jugular

Internal jugular

Subclavian

Right brachiocephalic

Facial

Lingual

Superior thyroid

Superior vena cava

Hepatic Portal System (page 196)

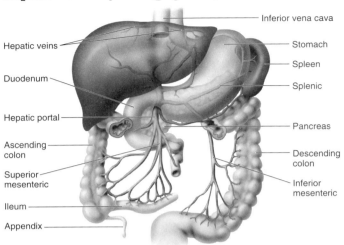

- Inferior vena cava
- Hepatic veins
- Stomach
- Spleen
- Duodenum
- Splenic
- Hepatic portal
- Pancreas
- Ascending colon
- Descending colon
- Superior mesenteric
- Inferior mesenteric
- Ileum
- Appendix

Male Reproductive System (page 211)

FRONT VIEW

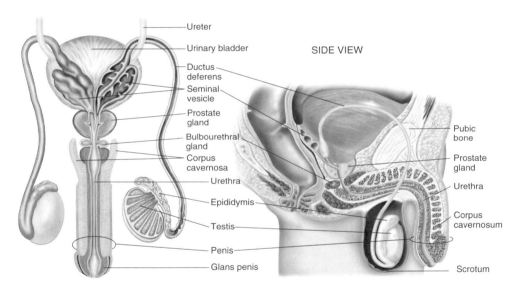

SIDE VIEW

- Ureter
- Urinary bladder
- Ductus deferens
- Seminal vesicle
- Prostate gland
- Bulbourethral gland
- Corpus cavernosa
- Urethra
- Epididymis
- Testis
- Penis
- Glans penis
- Pubic bone
- Prostate gland
- Urethra
- Corpus cavernosum
- Scrotum

Female Reproductive System (page 211)

FRONT VIEW

SIDE VIEW

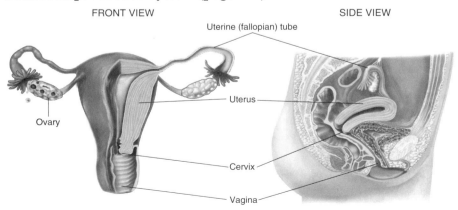

- Uterine (fallopian) tube
- Ovary
- Uterus
- Cervix
- Vagina

Vocabulary

1. Perfusion: The circulation of blood within an organ or tissue in adequate amounts to meet the cells' current needs. (page 197)
2. Aerobic metabolism: A biochemical process that occurs in the presence of oxygen and results in the production of energy in the form of ATP; also called cellular respiration. (page 129)
3. Autonomic nervous system: The part of the nervous system that regulates many body functions that are not under voluntary control. (page 171)
4. Pleural space: Potential space between the parietal and visceral pleura. (page 203)
5. Homeostasis: The maintenance of a relatively stable internal physiologic environment. (page 119)
6. pH: The measure of acidity or alkalinity of a solution. (page 213)
7. Solutes: Particles, such as salts, that are dissolved in a solvent. (page 126)
8. Endocrine system: A complex message and control system that integrates many body functions, including the release of hormones. (page 173)
9. Peripheral nervous system: The part of the nervous system that consists of 31 pairs of spinal nerves and 12 pairs of cranial nerves. These may be sensory or motor nerves. (page 168)
10. Epiglottis: The leaf-shaped valve that allows air to pass into the trachea but prevents food or liquid from entering the airway. (page 202)
11. Metabolism: Chemical reactions that occur in the body. (page 128)
12. Brainstem: The area of the brain that lies deep within the cranium and is the best-protected part of the central nervous system. It controls vital body functions. (page 163)

Fill-in

1. smooth (page 130)
2. Neurons, dendrites, axons (page 130)
3. retroperitoneal (page 144)
4. shoulder, glenoid fossa (page 146)
5. osteoblasts, osteoclasts (page 154)
6. hormones (page 173)
7. Antidiuretic hormone, oxytocin (page 175)
8. automaticity (page 185)
9. Cardiac output (page 187)
10. Peristalsis (page 209)
11. acid, base (page 213)

True/False

1. T   (page 125)
2. F   (page 128)
3. F   (page 132)
4. T   (page 135)
5. F   (page 139)
6. T   (page 143)
7. T   (page 161)
8. F   (page 176)
9. T   (page 184)
10. F   (page 207)

Short Answer

1. Plasma is a sticky yellow fluid that carries the blood cells and nutrients.

   Red blood cells give blood its red color and carry oxygen.

   White blood cells play a role in the body's immune defense mechanism against infection.

   Platelets are essential in the formation of blood clots. (pages 178 to 181)

2. Intracellular fluid exists within the individual cells and equals approximately 40% to 45% of total body weight. Makes up 75% of all body fluid.

   Extracellular fluid exists outside of the cell membrane and equals approximately 15% to 20% of the total body weight, or 25% of all body fluid.

   Intravascular fluid is the fluid portion of the blood. It is found within the blood vessels and accounts for 4.5% of total body weight. It is part of the extracellular fluid.

   Interstitial fluid is located outside of the blood vessels in the spaces between the body's cells. Accounts for approximately 10.5% of total body weight. It is part of the extracellular fluid. (page 212)

3. Growth hormone stimulates growth in most tissues, especially the long bones in the extremities.

   Thyroid-stimulating hormone controls the release of thyroid hormone from the thyroid gland into the bloodstream.

Adrenocorticotropic hormone is essential for the development of the cortex of the adrenal gland and its secretions of corticosteroids.

Reproductive-regulating hormones LH and FSH regulate the production of both eggs and sperm. (page 175)

4.   I Olfactory: sense of smell

    II Optic: sense of vision

   III Oculomotor: innervates muscles that move the eye and eyelid

   IV Trochlear: allows downward gaze of eye

    V Trigeminal: sensation to the scalp, forehead, face, lower jaw; movement of the muscles of chewing, the throat, and the inner ear

   VI Abducens: lateral movement of the eye

  VII Facial: facial expression

 VIII Vestibulocochlear: sense of hearing and balance

   IX Glossopharyngeal: sense of taste

    X Vagus: motor function to the pharynx and larynx; parasympathetic stimulation

   XI Spinal accessory: motor innervation to the muscles of the soft palate, pharynx, and shoulder

  XII Hypoglossal: motor function to the tongue

Word Fun

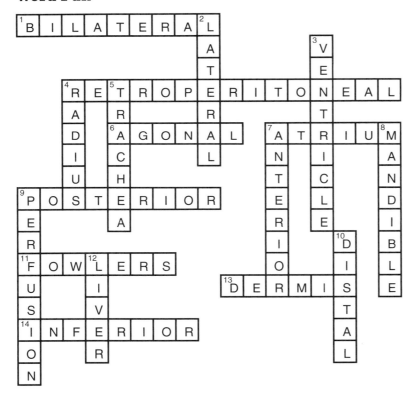

Ambulance Calls

1. Lacerated liver, gall bladder, small intestine, large intestine, pancreas, diaphragm, right lung if the pathway is up, right kidney depending on length of knife; you could also have involvement of the other four quadrants depending on the direction of travel of the blade. The description would be a puncture wound or stab wound.

2. The patient has angulation and deformity, possibly with crepitus, to the left forearm proximal to his left wrist or distal to his left elbow.

3. Deformity to left tibia/fibula with swelling. Possible fracture.

4. The patient has a possible posterior skull fracture. He also has swelling and deformity to the right forearm proximal to the wrist and distal to the elbow, indicating a possible fracture. There is an obvious open femur fracture with bone ends protruding through the skin.

Chapter 6

Matching

1. Y (page 257)	**14.** X (page 251)
2. M (page 250)	**15.** S (page 259)
3. L (page 252)	**16.** J (page 244)
4. Z (page 253)	**17.** H (page 252)
5. O (page 244)	**18.** N (page 258)
6. R (page 252)	**19.** Q (page 244)
7. V (page 255)	**20.** G (page 252)
8. T (page 245)	**21.** P (page 258)
9. A (page 249)	**22.** F (page 244)
10. W (page 245)	**23.** U (page 249)
11. D (page 254)	**24.** B (page 255)
12. I (page 262)	**25.** C (page 244)
13. K (page 259)	**26.** E (page 245)

Multiple Choice

1. D (page 245)

2. C – Generic medications have the same active ingredients in the same concentrations as their brand name counterparts. (page 244)

3. A – Causing an increase in the strength and rate of contractions (B, C) will have an adverse affect on the heart as it increases the oxygen demand and worsens the pain. (page 244)

4. A (page 245)

5. A (page 256)

6. B (page 256)

7. C (page 256)

8. D (page 250)

9. D (page 251)

10. B (page 252)

11. B (page 255)

12. D (page 256)

13. C (page 258)

14. D (page 258)

15. B (page 261)

16. B (page 262)

17. C (page 265)

18. D (page 266)

19. B (page 270)

Vocabulary

1. Trade name: The brand name that a manufacturer gives to a drug. (page 245)

2. Generic name: The original chemical name of a drug. (page 245)

3. OTC: Over-the-counter: Medications that can be purchased without a prescription. (page 245)

4. Solution: A liquid mixture of one or more substances that cannot be separated by filtering or allowing the mixture to stand. (page 251)

5. Suspension: A mixture of ground particles distributed evenly throughout a liquid. (page 252)

6. Sublingual: Under the tongue. (page 255)

7. Metered-dose inhaler (MDI): A miniature spray canister, used to direct substances small enough to be inhaled through the mouth and into the lungs. An MDI delivers the same amount of medication each time it is used. (page 252)

Fill-in

1. Drugs (page 244)

2. *U.S. Pharmacopeia* (page 245)

3. sublingually (page 255)

4. legally, morally, ethically (page 247)

5. solutions (page 251)

6. soluble (page 257)

7. agonists, antagonists (page 259)

True/False

1. T (page 245)   **5.** F (page 255)

2. T (page 247)   **6.** T (page 263)

3. F (page 250)   **7.** F (page 261)

4. T (page 272)   **8.** F (page 272)

Short Answer

1. -Intravenous

-Intramuscular

-Transcutaneous

-Oral

-Intraosseous

-Inhalation

-Sublingual

-Subcutaneous

-Per rectum (pages 255 to 256)

2. 1. Obtain an order from medical control.

2. Verify the proper medication and prescription.

3. Verify the form, dose, and route.

4. Check the expiration date and condition of medication.

5. Reassess vital signs, especially heart rate and blood pressure, at least every 5 minutes or as the patient's condition changes.

6. Document. (page 263)

3. -Nature of the absorbing surface

-Blood flow to the site of administration

-Solubility of the drug

-pH

-Drug concentration

-Dosage form

-Routes of drug administration

-Bioavailability

-Diffusion

-Osmosis

-Filtration

4. Epinephrine: (i) cardiac arrest, anaphylactic shock, (c) caution with hypertension, hyperthyroidism, angle-closure glaucoma (d) 1 mg IV every 3-5 minutes

Atropine sulfate: (i) symptomatic bradycardia, asystole, organophosphate poisoning, (c) angle-closure glaucoma, tachycardia (d) 0.5-1 mg IV every 5-15 minutes

Lidocaine HCl: (i) V-fib or pulseless V-tach, (c) hypersensitivity to local anesthetics, bradycardia, (d) 1.0-1.5 mg/kg IV every 5-10 minutes

Morphine sulfate: (i) pain management (c) hypersensitivity to opiates, acute bronchial asthma, CNS depression, head injury with increased ICP, undiagnosed abdominal pain, (d) 2-4 mg over 1-5 minutes every 5-30 minutes. (pages 266 to 271)

Word Fun

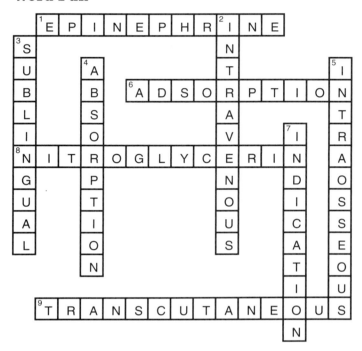

Ambulance Calls

1. Place the patient in the position of comfort.
   Give 100% oxygen via nonrebreathing mask.
   Start IV of NaCl
   Monitor vital signs and EKG
   Administer aspirin po and nitroglycerin SL
   Consider morphine sulfate for pain relief
   Rapid transport

2. Place patient in position of comfort.
   Give 100% oxygen via nonrebreathing mask.
   Start IV of NaCl
   Monitor vital signs and EKG
   Administer albuterol
   Consider epinephrine SC
   Continue to frequently monitor her airway.
   Rapid transport

3. Place patient in position of comfort.
   Give 100% oxygen via nonrebreathing mask.
   Check blood pressure!
   Check expiration date on nitroglycerin.
   Start IV NaCl
   Monitor vital signs and EKG
   Administer aspirin.
   Contact medical control for additional nitroglycerin
   Consider morphine sulfate for pain
   Rapid transport

Chapter 7: Intravenous Access

Matching

1. L	(page 287)	**8.** C	(page 286)	**15.** B	(page 287)
2. H	(page 288)	**9.** R	(page 289)	**16.** D	(page 289)
3. G	(page 286)	**10.** T	(page 290)	**17.** O	(page 293)
4. Q	(page 289)	**11.** E	(page 287)	**18.** J	(page 295)
5. I	(page 287)	**12.** F	(page 291)	**19.** M	(page 291)
6. P	(page 294)	**13.** S	(page 293)	**20.** K	(page 289)
7. N	(page 287)	**14.** A	(page 287)		

Multiple Choice

1. D (page 286)

2. C – Muscle cramps are a result of hypocalcemia. A, B, and D are signs of hypercalcemia. (page 287)

3. B – Poor skin turgor is a sign of dehydration. Other choices are all signs of overhydration. (page 292)

4. C – Hemorrhage causes dehydration. A, B, and D cause overhydration. (page 292)

5. D (pages 300 to 301)

6. A (page 304)

7. B (page 306)

8. D (page 307)

9. B (page 309)

10. C (page 310)

11. B – Phlebitis is a local reaction to IV therapy. A, C, and D are all systemic reactions. (page 313)

12. D – Vasovagal reaction, allergic reaction, and air embolus are all systemic complications of IV therapy. Infiltration is a local reaction. (page 316)

Vocabulary EMT-I vocab explorer web

1. Cannulation: The insertion of a hollow tube into a vein to allow for fluid flow. (page 321)

2. Crystalloid solution: A type of intravenous solution that contains compounds that quickly disassociate in solution and can cross membranes; considered the best choice for prehospital care of injured patients who need fluids to replace lost body fluids. (page 294)

3. Colloid solution: A type of intravenous solution that contains molecules (usually proteins) that are too large to pass out of the capillary membranes and therefore remain in the vascular compartment. (page 295)

4. Infiltration: The escape of fluid into the surrounding tissues. (page 314)

5. Tonicity: The osmotic pressure of a solution, based in the relationship between sodium and water inside and outside the cell, that takes advantage of their chemical and osmotic properties to move water to areas of higher sodium concentration. (page 288)

6. Angiocath: An over-the-needle catheter. (page 302)

7. Contaminated stick: The puncture of an emergency care provider's skin with a catheter that was used on a patient. (page 302)

8. Drip chamber: The area of the administration set where fluid accumulates so that the tubing remains filled with fluid. (page 298)

9. Intraosseous: Within a bone. (page 309)

10. "Piggyback" administration: The addition of a second IV administration set to a primary line via an access port. (page 297)

Fill-in

1. IV therapy (page 286)

2. Sodium (page 287)

3. Filtration (page 288)

4. depolarization (page 288)

5. tonicity (page 288)

6. distally, medially (page 300)

7. shorter (page 302)

8. Infiltration, occlusion (page 314)

9. joint (page 315)

10. ruptured (page 319)

True/False

1. T   (page 292)

2. F   (page 294)

3. F   (page 298)

4. T   (page 300)

5. T   (page 301)

6. T   (page 304)

7. F   (page 304)

8. T   (page 309)

9. T   (page 317)

10. F   (page 317)

11. F   (page 312)

Short Answer

1. It is a selective barrier. It chooses which compounds to allow across, depending on the needs of the cell. The selective permeability of the cell membrane is a result of its composition. It is a phospholipid bilayer. The hydrophilic outer layer is made up of a phosphate group, and the hydrophobic inner layer is made up of lipids or fatty acids. It is a very important barrier in fluid movement and acid/base balance. (page 286)

2. Isotonic solution: Same concentration of sodium as the cell. Water does not shift, and no change is seen in the shape of the cell.

Hypertonic solution: Greater concentration of sodium than the cell. Water is drawn out of the cell, and the cell collapses from increased extracellular osmotic pressure.

Hypotonic solution: Lower concentration of sodium than the cell. Water flows into the cell, causing the cell to swell and possible burst from increased intracellular osmotic pressure. (page 289)

3. 1. Always wear gloves! BSI precautions cannot be emphasized strongly enough.

   2. Choose a solution. Check the solution for clarity and the expiration date and to ensure it is the correct one.

   3. Choose an administration set appropriate for the needs of the patient.

   4. Choose an appropriate IV site.

   5. Choose an appropriately sized catheter.

   6. Recheck your work before you go any further.

   7. Tear tape for securing the IV site.

   8. Have blood tubes close by.

   9. Set up the Luer adapter and the Vacutainer barrel, or have a syringe close by for drawing blood, if indicated.

   10. Have a couple of catheters ready for insertion.

   11. Open an alcohol wipe.

   12. Have 4″ x 4″ pieces of gauze ready for catching blood.

   13. Then, and only then, apply a constricting band. (It is the last thing done before inserting the IV.)

   14. Insert the catheter and draw blood, if indicated.

   15. Hook up the IV tubing and adjust the flow.

   16. Secure the site and the blood tubes.

   17. Administer medication if necessary.

   18. Adequately dispose of sharps.

   19. Document every procedure. (page 296)

4. 1. Chose the appropriate fluid and examine for clarity and expiration date. Make sure there are no particles floating in the fluid and that the fluid is appropriate for the patient's condition.

2. Choose the appropriate drip set and attach it to the fluid.

3. Fill the drip chamber by squeezing it together.

4. Flush or "bleed" the tubing to remove any air bubbles by opening the roller clamp.

5. Tear tape prior to venipuncture.

6. Apply gloves prior to contact with the patient.

7. Apply the constricting band above the intended site.

8. Clean the area using aseptic technique.

9. Chose the appropriate sized catheter, and twist the catheter to break the seal.

10. Insert the catheter at approximately a 45° angle with the bevel up while applying distal traction with the other hand.

11. Observe for flashback.

12. Occlude the catheter to prevent blood leaking while removing the stylet.

13. Immediately dispose of sharps in the proper container.

14. Attach the prepared IV line.

15. Remove the constricting band.

16. Open the IV line and ensure fluid is flowing and the IV is patent.

17. Secure the catheter with tape.

18. Secure the tubing and adjust flow rate while monitoring the patient. (pages 305 to 306)

5. $$\frac{? \text{ gtt}}{\text{min}} = \frac{60 \text{ gtt}}{\text{mL}} \times \frac{100 \text{ mL}}{90 \text{ min}}$$

$$\frac{? \text{ gtt}}{\text{min}} = \frac{2 \text{ gtt}}{\text{mL}} \times \frac{100 \text{ mL}}{3 \text{ min}}$$

$$\frac{? \text{ gtt}}{\text{min}} = \frac{2 \text{ gtt}}{\text{L}} \times \frac{100}{3} = 200 \text{gtt}/3 \text{ min} = 67 \text{ gtt/min} \text{ (page 312)}$$

6. -The gauge of the needle

-The site

-The type of fluid you are administering

-The rate the fluid IS running (page 313)

Word Fun

Ambulance Calls

1. The patient should receive an IV of normal saline or lactated Ringer's in a large vein line such as those in the antecubital area. The catheter should be the largest that the vein will hold, 14g to 16g. The flow should be titrated to the patient's blood pressure and level of consciousness. Careful monitoring for signs of pulmonary edema is mandatory.

2. You should attempt IV access in 3 tries or 90 seconds. If unable to gain IV access, you should move on to IO access. The IO should be placed and secured in the proximal tibia. Patency should be verified, and crystalloid fluid should be infused.

Skill Drills

Skill Drill 7-1: Spiking the Bag

1. Pull on the rubber pigtail on the end of the IV bag to remove it. Remove the protective cover from the piercing spike.

2. Slide the spike into the IV bag port until you see fluid enter the drip chamber.

3. Allow the solution to run freely through the drip chamber and into the tubing to prime the line and flush the air out of the tubing.

4. Twist the protective cover on the opposite end of the IV tubing to allow air to escape. Do not remove this cover yet. Let the fluid flow until air bubbles are removed from the line before turning the roller clamp wheel to stop the flow.

5. Check the drip chamber; it should be only half filled. If the fluid level is too low, squeeze the chamber until it fills; if the chamber is too full, invert the bag and the chamber and squeeze the chamber to empty the fluid back into the bag. Hang the bag in an appropriate location. (page 299)

Skill Drill 7-2: IV Therapy

1. Choose the appropriate fluid and examine for clarity and check the expiration date.

2. Choose the appropriate drip set and attach it to the fluid.

3. Fill the drip chamber by squeezing it together.

4. Flush or "bleed" the tubing to remove any air bubbles by opening the roller clamp.

5. Tear tape prior to venipuncture, or have a commercial device available.

6. Apply gloves prior to contact with patient. Palpate a suitable vein.

7. Apply the constricting band above the intended IV site.

8. Clean the area using an aseptic technique. Use an alchohol pad to cleanse in a circular motion from the inside out. Use a second wipe straight down the center.

9. Choose the appropriate sized catheter and examine it for any imperfections.

10. Insert the catheter at an approximately 45° angle with the bevel up while applying distal traction with the other hand.

11. Observe for "flashback" as blood enters the catheter.

12. Occlude the catheter to prevent blood leaking while removing the stylet.

13. Immediately dispose of all sharps in the proper container.

14. Attach the prepared IV line.

15. Remove the constricting band.

16. Open the IV line to ensure fluid is flowing and the IV is patent. Observe for any swelling or infiltration around the IV site.

17. Secure the catheter with tape or a commercial device.

18. Secure IV tubing and adjust the flow rate while monitoring the patient. (pages 307 to 308)

Skill Drill 7-4: Determining if an IV is Viable

1. 10-mL syringe

2. alcohol wipe, Depress, port

3. Pinch, IV fluid

4. full, IV site, line, pressure, flow, dislodge, opposite, same (page 315)

Chapter 8: Medication Administration

Matching

1. N (page 331)	**8.** D (page 331)
2. H (page 328)	**9.** M (page 340)
3. L (page 328)	**10.** G (page 349)
4. J (page 331)	**11.** I (page 340)
5. C (page 335)	**12.** K (page 352)
6. B (page 328)	**13.** E (page 340)
7. F (page 337)	**14.** A (page 336)

Multiple Choice

1. B (page 328)	**6.** D (page 349)
2. C (page 331)	**7.** A (page 352)
3. A (page 340)	**8.** B (page 332)
4. D (pages 343–345)	**9.** C (page 335)
5. C (pages 347–349)	**10.** D (page 336)

Vocabulary

1. Bolus: A term meaning "in one mass;" in medication administration, a single dose given by the IV route, of a small or large quantity of the drug. (page 349)
2. Concentration: The total weight of a drug contained in a specific volume of liquid. (page 332)
3. Medical asepsis: A term applied to the practice of preventing contamination of the patient by using aseptic technique. (page 335)
4. Nebulizer: A device for producing a fine spray or mist that is used to deliver inhaled medications. (page 336)
5. Ampule: Small sealed glass containers with sterilized contents. (page 340)
6. Vial: Small glass bottles for medications; may contain single or multiple doses. (page 340)

Fill-in

1. weight, volume (page 329)
2. 0°, 100° (page 331)
3. kilograms (page 334)
4. protocol, medical direction (page 334)
5. inhalation (page 336)
6. Enteral, parenteral (pages 337 to 340)
7. Intravenous (page 340)
8. Ampules, vials (page 340)
9. Drug reconstitution (pages 340 to 341)
10. Prefilled syringes (page 343)

True/False

1. T (page 329)
2. F 1 kilogram weighs 2.2 lb (page 333)
3. F The desired dose is the physician's order. (page 331)
4. T (page 332)
5. F Albuterol is a common inhaled medication; however, the most common inhaled medication is oxygen. (page 336)
6. F BSI is needed with every patient contact. (page 338)
7. F Gauge measures the diameter of the needle. (page 340)

8. T   (page 343)

9. T   (page 347)

10. T   (page 349)

Short Answer

1. 1. Right patient

   2. Right drug

   3. Right dose

   4. Right route

   4. Right time

   6. Right documentation

2. -BSI

   -Determine need based on patient presentation

   -Focused history and physical

   -Contact medical control

   -Check for clarity, expiration, and concentration

   -Advise the patient of possible discomfort

   -Assemble equipment

   -Cleanse area

   -Pinch the skin surrounding the area and insert needle at 45° angle

   -Pull back plunger to aspirate for blood

   -If no blood is present, inject the medication and remove the needle and place it in the sharps container

   -Disperse medication by rubbing in a circular motion

   -Properly store any unused medication

   -Monitor the patient

3. Vastus lateralis: lateral thigh

   Rectus femoris: anterior thigh

   Gluteus maximus: buttocks

   Deltoid: shoulder

4. -BSI

   -Determine need based on patient presentation

   -Focused history and physical

   -Contact medical control

   -Explain procedure to the patient

   -Assemble equipment. Draw up medication. Expel air. Draw up 20 mL normal saline for flush.

   -Cleanse injection port with alcohol

   -Insert needle into port and pinch off IV tubing proximal to port

   -Administer the correct dose at the appropriate rate

   -Place needle and syringe in sharps container

   -Unclamp line and flush

   -Adjust line to correct rate

   -Properly store any unused medication

   -Monitor patient

Word Fun

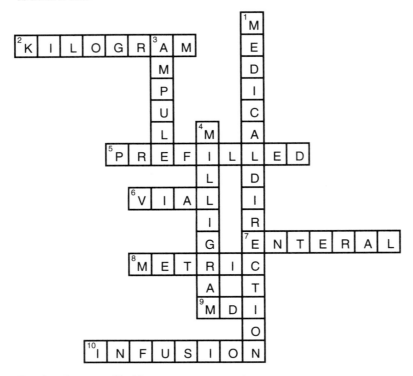

Ambulance Calls

1. 175 / 2.2 = 80.2 or 80 kg

   Drug is packaged 100 mg in 10 mL. To give 1 mg/kg (80mg), give 8 mL as IV bolus

   Infusion:

   #1 concentration: 2000 mg of lidocaine / 500 mL normal saline = 4 mg/mL

   #2 ordered dose: 2 mg/min

   2 mg / 4 mg/mL = 0.5 mL

   #3 0.5 mL/min x 60 gtt/mL

   30 gtt/min

2. 88 / 2.2 = 40 kg

   20 mL x 40 kg = total bolus of 800 mL

3. 1. Aspirin is administered PO.

   2. Nitroglycerin is administered SL.

   3. Morphine is administered IV.

Skill Drills

Skill Drill 8-1: Administering Medication Via Small-Volume Nebulizer

1. Check the medication and the expiration date.
2. Add premixed medication to the bowl of the nebulizer.
3. Connect the T piece with the mouthpiece to the top of the bowl, connect it to the oxygen tubing, and set the flowmeter at 6 L/min.
4. Instruct the patient to breathe as deeply as possible and hold his or her breath for 3 to 5 seconds before exhaling. Monitor the patient for effects. (page 337)

Skill Drill 8-3: Drawing Medication From a Vile

1. expiration date

2. air

3. rubber stopper, Expel, plunger

4. Withdraw

5. one-handed (page 344)

Skill Drill 8-4: Administering Medication Via the Subcutaneous Route

1. Check the medication to be sure that it is the correct one, that it is not cloudy or discolored, and that the expiration date has not passed.

2. Assemble and check the equipment.

3. Using aseptic technique, cleanse the injection area.

4. Pinch the skin surrounding the area, and insert the needle at a 45° angle. Pull back on the plunger to aspirate for blood. If there is no blood, inject the medication, remove the needle, and hold pressure over the area.

5. To disperse the medication, rub the area in a circular motion. Monitor the patient's condition. (page 346)

Skill Drill 8-6: Administering Medication Via the Intravenous Bolus Route

1. Assemble, check, injection port, protective cap

2. IV tubing, dose, rate

3. Unclamp, 20-mL bolus, flow rate (page 350)

Chapter 9: Airway Management and Ventilation

Matching

1. N	(page 369)	**16.** CC	(page 412)
2. Z	(page 372)	**17.** E	(page 378)
3. X	(page 374)	**18.** H	(page 409)
4. U	(page 398)	**19.** C	(page 369)
5. R	(page 370)	**20.** B	(page 372)
6. P	(page 378)	**21.** M	(page 382)
7. S	(page 412)	**22.** F	(page 370)
8. A	(page 371)	**23.** Q	(page 409)
9. T	(page 380)	**24.** V	(page 378)
10. AA	(page 422)	**25.** O	(page 371)
11. W	(page 369)	**26.** BB	(page 407)
12. G	(page 407)	**27.** D	(page 381)
13. Y	(page 372)	**28.** L	(page 412)
14. J	(page 417)	**29.** DD	(page 398, 400)
15. I	(page 371)	**30.** K	(page 380)

Multiple Choice

1. B	(page 368)	**8.** A	(page 380)	**15.** B	(page 439)
2. C	(page 368)	**9.** D	(page 382)	**16.** C	(page 439)
3. C	(page 369)	**10.** B	(page 402)	**17.** B	(page 439)
4. A	(page 370)	**11.** D	(page 407)	**18.** B	(page 439)
5. A	(page 372)	**12.** C	(page 417)	**19.** A	(page 445)
6. C	(page 368)	**13.** B	(page 423)	**20.** C	(page 445)
7. D	(page 373)	**14.** B	(page 422)		

Vocabulary

1. Pin-indexing system: A system established for portable cylinders to ensure that a regulator is not connected to a cylinder containing the wrong type of gas. (page 408)

2. Combitube: A dual-lumen airway that is inserted blindly. You can ventilate the patient whether the tube is placed in the esophagus or the trachea. (page 430)

3. Hering–Breuer reflex: The nervous system mechanism that terminates inhalation and prevents lung overexpansion. (page 372)

4. Sellick manuever: A technique used to prevent gastric distention in which pressure is applied on the cricoid cartilage. (page 369)

Fill-in

1. hypoxic drive (page 375)

2. Pulsus paradoxus (page 377)

3. metabolic (page 381)

4. tongue (page 389)

5. 40 L/min, 300 mm Hg (page 398)

6. burn, explode, combustion (page 411)

True/False

1. T   (page 374)

2. T   (page 382)

3. F   (page 385)

4. T   (page 388)

5. T   (page 391)

6. F   (page 396)

7. T   (page 425)

8. T   (page 430)

9. T   (page 438)

Short Answer

1. -Circulating bicarbonate

-Respiratory component

-Renal component (page 379)

2. tank pressure in psi − 200 psi [safe residual pressure] × cylinder constant flow rate in liters per minute (page 408)

3. 1. Mouth to mask

2. 2-person BVM

3. Flow restricted, oxygen powered ventilation device

4. 1-person BVM (page 414)

4. 1. Pediatric patients

2. Patients less than 5′ or greater than 7′ tall

3. Known pathologic conditions of the esophagus

4. Ingestion of caustics (page 431)

5. 1. BSI

2. Preoxygenate the patient

3. Check, prepare, and assemble equipment

4. Place the patient's head in sniffing position

5. Insert blade into right side of mouth and displace tongue to left

6. Gently lift until you see the glottic opening

7. Insert the ET tube between the cords

8. Remove the laryngoscope

9. Remove the stylet from the tube

10. Inflate the distal cuff and detach the syringe

11. Attach the end-tidal CO_2 detector

12. Attach the BVM and ventilate; auscultate apices, bases, and epigastrium

13. Secure the tube

14. Place bite block in the patient's mouth (page 445)

6. -Unrecognized esophageal intubation

-Induction of emesis and aspiration

-Hypoxia resulting from prolonged intubaton attempts

-Damage to teeth, soft tissue, and intraoral structures (page 460)

Word Fun

```
1G
 A      2V A L 3L E C U L A
 S          A
 T          R
 R          Y
 I          N
 C  4L A R Y N G O 5S C O P E
 T          O      T
 U          S      Y
 B          P      L
6S E L L I C K M A N E U V E R
            S      T
            M
```

Ambulance Calls

1. -Initiate ventilations by opening the airway, inserting an adjunct, and ventilating with a BVM and 100% oxygen

   -Begin chest compressions

   -Attach EKG and defibrillate if the patient is in a shockable rhythm

   -Prepare for ET intubation

   -Rapid transport

2. -Open the airway and suction of necessary

   -Insert an oral adjunct

   -Ventilate patient with BVM and 100% oxygen

   -Intubate with endotracheal tube (combitube is contraindicated)

   -Rapid transport

3. -Maintain c-spine control

   -Suction if needed

   -Ventilate with BVM and 100% oxygen while c-spine and jaw thrust is maintained

   -Insert a Combitube to protect the airway

   -Continue to ventilate until patient is extricated

Chapter 10: Patient Assessment

Matching

1. R (page 502)		**10.** L (page 532)	
2. D (page 513)		**11.** Q (page 532)	
3. N (page 520)		**12.** J (page 513)	
4. O (page 521)		**13.** G (page 513)	
5. B (page 513)		**14.** E (page 509)	
6. H (page 520)		**15.** F (page 532)	
7. M (page 511)		**16.** I (page 512)	
8. A (page 521)		**17.** K (page 509)	
9. P (page 501)		**18.** C (page 521)	

Multiple Choice

1. C – Level of responsiveness is determined during the initial assessment. (page 497)
2. D – Possible dangers you may observe in scene size-up also include leaking gasoline or diesel fuel, hostile bystanders/potential for violence, fire or smoke, possible hazardous or toxic materials, and other dangers at crash or rescue scenes and crime scenes. (page 497)
3. D (page 499)
4. B – Gunshot wounds (D) are penetrating trauma. (page 499)
5. C – Falls (D) may result in blunt or penetrating trauma but are not classified as either. page 500)
6. D (page 499)
7. A – The geographic location is irrelevant to the injury. (page 500)
8. C – As the speed of a crash increases, the forces that are exerted on the patient increase as well. (page 500)
9. D (page 500)
10. D (page 501)
11. B – The amount of force is directly related to the distance fallen; however, the other factors play a significant role in the extent of injury. (page 501)
12. D (page 501)
13. B – Rain is only a factor when it is raining in such a manner as to interfere with patient care. (page 502)
14. B – The pupils are assessed during the detailed exam. (page 504)
15. C – Mental status is the best indicator of cerebral perfusion. (page 508)
16. D – An altered mental status may also be caused by stroke, cardiac problems, or drug use. (page 509)
17. A – Tightness in the chest is a symptom. (page 511)
18. B – The tongue becomes an obstruction because of the relaxation of the muscles. (page 511)
19. D (page 511)
20. D (page 512)
21. B (page 512)
22. A – Use a gloved hand and a sterile dressing over the wound, then bandage. (page 512)
23. C (page 513)
24. D (page 513)
25. D – When assessing for changes in skin color in deeply pigmented skin, also check the fingernail beds. (page 513)
26. D – Other conditions that may slow capillary refill but are not related to the body's circulation include frostbite and the patient's gender. (page 513)
27. D (page 514)
28. B – Only apply an AED if the patient is unresponsive, apneic, and pulseless. (page 513)
29. C (page 514)
30. C – A, B, and D are all treatments. (page 515)
31. D (page 517)

32. B   (page 518)

33. C   (page 519)

34. B – AVPU (A) evaluates level of responsiveness in the initial assessment, OPQRST (C) evaluates pain, and SAMPLE (D) gains the necessary history. (page 520)

35. C – Once the c-collar is in place it should not be removed and does not allow for palpation of the neck and cervical spine. (page 521)

36. A – B and C evaluate sensation, not motor function. (page 524)

37. C   (page 525)

38. C – Evaluating whether the patient can move is irrelevant. When assessing a complaint of dizziness, also evaluate the rate and quality of respirations, monitor the level of consciousness and orientation, and check the head for signs of trauma. (page 528)

39. B – If the impact is minor and ABCs are intact with no other complaint, patients do not require a rapid trauma assessment and rapid transport. (page 529)

40. C   (page 532)

41. B   (page 532)

42. C   (page 533)

43. D – When assessing a chief complaint of chest pain, also evaluate blood pressure and look for trauma to the chest. (page 535)

44. D   (page 536)

45. B   (page 537)

46. D – When performing the detailed physical exam, depending on what you learn, you should also be prepared to perform spinal immobilization, provide transport to an appropriate facility, or call for ALS backup. (page 541)

47. C   (page 539)

48. D   (page 546)

49. B   (page 548)

50. A   (page 549)

51. D   (page 546)

52. B – A diagnosis cannot be made in the field. (page 553)

53. B   (page 550)

54. D – When reevaluating interventions, also take a moment to ensure that the airway is still open. (page 553)

55. D   (page 553)

56. D   (page 553)

57. C   (page 559)

58. B   (page 561)

Vocabulary

1. Blunt trauma: A mechanism of injury in which force occurs over a broad area and the skin is not usually broken. (page 499)

2. Penetrating trauma: A mechanism of injury in which force occurs at a small point of contact between the skin and the object. The skin is broken and the potential for infection is high. (page 500)

3. Mechanism of injury: The way in which traumatic injuries occur; the forces that act on the body to cause damage. (page 499)

4. Capillary refill: A test that evaluates distal circulatory system function by squeezing (blanching) blood from an area such as a nail bed and watching the speed of its return after releasing the pressure. (page 513)

5. Golden Hour: The time from injury to definitive care, during which treatment of shock or traumatic injuries should occur because survival potential is the best. (page 517)

Fill-in

1. patient assessment (page 495)

2. body substance isolation (page 497)

3. victim (page 497)

4. safety (page 498)

5. properly (page 500)

6. three (page 501)

7. entrance wound, exit wound (page 501)

8. triage (page 502)

9. general impression (page 505)

10. life-threatening (page 506)

11. patency (page 511)

12. reevaluate (page 511)

13. wrist (page 513)

14. initial assessment (page 515)

15. medications (page 514)

16. obstruction, cardiac failure, infection (page 547)

17. chaos, mentally triage (page 557)

18. potentially critical (page 558)

19. dynamic (page 560)

True/False

1. F	(page 509)	**10.** T	(page 515)
2. T	(page 541)	**11.** T	(page 520)
3. F	(page 501)	**12.** F	(page 519)
4. T	(page 513)	**13.** T	(page 543)
5. F	(page 553)	**14.** T	(page 546)
6. T	(page 534)	**15.** T	(page 553)
7. T	(page 517)	**16.** F	(page 554)
8. F	(page 513)	**17.** F	(page 555)
9. T	(page 512)	**18.** F	(page 557)

Short Answer

1. The characteristics of the penetrating object, the amount of force or energy, and the part of the body affected. (page 500)

2. To identify and initiate treatment of immediate or potential threats to life. (page 505)

3. Immediate assessment of the environment, the patient's presenting signs and symptoms, and the patient's chief complaint. (page 505)

4. A-Airway.

B-Breathing,

C-Circulation (page 508)

5. With focal pain, a patient is able to identify a single place or point of pain. With diffuse pain, patients are unable to point to a single location. Instead, they often move their finger around in a circle as they are asked to point to the pain. (page 532)

6. Orientation to person, place, time, and event. Person (name) evaluates long-term memory. Place and time evaluate intermediate-term memory. Event evaluates short-term memory. (page 509)

7. 1. Identify the patient's chief complaint.

2. Understand the circumstances surrounding the chief complaint.

3. Direct further physical examination. (page 517)

8. Deformities, Contusions, Abrasions, Punctures/Penetrations, Burns, Tenderness, Lacerations, Swelling (page 520)

9. -Ejection from a vehicle

-Death in the passenger compartment

-Fall greater than 15 to 20 feet

-Vehicle rollover

-High-speed vehicle collision

-Vehicle-pedestrian collision

-Motorcycle crash

-Unresponsiveness or altered mental status following trauma

-Penetrating head, chest, or abdominal trauma (page 518)

10. 1. Adequate foundation of knowledge

2. Ability to focus on specific and multiple elements of data

3. Ability to identify and organize data and form concepts

4. Ability to differentiate between relevant and irrelevant data

5. Ability to analyze and compare similar situations

6. Ability to recall contrary situations

7. Ability to articulate assessment-based decisions and construct arguments

11. 1. Read the patient

2. Read the scene

3. React

4. Reevaluate

5. Revise the management plan

6. Review performance at the run critique (page 563)

Word Fun

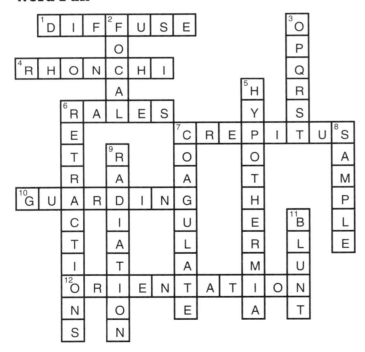

Ambulance Calls

1. -Maintain cervical spine control

-Immediately manage the airway by suction and oxygen

-Rapid survey and transport

-This patient is a load-and-go based on:

-Mechanism of injury

-Level of consciousness

-Airway compromise

-Damage to vehicle indicates possible occult injuries

2. -Assess level of responsiveness and the patient's orientation by asking her:
- the day of the week
- her name
- where she is
- if she knows why you are there

-Apply high-flow oxygen via nonrebreathing mask

-Complete a focused history and physical exam

-Transport the patient in a position of comfort

-Ask family members:
- What is her normal mental status?
- When did this start?
- Does she have any past history?
- Is she taking any new medications?
- Has she taken her medications?
- Has she eaten today?
- Anything else that might be pertinent based on your scene survey

3. -He is a rapid transport based on his altered mental status.

-En route, you should reassess all vital signs and interventions.

-Complete a detailed physical exam.

-Splint any fractures and bandage any minor wounds.

-Reassess vital signs at least every 5 minutes.

-Call in your radio report to the receiving facility.

-Reassess, reassess, reassess!

Skill Drills

Skill Drill 10-1: Performing a Rapid Trauma Assessment

1. Check ABCs, continue spinal immobilization, and assess mental status. Assess the head.

2. Assess the neck.

3. Apply a cervical collar.

4. Assess the chest, including breath sounds.

5. Assess the abdomen.

6. Assess the pelvis.

7. Assess the extremities.

8. Log roll the patient and assess the back.

9. Fully immobilize the spine and assess baseline vitals and SAMPLE history. (pages 522 to 523)

Skill Drill 10-2: Performing a Rapid Medical Assessment: Unresponsive Patient

1. Assess the head.

2. Assess the neck.

3. Assess the chest.

4. Assess the abdomen.

5. Assess the pelvis.

6. Assess the extremities.

7. Assess the back. (pages 538 to 539)

Skill Drill 10-3: Performing the Detailed Physical Exam

1. Observe the face.

2. Inspect the eyelids and the area around the eyes.

3. Examine the eyes for redness, contact lenses. Check pupil function.

4. Look behind the ear for Battle's sign.

5. Check the ears for drainage or blood.

6. Observe and palpate the head.

7. Palpate the zygomas.

8. Palpate the maxillae.

9. Palpate the mandible.

10. Assess the mouth.

11. Check for unusual breath odors.

12. Inspect the neck.

13. Palpate the neck, front and back.

14. Observe for jugular vein distention.

15. Inspect the chest and observe breathing motion.

16. Gently palpate the ribs.

17. Listen to anterior breath sounds (midaxillary, midclavicular).

18. Listen to posterior breath sounds (bases, apices).

19. Observe the abdomen and pelvis.

20. Gently palpate the abdomen.

21. Gently compress the pelvis from the sides.

22. Gently press the iliac crests.

23. Inspect the extremities; assess distal circulation and motor sensory function. Assess for the presence of edema and pitting edema.

24. Assess the back, unless the patient is immobilized. Complete assessment of the respiratory system. Complete assessment of the cardiovascular system. (pages 544 to 545)

Chapter 11: Communications and Documentation

Matching

1. M (page 580)
2. G (page 581)
3. J (page 582)
4. K (page 582)
5. H (page 582)
6. L (page 581)
7. I (page 581)
8. C (page 583)
9. A (page 581)
10. F (page 584)
11. E (page 584)
12. D (page 580)
13. B (page 594)

Multiple Choice

1. D (page 580)
2. A (page 582)
3. D (page 581)
4. B (page 582)
5. B (page 583)
6. D (page 583)
7. D (page 584)
8. C – This is true of the duplex mode (C). (page 584)
9. C – (page 584)
10. D – Principle EMS-related responsibilities of the FCC also include licensing base stations and assigning appropriate radio call signs for those stations, and establishing licensing standards and operating specifications for radio equipment used by EMS providers. (page 586)
11. D – The dispatchers do not provide care; they provide instructions for care. Responsibilities of the dispatcher also include coordinating EMS response units with other public safety services until the incident is over. (page 585)
12. D (page 587)
13. D – The determination of the level and type of response necessary is also based on the need for additional EMS units, fire suppression, rescue, a HazMat team, air medical support, or law enforcement. (page 587)
14. B – There is no way to know when the unit will arrive (B). The nature and severity of the injury, illness, or incident, special directions, or advisories, and the time at which the unit(s) are dispatched are also given. (page 588)
15. D – (page 588)
16. A – The patient report also commonly includes your unit identification and level of services, the receiving hospital, the patient's chief complaint or your perception of the problem and its severity, a brief report of physical findings, and a brief summary of care given and any patient response. (page 589)
17. B (page 589)
18. D (page 589)
19. D (page 591)
20. A (page 589)
21. D (page 589)
22. A (page 589)
23. A – If the patient wishes to be transported, you do not need permission (B). Dispatch coordinates the request of assistance from other agencies (C). You must have permission to restrain a patient but not to immobilize (D). (page 589)
24. D (page 589)
25. A – It is very important to report changes, especially if the status is worse (B). You must check vital signs every 5 minutes in critical patients and every 15 minutes for stable patients (C). All treatments should be reassessed for the patient's response to care (D). (page 591)

26. C – As long as it is not on the road creating a hazard, there is no need to report an abandoned vehicle. (page 591)

27. D   (page 591)

28. B   (page 593)

29. D   (page 593)

30. D – Components of the oral report also include a summary of the information you gave in your radio report, the patient's response to treatment, and any other information gathered that was not important enough to report sooner. (page 594)

31. D – (page 594)

32. C – Always face the person (A). Never shout (B). Never use baby talk (D). (page 595)

33. C – Sign language only works for hearing-impaired patients, for obvious reasons (A). Stay in physical contact (B). If the patient can walk to the ambulance, place his or her hand on your arm, taking care not to rush (D). (page 599)

34. A – Use simple terms and phrases, not medical terms (B). Never shout (C). Positioning yourself so the patient can read your lips only works if the patient knows the language (D). (page 600)

35. B – This (B) is administrative information. (page 600)

36. A – B, C, and D are all patient information. (page 600)

37. D – Functions of the prehospital care report also include legal documentation, administrative functions, and evaluation and continuous quality improvement. (page 600)

38. D   (page 600)

39. A – Include pertinent negative findings as well as pertinent positive findings (B). Never record conclusions, only findings (C). Avoid radio codes and use only standard abbreviations (D). (page 602)

40. D – You may also be required to file special reports for incidents involving certain infectious diseases. (page 606)

Vocabulary

1. Simplex: Single frequency radio; transmissions can occur in either direction but not simultaneously in both. When one party transmits, the other can only receive, and the party that is transmitting is unable to receive. (page 584)

2. Standing orders: Written documents, signed by the EMS system medical director, that outline specific directions, permissions, and sometimes prohibitions regarding patient care; also called protocols. (page 592)

3. Federal Communications Commission (FCC): The federal agency that has jurisdiction over interstate and international telephone and telegraph services and satellite communications, all of which may involve EMS activity. (page 586)

4. Duplex: The ability to transmit and receive simultaneously. (page 584)

5. Prehospital care report: A written record of the incident that describes the nature of the patient's injuries or illness at the scene and the treatment provided. (page 600)

Fill-in

1. patient care report (page 580)

2. transmitter, receiver (page 580)

3. dedicated line (page 581)

4. trunking (page 581)

5. telemetry (page 582)

6. cell phones (page 583)

7. Pagers (page 587)

8. importance (page 587)

9. medical control (page 588)

10. slander (page 589)

11. medical control (page 589)

12. repeat (page 590)

13. standing orders (page 592)

14. eye contact (page 594)

15. honest (page 598)

16. interpreter (page 600)

17. minimum data set (page 600)

18. accurate, legible, timely, unaltered (page 603)

19. accurate, detailed, timely (page 606)

20. Competent (page 604)

True/False

1. T (page 580)   **8.** F (page 584)

2. T (page 581)   **9.** T (page 588)

3. T (page 583)   **10.** F (page 591)

4. F (page 582)   **11.** F (page 593)

5. T (page 581)   **12.** F (page 593)

6. T (page 580)   **13.** T (page 606)

7. F (page 582)   **14.** T (page 596)

Short Answer

1. 1. Allocating specific radio frequencies for use by EMS providers

2. Licensing base stations and assigning appropriate radio call signs for thosestations

3. Establishing licensing standards and operating specifications for radio equipment used by EMS providers

4. Establishing limitations for transmitter power output

5. Monitoring radio operations (page 586)

2. -Monitor the channel before transmitting.

-Plan your message.

-Press the push-to-talk (PTT) button.

-Hold the microphone 2 to 3 inches from your mouth and speak clearly.

-Identify the person or unit you are calling, then identify your unit as the sender.

-Acknowledge a transmission as soon as you can.

-Use plain English.

-Keep your message brief.

-Avoid voicing negative emotions.

-When transmitting a number with two or more digits, say the entire number first, then each digit separately.

-Do not use profanity on the radio.

-Use EMS frequencies only for EMS communications.

-Reduce background noise.

-Be sure other radios on the same frequency are turned down. (page 592)

3. 1. Continuity of care

2. Legal documentation

3. Education

4. Administrative

5. Research

6. Evaluation and continuous quality improvement (page 600)

4. 1. Traditional written form with check boxes and a narrative section

2. Computerized, using electronic clipboard or similar device (page 602)

5. -Draw a single line through the error

-Write the appropriate information

-Initial and date (page 604)

6. -Mechanism of injury

-Patient's behavior

-First aid prior to arrival of EMS

-Safety-related information

-Information of interest to crime scene investigators

-Disposition of valuable personal property (page 603)

Word Fun

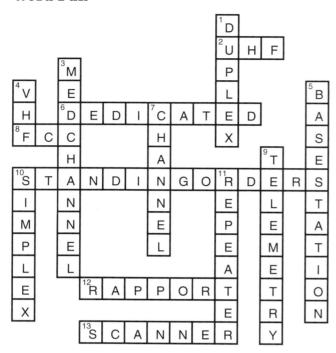

Ambulance Calls

1. -Dispatch the closest ambulance for an emergency response.
   -Call for assistance from the fire department and local law enforcement.
   -Try to calm the caller down to obtain additional information.
   -If the caller is still of no help, ask her to get someone else to the phone.
   -Relay any additional information to the responding units.

2. -Obtain a general impression of the patient as you approach.
   -Squat down to be on the same level and smile.
   -Speak slowly and distinctly, and make sure you are positioned in front of the patient.
   -Use sign language, or point to the child's leg and shrug your shoulders with palms up to ask what's wrong.
   -Use a teacher as an "interpreter" to explain to the child what you will do.
   -Remember to maintain eye contact and smile to reduce anxiety.

3. -Explain who you are.
   -Keep in physical contact with the patient.
   -Explain each procedure you will perform.
   -Transport the dog along with the patient.

Chapter 12: Trauma Systems and Mechanism of Injury

Matching

1. H (page 622)   **5.** C (page 622)
2. G (page 624)   **6.** A (page 623)
3. F (page 621)   **7.** D (page 636)
4. E (page 623)   **8.** B (page 621)

Multiple Choice

1. A   (page 619)
2. B – Thermal energy causes burns. (page 620)
3. C – (page 621)
4. C – Energy can be neither created nor destroyed. (page 621)
5. C (page 622)
6. B (page 622)
7. A (page 622)
8. D – Rear-end and rotational are types of motor vehicle crashes as well. (page 623)
9. C (pages 623 to 624)
10. C (page 623)
11. D (page 623)
12. C (page 624)
13. A (page 624)
14. C (page 625)
15. B (page 625)
16. D – Significant mechanisms of injury also include severe deformities of the frontal part of the vehicle, with or without intrusion to the passenger compartment. (page 626)
17. A – Other passengers have likely experienced the same amount of force that caused the passenger's death. (page 626)
18. D (page 627)
19. B – You should still suspect that other serious injuries to the extremities and to internal organs have occurred. (page 627)
20. C (page 628)
21. C (page 630)
22. B – The cervical spine has little tolerance for lateral bending. Approximately 25% of all severe injuries to the aorta that occur in motor vehicle crashes are a result of lateral collisions. (page 630)
23. D (page 629)
24. B (page 633)
25. C – Rollover crashes are particularly dangerous for both restrained and, to a greater degree, unrestrained passengers because these crashes provide multiple opportunities for second and third collisions. (page 632)
26. C (page 634)
27. B (page 635)
28. D (page 635)
29. D (page 636)
30. B – This is one reason that exit wounds are often many times larger than entrance wounds. (page 637)
31. B (page 636)
32. B (page 634)
33. A (page 638)
34. C (page 638)

Vocabulary

1. Newton's First Law: Objects at rest tend to stay at rest, and objects in motion tend to in motion unless acted upon by some force. (page 620)
2. Newton's Second Law: Force equals mass times acceleration (F = *ma*). (page 620)
3. Newton's Third Law: For every action, there is an equal and opposite reaction. (page 621)
4. Mesentery: The peritoneal fold that surrounds the small intestine and connects to the posterior abdominal wall; also the membranous fold that attaches other organs to a body wall. (page 630)

Fill-in

1. Injuries (page 618)
2. injury patterns, injury events (page 618)
3. index of suspicion (page 618)
4. Traumatic injury (page 620)
5. $KE = 1/2mv^2$ (page 621)
6. Polaroids (page 626)
7. deceleration (page 627)
8. submarining (page 627)
9. serious injury, death (page 627)
10. Rear-end impacts (page 630)
11. Lap belts (page 633)
12. minimally (page 633)
13. skull fractures, contusions, lacerations (page 636)

True/False

1. T	(page 621)		6. T	(page 630)	
2. F	(page 621)		7. T	(page 631)	
3. F	(page 621)		8. T	(page 634)	
4. T	(page 623)		9. T	(page 635)	
5. T	(page 627)		10. T	(page 618)	

Short Answer

1. Potential energy is the product of mass (weight), force of gravity, and height and is mostly associated with the energy of falling objects. (page 622)
2. 1. Collision of the car against another car or other object
   2. Collision of the passenger against the interior of the car
   3. Collision of the passenger's internal organs against the solid structures of the body (pages 623 to 624)
3. 1. The height of the fall
   2. The surface struck
   3. The part of the body that hits first, followed by the path of energy displacement (page 635)
   4. A bullet, because of its speed, creates pressure waves that emanate from its path, causing distant damage. (pages 636 to 637)
4. The size (mass) and speed (velocity) of the projectile affect the potential damage. If the mass is doubled, the potential energy is doubled. If the velocity is doubled, the potential energy is quadrupled. (page 637)
5. -injury prevention
   -effective education
   -treatment, transport, and trauma triage
   -rehabilitation
   -data collection (page 618)

7. -extended transport time by ground

-mass casualties

-extrication times are prolonged with critically injured patients

-long distances to an appropriate facility (page 619)

8. Front end: Head, spine, chest (rib fractures, flail chest, pneumothorax, hemothorax, contusions, great vessel injury), abdomen (solid organ, hollow organ, diaphragm), fractured pelvis, posterior hip and knee dislocation, lower extremity fractures, pelvic and acetabular fractures

Rear-end: Whiplash, c-spine, spine, pelvis, acceleration injury to brain

Lateral: C-spine, lateral whiplash, shearing of the brain, rib fracture, flail chest, pneumothorax, liver and spleen lacerations, aortic tears, fractured pelvis, fractured clavicle, femur and humerus fractures (pages 629 to 631)

9. 1. Vehicle vs. pedestrian

2. Pedestrian rotates onto hood

3. Pedestrian rolls onto the ground (page 635)

Word Fun

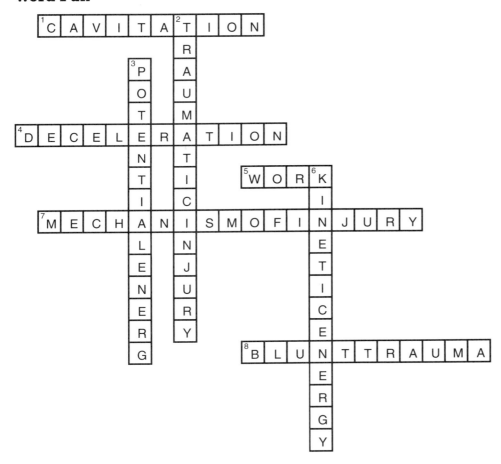

Ambulance Calls

1. -Maintain cervical spine control.

-Apply high-flow oxygen.

-Keep a high index of suspicion for life-threatening injuries.

-Monitor vital signs.

-Monitor ECG

-Consider IV therapy

-Rapid transport

2. -Maintain cervical spine control.

-Apply high-flow oxygen.

-Fully immobilize the patient and splint the leg.

-Monitor vital signs.

-Consider IV placement and analgesic therapy

-Normal transport

3. -Apply high-flow oxygen via NRB mask

-Consider spinal immobilization

-Monitor vital signs

-Establish IV access and bolus 20 ml/kg crystalloid as needed to maintain perfusion

-EKG monitoring

-Consider endotracheal intubation if the respiratory status or LOC decreases

-Rapid transport

4. -Apply high-flow oxygen

-Stabilize object in place with bulky dressings

-Monitor vital signs

-Monitor ECG

-Initiate IV therapy

-Transport in a supine position

-Rapid transport because of abdominal penetration

Chapter 13: Patient Hemorrhage and Shock

Matching

1. G   (page 647)
2. J   (page 646)
3. I   (page 660)
4. K   (page 661)
5. N   (page 650)
6. Q   (page 664)
7. A   (page 651)
8. F   (page 661)
9. P   (page 660)
10. O   (page 664)
11. B   (page 648)
12. C   (page 660)
13. E   (page 654)
14. R   (page 651)
15. H   (page 664)
16. L   (page 649)
17. M   (page 660)
18. D   (page 651)

Multiple Choice

1. D   (page 646)
2. B   (page 646)
3. C – The lungs (A) and kidneys (B) require a constant blood supply. (page 646)
4. D   (page 647)
5. B   (page 647)
6. B   (page 648)
7. D – The patient may also present with an altered mental status, cool clammy skin, and cyanosis. (page 649)
8. C   (page 649)
9. D   (pages 649 to 650)
10. A   (page 651)
11. B   (page 650)
12. A   (page 651)
13. A   (page 651)
14. A   (page 651)
15. B   (page 651)
16. D – Contraindications also include acute heart failure, groin injuries, and major head injuries. (page 654)
17. C   (page 656)
18. D – Never cover a tourniquet (B). Wide padding may actually help protect the tissues and help with arterial compression (C). (page 658)
19. B   (page 658)
20. B   (page 664)
21. D   (pages 663 to 664)
22. C   (page 664)
23. C   (page 664)
24. A   (page 664)

Labeling

Perfusion (page 646)

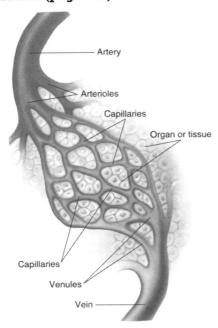

Artery

Arterioles

Capillaries

Organ or tissue

Capillaries

Venules

Vein

Arterial Pressure Points (page 653)

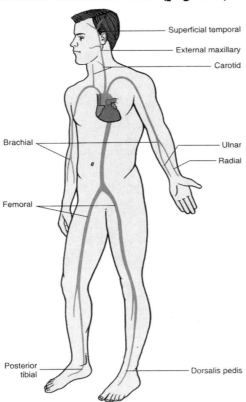

Superficial temporal

External maxillary

Carotid

Brachial

Ulnar

Radial

Femoral

Posterior tibial

Dorsalis pedis

Cardiovascular System (page 659)

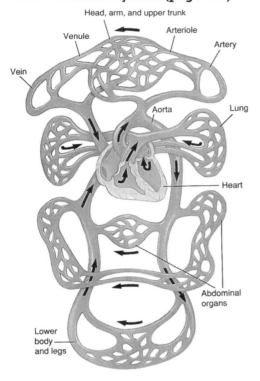

Vocabulary

1. Perfusion: Circulation of blood within an organ or tissue in adequate amounts to meet the cells' current needs for oxygen, nutrients, and waste removal. (page 646)

2. Shock: A condition in which the circulatory system fails to provide sufficient circulation for every body part to perform its function. Low blood volume results in inadequate perfusion, also known as hypovolemic shock. (page 647)

3. Autonomic nervous system: The part of the nervous system that regulates involuntary functions, such as digestion and sweating. (page 661)

4. Pressure point: A point where a blood vessel lies near a bone; useful when direct pressure and elevation do not control bleeding. (page 652)

5. Pulse pressure: Difference between the systolic and diastolic blood pressures. (pages 662 to 663)

Fill-in

1. perfusion (page 646)
2. autonomic nervous system (page 647)
3. 4 to 6 minutes (page 647)
4. 20% (page 648)
5. signs and symptoms (page 648)
6. Hemostats (page 654)
7. skull fracture (page 658)
8. nonessential, essential (page 659)
9. 80 mm Hg (page 660)
10. cellular ischemia (page 660)
11. inotropic (page 668)
12. body temperature (page 665)
13. 80 to 90 mm Hg (page 668)

True/False

1. F   (page 649)
2. F   (page 648)
3. F   (page 653)
4. T   (page 651)
5. F   (page 658)
6. F   (page 651)
7. T   (page 656)
8. F   (page 666)
9. T   (page 668)

Short Answer

1. 1. Direct pressure and elevation
   2. Pressure dressings
   3. Pressure points (for upper and lower extremities)
   4. Splints
   5. Air splints
   6. PASG
   7. Tourniquets (page 653)

2. The body can still compensate for blood loss by using internal mechanisms.

   The blood pressure begins to fall.

   Occurs when the blood volume drops more than 15% to 25%.

   Compensatory mechanisms begin to fail. (page 662)

3. Shock has progressed to a terminal stage.

   Blood pressure is abnormally low.

   Even if the cause is treated and reversed, vital organ damage cannot be repaired, and the patient will die. (pages 662 to 663)

Word Fun

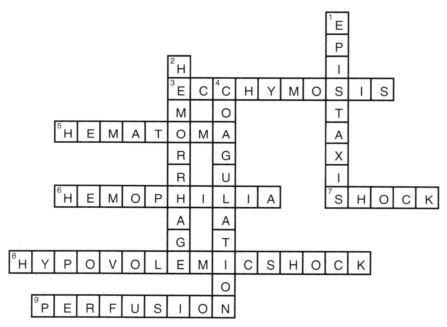

Ambulance Calls

1. -Control bleeding with direct pressure, elevation, pressure point, and a tourniquet as a LAST resort.
   -Apply high-flow oxygen
   -Place patient in a position of comfort
   -Monitor vital signs
   -Rapid transport

2. -High-flow oxygen
   -Maintain c-spine immobilizations and place patient in Trendelenburg's position
   -Cover to keep warm
   -Consider the mechanism of injury
   -Monitor vital signs.
   -Establish IV access
   -Monitor ECG
   -Rapid transport

3. -Control bleeding with direct pressure, elevation, pressure point, or tourniquet as a LAST resort.

-Apply high-flow oxygen and treat for shock as signs and symptoms present.

-Monitor vital signs.

-Establish IV access.

-Monitor EKG.

-Normal transport unless patient shows signs and symptoms of shock.

Skill Drills

Skill Drill 13-1: Controlling External Bleeding

1. direct pressure, level, heart, fracture

2. pressure dressing

3. pressure point, direct pressure, (page 652)

Skill Drill 13-2: Applying a Pneumatic Antishock Garment (PASG)

1. Rapidly expose and examine the areas to be covered by the PASG. Pad any exposed bone ends. Apply the garment so that the top is below the lowest rib.

2. Close and fasten both leg compartments and the abdominal compartment.

3. Open the stopcocks.Auscultate breath sounds for pulmonary edema before inflation of any compartment.

4. Inflate with the foot pump until the patient's blood pressure reaches 90 to 100 mm Hg or the velcro crackles. Monitor radial pulses.

5. Check the patient's blood pressure again. Monitor vital signs. (page 655)

Skill Drill 13-4: Treating Shock

1. Keep the patient supine, open the airway, and check breathing and pulse.

2. Control obvious external bleeding.

3. Splint any broken bones or joint injuries.

4. Give high-flow oxygen if you have not already done so, and place blankets under and over the patient.

5. If no fractures are suspected, elevate the legs 6 to 12 inches. (page 667)

Chapter 14: Burns and Soft-Tissue Injuries

Matching

1. G (page 678)	**7.** E (page 681)
2. B (page 678)	**8.** J (page 686)
3. D (page 678)	**9.** A (page 683)
4. F (page 678)	**10.** C (page 682)
5. I (page 678)	**11.** K (page 688)
6. L (page 681)	**12.** H (page 686)

Multiple Choice

1. C (page 678)

2. B (page 678)

3. B (page 678)

4. A (page 678)

5. B (page 679)

6. C (page 680)

7. B (page 680)

8. B (page 680)

9. D (page 680)

10. C (page 680)

11. C (page 681)

12. C (page 681)

13. B (page 681)

14. A (page 681)

15. D (page 681)

16. B (page 683)

17. D (page 684)

18. D (page 684)

19. A (page 681)

20. D (page 684)

21. D (page 685)

22. B (page 686)

23. C – Never touch exposed organs (A). Use moist sterile dressings (B). Never use adherent dressings (C). (page 688)

24. C – Hypovolemic shock (A) does not result from air being sucked in. Tracheal deviation (B) results from a tension pneumothorax. Subcutaneous emphysema (C) results from air outside the vessels. (page 690)

25. D (page 691)

26. D (page 691)

27. D (page 691)

28. C (page 691)

29. D – Factors in helping to determine the severity of a burn also include whether or not there are any preexisting medical conditions or other injuries and if the patient is younger than 5 years of age or older than 55 years of age. (page 692)

30. C (page 693)

31. B (page 693)

32. C (page 693)

33. D (page 693)

34. D – Significant airway burns may also be associated with soot around the nose and mouth. (page 694)

35. A (page 694)

36. D (page 700)

37. C (page 702)

38. B – Personal safety always comes first. (page 703)

39. D (page 703)

40. D (page 705)

41. A (page 706)

42. C (page 706)

43. D (page 707)

44. D – Apply high-flow oxygen (A). Be prepared to defibrillate (B). (page 704)

45. A – An occlusive dressing must be airtight; gauze pads (A) are not. (page 707)

46. D (page 708)

47. D (page 699)

Labeling EMT-I anatomy review web

Skin (page 679)

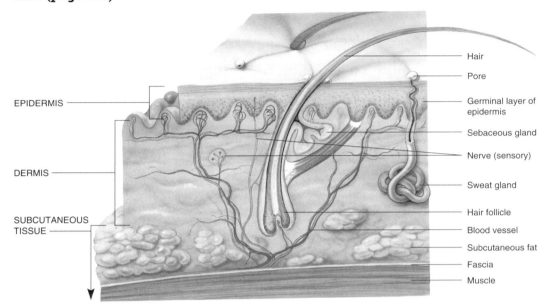

EPIDERMIS

DERMIS

SUBCUTANEOUS TISSUE

Hair

Pore

Germinal layer of epidermis

Sebaceous gland

Nerve (sensory)

Sweat gland

Hair follicle

Blood vessel

Subcutaneous fat

Fascia

Muscle

Classifications of Burns (page 693)

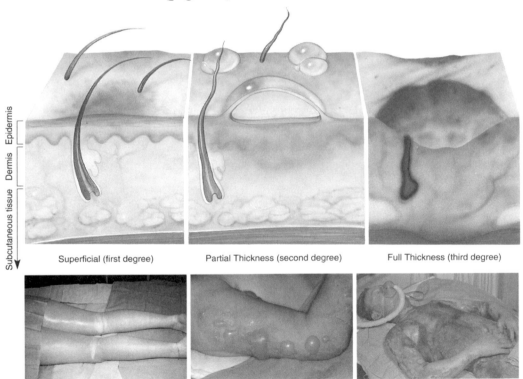

Epidermis   Dermis   Subcutaneous tissue

Superficial (first degree)

Partial Thickness (second degree)

Full Thickness (third degree)

Rule of Nines (page 694)

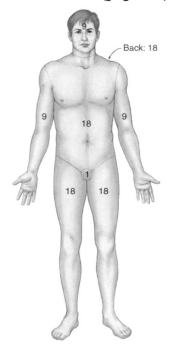

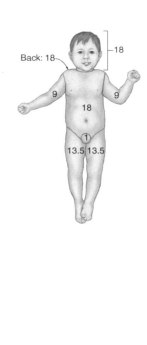

Vocabulary EMT-I vocab explorer web

1. Partial-thickness burn: A burn affecting the epidermis and some portion of the dermis; characterized by red moist mottled skin with blisters. (page 693)
2. Closed injury: Injury in which damage occurs beneath the skin or mucous membrane but the surface remains intact. (page 679)
3. Evisceration: An open wound in the abdominal cavity in which organs protrude through the wound. (page 688)
4. Compartment syndrome: Swelling in a confined space that produces dangerous pressure. (page 681)
5. Contamination: The presence of infective organisms or foreign bodies such as dirt, gravel, or metal. (page 681)
6. Tetany: Intermittent tonic spasms that involve the extremities. (page 702)
7. Eschar: Thick, coagulated crust or slough of leathery skin that develops following a burn. (page 691)

Fill-in

1. moist (page 679)
2. cool (page 679)
3. dermis (page 678)
4. subcutaneous (page 678)
5. constrict (page 679)
6. bacteria, water (page 679)
7. dermis (page 678)
8. temperature (page 679)
9. epidermis, dermis (page 678)
10. radiated (page 679)
11. shortening (page 690)
12. early intubation (page 692)
13. airway, respiratory (page 694)
14. dry chemicals (page 700)
15. hands, wrists, feet (page 703)

True/False

1. T   (page 693)
2. F   (page 693)
3. T   (page 693)
4. T   (page 694)
5. T   (pages 693 to 694)
6. T   (page 692)
7. F   (page 695)
8. F   (page 698)
9. T   (page 698)
10. T   (page 699)
11. T   (page 703)
12. T   (page 706)
13. T   (page 704)
14. T   (page 707)
15. T   (page 707)
16. F   (page 707)
17. F   (page 708)
18. T   (page 708)
19. F   (page 680)
20. F   (page 681)

Short Answer

1. 1. superficial
   2. partial-thickness
   3. full-thickness (page 693)

2. 1. closed
   2. open
   3. burns (page 679)

3. I: ice
   C: compression
   E: elevation
   S: splinting (page 681)

4. -Full- or partial-thickness burns covering more than 20% of total body surface area
   -Burns involving the hands, feet, face, airway, or genitalia (page 695)

5. Brush off dry chemicals and/or remove clothing, then flush the burned area with large amounts of water.(page 700)

6. First, there may be deep tissue injury not visible on the outside. Second, there is a danger of cardiac arrest from the electrical shock. (page 703)

7. A wound caused by a penetrating object into the chest that causes air to enter the chest. The air enters the chest area through the wound, but remains in the pleural space and the lung does not expand. With exhalation, air passes back through the wound, making a "sucking" sound. (page 686)

8. 1. Control bleeding
   2. Protect from further damage
   3. Prevent further contamination and infection (page 707)

9. 1. Abrasions
   2. Lacerations
   3. Avulsions
   4. Penetrating (page 681)

10. 1. Depth (superficial/partial/full)
   2. Extent (% of body burned)
   3. Involvement of critical areas (face, upper airway, hands, feet, genitalia)
   4. Preexisting medical conditions or other injuries
   5. Age of younger than 5 years or older than 55 years (page 692)

11. 4 mL $\times$ patient's weight in kilograms $\times$ BSA = total fluid replacement
   -Give $\frac{1}{2}$ of this over the first 8 hours
   -Give $\frac{1}{4}$ over the next 8 hours
   -Give last $\frac{1}{4}$ over the next 8 hours

12. -Pain
   -Blistering/sloughing
   -Musculoskeletal injury
   -Abnormal breath sounds:
     •hoarseness
     •dyspnea
     •dysphagia
     •dysphasia
   -burned hair
   -nausea/vomiting
   -altered LOC
   -edema
   -paresthesia
   -possible hemorrhage
   -chest pain

13. -Damage from heat inhalation

    -Damage from systemic toxins

    -Damage from smoke inhalation

14. Alpha, beta, and gamma (page 705)

Word Fun

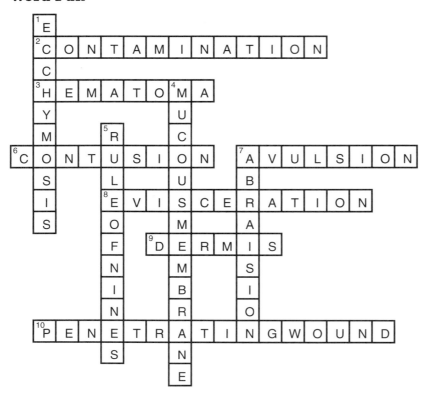

Ambulance Calls

1. -Take BSI precautions

    -Apply direct pressure

    -Elevate the extremity and apply a pressure dressing

    -Try a pressure point if bleeding is not controlled (tourniquet as a last resort)

    -Once bleeding is controlled, splint the arm to decrease movement

    -Apply high-flow oxygen

    -Transport in position of comfort, normal response

    -Monitor vital signs

2. -BSI precautions

    -Quickly assess ABCs

    -Wrap foot with a pressure dressing to control bleeding

    -Transport in position of comfort

    -Standard transport

    -Monitor vital signs en route

    -Apply oxygen as needed

    -Be alert for signs of hypovolemic shock

3. -Apply high-flow oxygen, preferably humidified (dry oxygen may irritate the tissues further)

    -Cover burns with sterile dressings loosely

    -Rapid transport in position of comfort

    -Monitor airway and vital signs continuously

-Consider early endotracheal intubation

-Establish IV access

-Monitor ECG

-Protect from hypothermia

4. -High-flow oxygen by NRB if the patient will tolerate (may use blow-by technique otherwise)

-Bandage burns including bandages between the digits

-Monitor vital signs

-Establish IV access

-Monitor ECG

-Consider analgesics

-Consider possibility of child abuse

-Rapid transport

-May need special report documentation

Skill Drills

Skill Drill 14-1: Controlling Bleeding from a Soft-Tissue Injury

1. direct pressure, sterile dressing

2. roller

3. dressing, roller

4. Splint (page 686)

Skill Drill 14-2: Sealing a Sucking Chest Wound

1. supine, high-flow oxygen

2. occlusive

3. local protocol, leaving open (page 687)

Skill Drill 14-3: Stabilizing an Impaled Object

1. move, remove

2. bleeding, stabilize, soft dressings, gauze, tape

3. rigid, movement (page 689)

Skill Drill 14-4: Caring for Burns

1. Follow BSI precautions to help prevent infection.
Remove the patient from the burning area; extinguish or remove hot clothing and jewelry as needed.
If the wound(s) is still burning or hot, immerse the hot area in cool sterile water or cover with a cool wet dressing.

2. Give supplemental oxygen and continue to assess the airway.

3. Estimate the severity of the burn, then cover the area with a dry sterile dressing or clean sheet.
Assess and treat the patient for any other injuries.

4. Prepare for transport.
Treat for shock if needed.

5. Cover the patient with blankets to prevent loss of body heat.
Transport promptly. (page 696)

Chapter 15: Thoracic Trauma

Matching

1. B   (page 716)
2. D   (page 716)
3. C   (page 718)
4. A   (page 718)
5. E   (page 717)
6. H   (page 719)
7. I   (page 721)
8. J   (page 732)
9. F   (page 719)
10. G   (page 721)

Multiple Choice

1. B   (page 717)
2. A   (page 716)
3. C   (page 718)
4. D   (page 720)
5. D – A, B, and C are signs. (page 721)
6. D   (page 721)
7. B – Flail segment (A) is a common cause of paradoxical motion. (page 721)
8. C   (page 721)
9. B   (page 722)
10. D   (page 722)
11. D   (page 722)
12. B   (page 723)
13. A   (page 723)
14. B   (page 724)
15. C   (page 725)
16. C   (page 722)
17. D   (page 725)
18. D   (pages 723)

19. D   (page 725)
20. D   (page 727)
21. D – It also includes tachycardia, low blood pressure, cyanosis, and decreased breath sounds on the injured side. (page 727)
22. D   (page 730)
23. C   (page 727)
24. B   (page 733)
25. A   (page 733)
26. D   (page 723)
27. A   (page 724)
28. C – Bruising of the lung (A) is called a pulmonary contusion. Broken ribs in two or more places (B) is called flail chest. (page 734)
29. D   (page 735)
30. D – Signs and symptoms of pericardial tamponade also include jugular vein distention and a decrease in the difference between the systolic and diastolic blood pressure. (page 733)
31. B   (page 733)

Labeling

Anterior Aspect of the Chest (page 716)

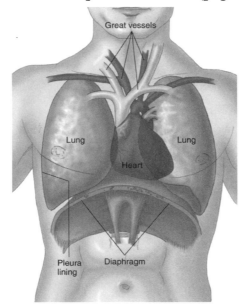

Ribs (page 717)

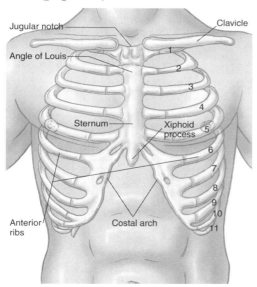

Jugular notch

Clavicle

Angle of Louis

1

2

3

4

Sternum

Xiphoid process

5

6

7

8

9

10

11

Anterior ribs

Costal arch

Flail Chest (page 724)

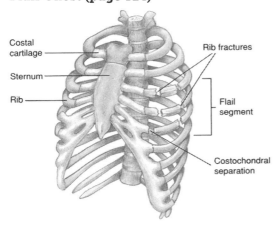

Costal cartilage

Rib fractures

Sternum

Rib

Flail segment

Costochondral separation

Hemothorax and Hemopneumothorax (page 731}

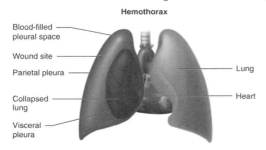

Hemothorax

Blood-filled pleural space

Wound site

Parietal pleura

Collapsed lung

Visceral pleura

Lung

Heart

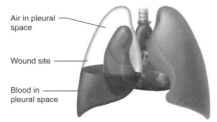

Hemopneumothorax

Air in pleural space

Wound site

Blood in pleural space

Vocabulary

1. Flail chest: A condition in which three or more ribs are fractured in two or more places, or in association with a fracture of the sternum, so that a segment of chest wall is effectively detached from the rest of the thoracic cage. (page 724)

2. Paradoxical motion: The motion of a portion of the chest wall that is detached in a flail chest; the motion of in during inhalation, out during exhalation is exactly the opposite of normal motion during breathing. (page 724)

3. Pericardial tamponade: Compression of the heart due to a buildup of blood or other fluid in the pericardial sac. (page 732)

4. Spontaneous pneumothorax: Pneumothorax that occurs when a weak area on the lung ruptures in the absence of major injury, allowing air to leak into the pleural space. (page 725)

5. Sucking chest wound: An opening or penetrating chest wall wound through which air passes during inspiration and expiration, creating a sucking sound. (page 727)

6. Tension pneumothorax: An accumulation of air or gas in the pleural cavity that progressively increases the pressure in the chest with potentially fatal results. (page 727)

7. Paper bag syndrome: Rupture of the lungs that occurs as the chest meets with blunt trauma after taking a deep breath, usually during a motor vehicle crash, similar to rupture of an air-filled paper bag. (page 726)

8. Chemoreceptors: Sensors that respond to chemical fluctuations such as a decreased oxygen concentration in the bloodstream. (page 718)

9. Bradypnea: Slow respirations (page 721)

Fill-in

1. posterior (page 717)
2. decreases (page 718)
3. sternum (page 716)
4. bronchi (page 717)
5. phrenic (page 718)
6. ribs (page 716)
7. diaphragm (page 716)
8. Pleura (page 717)
9. aorta (page 717)
10. contracts (page 718)
11. Chemical changes, carbon dioxide, oxygen, hydrogen ions (page 718)
12. bellows action (page 720)
13. C3, C4, and C5 (page 718)
14. cardiac output (page 720)
15. pulsus paradoxus (page 721)
16. hyperflexion (page 725)
17. sucking chest wound (page 727)
18. size (page 732)
19. ligamentum arteriosum (page 733)
20. carina (page 734)

True/False

1. T (page 721)
2. F (page 721)
3. T (page 727)
4. F (page 723)
5. F (page 726)
6. F (page 730)
7. F (page 716)
8. T (page 718)
9. F (page 733)
10. T (page 731)
11. F (page 724)
12. T (page 723)
13. F (page 724)
14. T (page 724)
15. T (page 724)
16. F (page 727)
17. T (page 731)
18. F (page 733)

Short Answer

1. -Pain at the site of injury

   -Pain localized at the site of injury that is aggravated by or increased with breathing

   -Dyspnea (difficulty breathing, shortness of breath)

-Hemoptysis (coughing up blood)

-Failure of one or both sides of the chest to expand normally with inspiration

-Rapid, weak pulse and low blood pressure

-Cyanosis around the lips or fingernails. (page 721)

2. -Assess the patient

-Prepare and assemble necessary equipment

-Obtain orders from medical control

-Locate appropriate site

-Make a one-way valve or flutter valve

-Insert the needle at 90°

-Remove the needle and dispose of in sharps container

-Secure catheter in place

-Monitor patient (page 727)

3. Tape a bulky pad against the segment of the chest. (page 724)

4. Sudden severe compression of the chest, causing a rapid increase of pressure within the chest. Characteristic signs include distended neck veins, facial and neck cyanosis, and hemorrhage in the sclera of the eye. (pages 734 to 735))

Word Fun

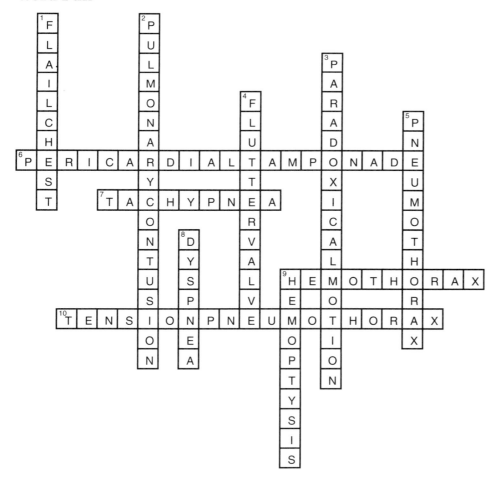

Ambulance Calls

1. -Immediately begin assisting ventilations with a BVM attached to 100% oxygen.

-Begin chest compressions.

-Perform endotracheal intubation.

-Establish IV access.

-ECG monitoring

-Continue CPR and continuously monitor the patient.

2. -Apply high-flow oxygen

-Monitor vital signs

-Monitor for development of tension

-ECG monitoring

-Circulatory support

-Consider needle thoracostomy

-Rapid transport in position of comfort

-Continue to monitor patient for signs of distress en route to the hospital

3. -Apply high-flow oxygen via nonrebreathing mask or BVM.

-Endotracheal intubation

-Establish IV access

-ECG monitoring

-Fully c-spine immobilize patient.

-Rapid transport

-Monitor vital signs en route.

4. -Rapid extrication from the vehicle

-Full spinal immobilization

-Inspect for paradoxical motion of the chest

-Monitor vital signs

-Apply high-flow oxygen via NRB mask

-Establish IV access

-ECG monitoring

-Allow patient to splint ribs with arm

-If flail segment is present, use a bulky dressing for a splint

-Monitor for changes in LOC and respiratory status

-If condition deteriorates, consider endotracheal intubation

Skill Drills

Skill Drill 15-1: Decompression of a Tension Pneumothorax

1. Assess

2. Prepare, assemble, medical control

3. Locate

4. Cleanse, aseptic

5. one-way, flutter

6. 90°

7. release, air, dispose, sharps container

8. catheter, Monitor, tension pneumothorax (pages 728 to 729)

Chapter 16: Abdomen and Genitalia Injuries

Matching

1. G (page 744)
2. D (page 744)
3. C (page 744)
4. H (page 751)

5. E (page 751)
6. B (page 750)
7. A (page 753)
8. F (page 744)

Multiple Choice

1. D (page 744)
2. D – The intestines are also hollow. (page 744)
3. C (page 744)
4. D (page 744)
5. B – The abdomen becomes distended and firm to the touch (A); normal bowel sounds diminish or disappear (C). (page 744)
6. D (page 744)
7. A (page 744)
8. C (page 746)
9. B (page 745)
10. A (page 745)
11. D (page 745)
12. C (page 745)
13. B – (A) and (C) are types of open injuries (page 745)
14. A (page 746)
15. B – (A) is a symptom (page 746)
16. B (page 746)
17. B (page 746)
18. D (page 747)
19. D (page 747)

20. D – Using diagonal shoulder safety belts alone can also cause rib fractures and other types of fractures. Far fewer head and neck injuries are seen when this belt is used in combination with a lap belt and a headrest. (page 748)
21. C (page 749)
22. D (page 749)
23. D – Only a surgeon can accurately assess the damage. (page 749)
24. D – Never attempt to replace abdominal contents (A), always keep organs moist (B), and never use any type of adherent dressing (C). (page 750)
25. A – (B), (C), and (D) are all hollow organs (page 751)
26. C (page 751)
27. D (page 752)
28. D (pages 752 to 753)
29. A (page 753)
30. B (page 754)
31. D (page 754)
32. D (page 755)
33. D (page 751)

Labeling EMT-I anatomy review web

Hollow Organs (page 744)

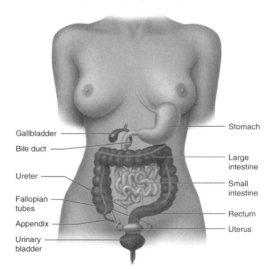

Gallbladder
Bile duct
Ureter
Fallopian tubes
Appendix
Urinary bladder
Stomach
Large intestine
Small intestine
Rectum
Uterus

Solid Organs (page 745)

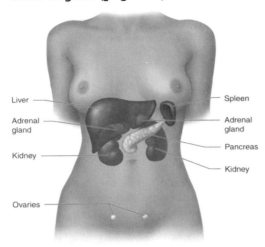

Liver
Adrenal gland
Kidney
Ovaries

Spleen
Adrenal gland
Pancreas
Kidney

Male Reproductive System (page 752)

FRONT VIEW

SIDE VIEW

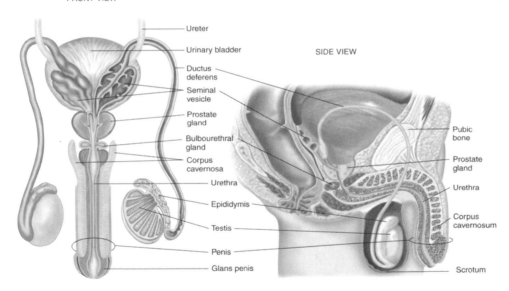

Ureter
Urinary bladder
Ductus deferens
Seminal vesicle
Prostate gland
Bulbourethral gland
Corpus cavernosa
Urethra
Epididymis
Testis
Penis
Glans penis

Pubic bone
Prostate gland
Urethra
Corpus cavernosum
Scrotum

Female Reproductive System (page 752)

FRONT VIEW

SIDE VIEW

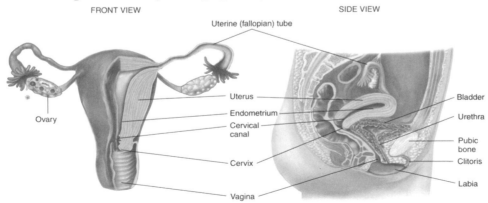

Uterine (fallopian) tube
Ovary
Uterus
Endometrium
Cervical canal
Cervix
Vagina

Bladder
Urethra
Pubic bone
Clitoris
Labia

Vocabulary

1. Closed abdominal injury: Any injury of the abdomen caused by a nonpenetrating instrument or force in which the skin remains intact; also called blunt abdominal injury. (page 745)

2. Open abdominal injury: Any injury of the abdomen caused by a penetrating or piercing instrument or force in which the skin is lacerated or perforated and the cavity is opened to the atmosphere; also called penetrating injury. (page 745)

3. Guarding: Contracting the stomach muscles to minimize the pain of abdominal movement; a sign of peritonitis. (page 745)

Fill-in

1. solid (page 744)
2. urinary (page 751)
3. retroperitoneal (page 751)
4. external signs (page 752)

5. peritonitis (page 744)
6. inflammatory response (page 744)
7. blunt injuries (page 745)
8. analgesics (page 755)

True/False

1. F (page 744)
2. T (page 746)
3. F (page 747)
4. T (page 744)

5. F (page 750)
6. F (page 751)
7. T (page 751)

Short Answer

1. -stomach
   -intestines
   -ureters
   -bladder
   -gallbladder
   -rectum (page 744)

2. -liver
   -spleen
   -pancreas
   -kidneys (page 745)

3. -pain
   -shock signs
   -bruises
   -lacerations
   -bleeding
   -tenderness
   -guarding
   -difficulty with movement because of pain (page 746)

4. 1. Inspect the patient's back and sides for exit wounds.
   2. Apply a dry sterile dressing to all open wounds.
   3. If the penetrating object is still in place, apply a stabilizing bandage around it to control external bleeding and to minimize movement of the object. (page 749)

5. 1. Cover with moistened sterile dressing.
   2. Secure dressing with bandage.
   3. Secure bandage with tape. (page 750)

6. 1. An abrasion, laceration, or contusion in the flank
   2. A penetrating wound in the region of the lower rib cage (the flank) or the upper abdomen
   3. Fractures on either side of the lower rib cage or of the lower thoracic or upper lumbar vertebrae (page 752)

Word Fun

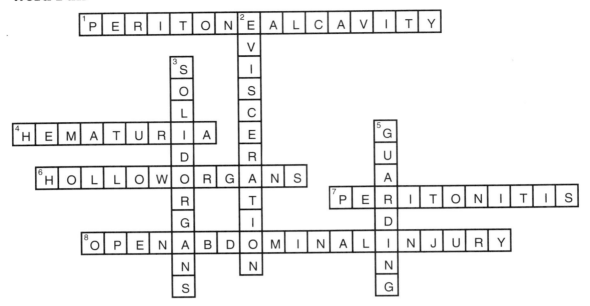

Ambulance Calls

1. Assess the ABCs.

Apply high-flow oxygen.

Control any bleeding.

Stabilize the knife in place with bulky dressings; DO NOT REMOVE.

Keep movement of patient to a bare minimum so as not to create further injury. (Sliding the patient very carefully onto a backboard may help to minimize movement.)

Monitor vital signs.

Establish IV access.

ECG monitoring

Rapid transport

Bandage minor lacerations en route.

2. C-spine immobilization

Apply high-flow oxygen.

Normal transport unless patient's condition changes

Continue your assessment en route.

Monitor vital signs and airway continuously.

Consider IV access

ECG monitoring

3. Apply high-flow oxygen via nonrebreathing mask.

Cover the abdominal contents with moist sterile gauze and an occlusive dressing.

Transport in the position of comfort (probably supine with knees bent).

Establish IV access

ECG monitoring

Rapid transport

Monitor vital signs and airway continuously

4. Patient 1

-Bandages to abrasions

-Ice pack to lip

-Monitor for changes

Patient 2

-Apply high-flow oxygen via NRB mask

-Monitor vital signs

-Establish IV access

-ECG monitoring

-Transport with knees flexed

Chapter 17: Head and Spine Injuries

Matching

1. D	(page 762)	**6.** C	(page 762)
2. E	(page 762)	**7.** B	(page 781)
3. H	(page 765)	**8.** I	(page 764)
4. G	(page 765)	**9.** J	(page 766)
5. A	(page 766)	**10.** F	(page 762)

Multiple Choice

1. D   (page 762)

2. B   (page 762)

3. C   (page 762)

4. C   (page 783)

5. A   (page 762)

6. B   (page 766)

7. D   (page 764)

8. D   (page 762)

9. C   (page 765)

10. A   (page 767)

11. D   (page 768)

12. D   (page 769)

13. B   (page 766)

14. D – Assess pulse and motor and sensory function in all extremities. (page 771)

15. B   (page 771)

16. A   (page 771)

17. A – Remember BSI. (page 775)

18. B   (page 774)

19. D   (page 774)

20. D   (page 774)

21. B   (page 774)

22. C   (page 774)

23. B   (page 779)

24. D   (page 779)

25. D – An intracerebral hemorrhage (B) is within the substance of the brain tissue itself. A subdural hematoma (C) is below the dura but outside the brain. (page 779)

26. B   (page 780)

27. B   (page 781)

28. D – Cyanosis (A) and hypoxia (B) are results of cerebral edema. Vomiting (C) results from increased intracranial pressure. (page 781)

29. C   (page 781)

30. C   (page 782)

31. D   (page 783)

32. C   (page 783)

33. B – BSI and scene safety always come first, but (B) is the best answer of the choices given. (pages 782 to 783)

34. D   (page 785)

35. A   (page 784)

36. C   (page 788)

37. A   (page 792)

Labeling

Brain (page 763)

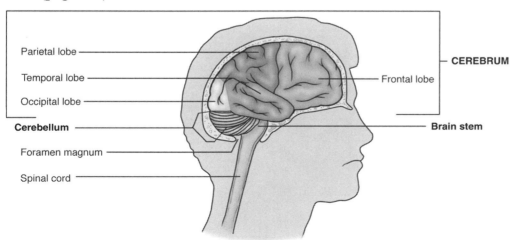

Parietal lobe

Temporal lobe

Occipital lobe

Cerebellum

Foramen magnum

Spinal cord

CEREBRUM

Frontal lobe

Brain stem

Connecting Nerves in the Spinal Cord (page 765)

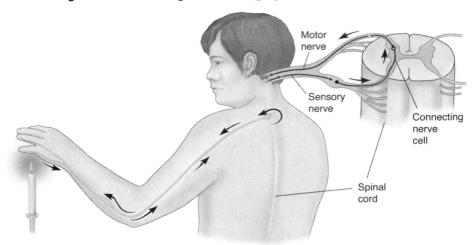

Skull (page 766)

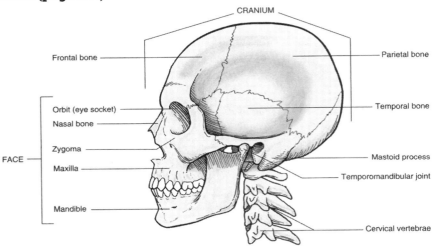

Spinal Canal (page 767)

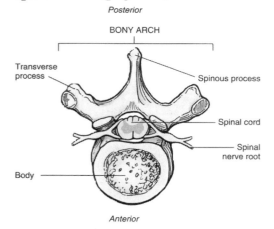

Vocabulary

1. Retrograde amnesia: The inability to remember events leading up to a head injury. (page 779)
2. Anterograde (posttraumatic) amnesia: Inability to remember events after an injury. (page 779)
3. Closed head injury: Injury usually associated with trauma in which the brain has been injured but the skin has not been broken and there is no obvious bleeding. (page 781)
4. Eyes-forward position: A position in which the head is gently lifted until the patient's eyes are looking straight ahead and the head and torso are in line. (page 770)
5. Open head injury: Injury to the head often caused by a penetrating object in which there may be bleeding and exposed brain tissue. (page 782)
6. Distracted: The act of pulling the spine along its length. (page 767)

Fill-in

1. motor (page 764)
2. meninges (page 762)
3. central (page 762)
4. 31 (page 764)
5. cranial (page 764)
6. intervertebral disks (page 766)
7. cranium, face (page 766)
8. arachnoid, pia mater (page 762)
9. sympathetic (page 765)
10. parasympathetic (page 765)
11. Decorticate posturing, decerebrate posturing (page 782)
12. large bore, isotonic (page 783)
13. doubles (page 784)

True/False

1. F (page 767)
2. F (page 765)
3. F (page 765)
4. T (page 765)
5. F (page 765)
6. F (page 771)
7. F (page 768)
8. T (page 784)

Short Answer

1. 1. Does your neck or back hurt?
   2. What happened?
   3. Where does it hurt?
   4. Can you move your hands and feet?
   5. Can you feel me touching your fingers? Your toes? (page 768)
2. 1. Muscle spasms in the neck
   2. Increased pain
   3. Numbness, tingling, or weakness
   4. Compromised airway or ventilations (page 771)
3. 1. Concussion
   2. Contusion
   3. Intracranial bleeding (page 779)
4. -Lacerations, contusions, or hematomas to the scalp
   -Soft area or depression on palpation
   -Visible fractures or deformities of the skull
   -Ecchymosis about the eyes or behind the ear over the mastoid process
   -Clear or pink cerebrospinal fluid leakage from a scalp wound, the nose, or the ear
   -Failure of the pupils to respond to light
   -Unequal pupil size
   -Loss of sensation and/or motor function
   -A period of unconsciousness
   -Amnesia
   -Seizures
   -Numbness or tingling in the extremities
   -Irregular respirations
   -Dizziness
   -Visual complaints
   -Combative or other abnormal behavior
   -Nausea or vomiting (page 782)
5. 1. Establish an adequate airway
   2. Control bleeding
   3. Assess the patient's baseline level of consciousness (page 783)
6. 1. Is the patient's airway clear?
   2. Is the patient breathing adequately?
   3. Can you maintain the airway and assist ventilations if the helmet remains in place?
   4. How well does the helmet fit?
   5. Can the patient move within the helmet?
7. Can the spine be immobilized in a neutral position with the helmet on? (page 788)

Word Fun

Crossword puzzle answers:

1. Down: BRAIN
2. Down: CONNECTMENT *(C-O-N-N-E-C-T-I-N-G)*
3. Down: MENINGES
4. Across: DISTRACTION
5. Across: SOMATIC NERVOUS SYSTEM
6. Down: RETROGRADE
7. Across: ANTEROGRADE AMNESIA
8. Across: CLOSED HEAD INJURY
9. Across: INTERVERTEBRAL DISK
10. Across: CEREBRAL EDEMA

Down answers also include: CEREBELLUM, MENINGES, CONVULSIVE NERVES, DERMAMNESIA

Ambulance Calls

1. -Apply a cervical collar and hold manual stabilization

-Use a short spinal extrication device

-Secure patient to long backboard

-Apply high-flow oxygen

-Monitor vital signs and continue with assessment

-Normal transport

2. -Cervical spine immobilization

-Maintain the airway/apply high-flow oxygen; suction as needed

-Cover the open laceration with gauze, being careful to gently press over the area to avoid further damage

-Put patient on long backboard and rapid transport

-Monitor vital signs en route

-Establish IV access

-Monitor ECG

-Consider intubation if condition deteriorates

3. -Leave the patient in his car seat

-Pad appropriately to immobilize the patient

-Use blow-by oxygen if the patient will tolerate it

-Monitor vital signs

-Continue assessment

-Rapid transport because of mechanism of injury and death in vehicle

4. -Rapid extrication

-Full spinal immobilization

-Apply oxygen at 15 L/min by NRB if tidal volume is adequate, otherwise intubate

-Monitor vital signs

-Establish IV access

-ECG monitoring

-Transport with head of spine board elevated

-Monitor of changes

-Be prepared for seizures or arrest

Skill Drills

Skill Drill 17-1: Performing Manual In-Line Stabilization

1. base, skull, side
2. index, long, palms, lift, neutral, move
3. support, cervical collar, manual support (page 770)

Skill Drill 17-2: Immobilizing a Patient to a Long Backboard

1. Apply and maintain **cervical** stabilization. Assess **distal functions** in all extremities.
2. Apply a **cervical collar**.
3. Rescuers kneel on one side of the patient and place hands on the **far side** of the patient.
4. On command, rescuers roll the patient **toward** themselves, quickly examine the **back**, slide the backboard **under** the patient, and **roll** the patient onto the board.
5. **Center** the patient on the board.
6. Secure the **upper torso** first.
7. Secure the **chest, pelvis**, and upper **legs**.
8. Begin to secure the patient's **head** using a **commercial immobilization** device or **rolled towels**.
9. Place tape across the patient's **forehead**.
10. Check all **straps** and readjust as needed. Reassess **distal** functions in all **extremities**. (pages 772 to 773)

Skill Drill 17-5: Application of a Cervical Collar

1. Apply in-line stabilization.
2. Measure the proper collar size.
3. Place the chin support first.
4. Wrap the collar around the neck and secure the collar.
5. Assure proper fit and maintain neutral in-line stabilization. (page 786)

Chapter 18: Musculoskeletal Care

Matching

1. G (page 800)   **7.** K (page 806)
2. J (page 801)   **8.** A (page 805)
3. D (page 801)   **9.** C (page 802)
4. I (page 802)   **10.** E (page 804)
5. F (page 802)   **11.** H (page 814)
6. B (page 804)

Multiple Choice

1. A (page 833)

2. B (page 801)

3. A – Minerals (B) and electrolytes (C) are stored in the bone marrow, which serves as a reservoir. (page 801)

4. B (page 802)

5. C (page 802)

6. B (page 802)

7. C – With a strain (B), no ligament or joint damage occurs. (page 803)

8. A (page 803)

9. D – The size of the zone of injury depends on the amount of kinetic energy the tissues absorb from forces acting in the body. (page 803)

10. A (page 804)

11. B (page 804)

12. C (page 804)

13. D (page 804)

14. B (page 804)

15. C (page 804)

16. D (page 805)

17. A (page 805)

18. C (page 806)

19. D (page 805)

20. A (page 805)

21. C (page 805)

22. B (page 805)

23. A (page 806)

24. C (page 806)

25. D (page 807)

26. C – Marked deformity occurs with dislocations and fractures. (page 808)

27. D (page 808)

28. D (page 809)

29. D (page 809)

30. D (pages 813 to 814)

31. C (page 314)

32. D (pages 815 to 819)

33. D (page 817)

34. B (page 819)

35. D – Hazards of improper splinting also include aggravation of the injury and injury to tissue, nerves, blood vessels, or muscles as a result of excessive movement of the bone or joint. (page 824)

36. B (page 824)

37. D (page 824)

38. D (page 829)

39. D (page 834)

40. C – With open fractures, the amount of blood loss may be even greater. (page 836)

41. B (page 836)

42. D (page 836)

43. C (page 836)

44. B (page 837)

45. A (page 839)

46. C (page 839)

Labeling

Human Skeleton (page 802)

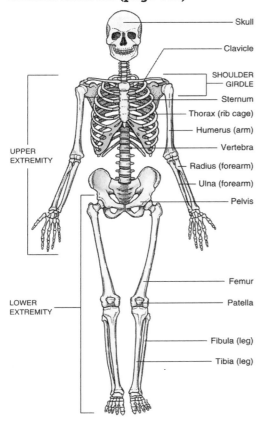

- Skull
- Clavicle
- SHOULDER GIRDLE
- Sternum
- Thorax (rib cage)
- Humerus (arm)
- Vertebra
- Radius (forearm)
- Ulna (forearm)
- Pelvis
- Femur
- Patella
- Fibula (leg)
- Tibia (leg)

UPPER EXTREMITY

LOWER EXTREMITY

Vocabulary

1. Acromioclavicular (A/C) joint: A simple joint where the bony projections of the scapula and the clavicle meet at the top of the shoulder. (page 825)
2. Compartment syndrome: An elevation of pressure within the fascial compartment, characterized by extreme pain, decreased sensation, pain on stretching of affected muscles, and decreased power; most frequently seen below the elbow or knee in children. (page 809)
3. Dislocation: Disruption of a joint in which ligaments are damaged and the bone ends are completely displaced. (page 807)
4. Nondisplaced fracture: A simple crack in the bone that has not caused the bone to move from its normal anatomic position; also called a hairline fracture. (page 804)
5. Position of function: A hand position in which the wrist is slightly dorsiflexed and all finger joints are moderately flexed. (page 831)
6. Sling: A bandage or material that helps support the weight of an injured upper extremity. (page 825)
7. Swathe: A bandage that passes around the chest to secure an injured arm to the chest. (page 826)

Fill-in

1. wasting (page 801)
2. red (page 801)
3. hinge (page 802)
4. clavicle (page 824)
5. mechanism of injury (page 808)
6. open fracture (page 808)
7. sciatic nerve (page 834)
8. femur (page 832)
9. crepitus (page 806)
10. reduce (page 807)
11. neurovascular status (page 809)
12. pulse, motor, sensory (page 818)

True/False

1. T   (page 813)   **6.** F   (page 814)

2. T   (page 813)   **7.** T   (page 811)

3. F   (page 814)   **8.** T   (page 809)

4. T   (page 814)   **9.** T   (page 811)

5. T   (page 814)

Short Answer

1. 1. Direct

   2. Indirect

   3. Twisting

   4. High-energy (page 804)

2. -Deformity

   -Tenderness (point)

   -Guarding

   -Swelling

   -Bruising

   -Crepitus

   -False motion

   -Exposed fragments

   -Pain

   -Locked joint (pages 805 to 807)

3. 1. Pulse

   2. Capillary refill

   3. Sensation

   4. Motor function (pages 811 to 812)

4. 1. Remove clothing from the area.

   2. Note and record the patient's neurovascular status distal to the site of the injury.

   3. Cover all wounds with a dry, sterile dressing before splinting.

   4. Do not move the patient before splinting.

   5. For a suspected fracture, immobilize the joints above and below the fracture.

   6. For a joint injury, immobilize the bones above and below the injured joint.

   7. Pad all rigid splints.

   8. Maintain manual immobilization to minimize movement of the limb and to support the injury site.

   9. Use a constant gentle manual traction to align the limb.

   10. If you encounter resistance to limb alignment, splint the limb in its deformed position.

   11. Immobilize all suspected spinal injuries in a neutral in-line position on a backboard.

   12. If the patient has signs of shock, align the limb in the normal anatomic position and provide transport.

   13. When in doubt, splint. (page 814)

5. 1. Stabilize the fracture.

   2. Align the limb.

   3. Avoid potential neurovascular compromise. (page 815)

Word Fun EMT-I vocab explorer web

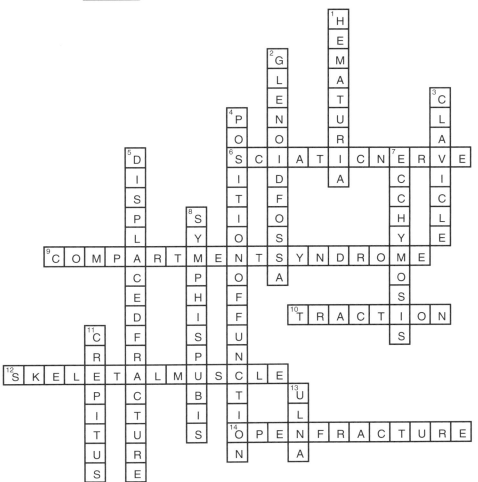

Ambulance Calls

1. -Evaluate ABCs and pulse/motor/sensation in all extremities

-Apply high-flow oxygen

-Splint fractured scapula with a sling and swathe

-Transport patient in position of comfort

-Consider c-spine immobilization if patient fell, was thrown, or complains of any neck pain

-Establish IV access

-Consider analgesics

-ECG monitoring

-Upgrade to rapid transport if patient shows any signs of altered mental status, respiratory distress/compromise, or circulatory compromise

2. -Splint the arm in position found, since circulation is intact

-Use a board splint for support with a sling and swathe

-Immobilize hand in the position of function

-Apply oxygen as needed

-Transport in the position of comfort

-Normal transport

-Monitor vital signs

3. -Treat for shock (hypovolemic)

-Apply high-flow oxygen

-Apply PASG with cervical spine immobilization

-Place patient in Trendelenburg's position

-Establish IV access.

-ECG monitoring

-Keep patient warm

-Rapid transport

-Continue to reassess constantly en route to the hospital.

4. -Apply oxygen as needed

-Monitor vital signs

-Splint the wrist and knee

-Establish IV access

-ECG monitoring

-Consider analgesics

-Apply cold packs to wrist and knee

-Elevate wrist and knee

-Transport

Skill Drills

Skill Drill 18-1: Assessing Neurovascular Pulse (page 810)

1. radial

2. posterior tibial

3. toenail

4. tip, index finger

5. tip, great toe

6. lateral side, foot

7. open, injured, Stop

8. make, fist

9. extend

10. flex, wiggle (page 810)

Skill Drill 18-2: Caring for Musculoskeletal Injuries

1. Cover open wounds with a dry, sterile dressing, and apply pressure to control bleeding.

2. Assess pulse, motor, and sensory functions. Apply a splint, and elevate the extremity about 6″ (slightly above the level of the heart).

3. Apply cold packs if there is swelling, but do not place them directly on the skin.

4. Position the patient for transport, and secure the injured area. (page 813)

Skill Drill 18-3: Applying a Rigid Splint (page 816)

1. gentle support, in-line traction

2. alongside, under

3. bindings

4. distal neurovascular (page 816)

Skill Drill 18-9: Splinting the Hand and Wrist

1. Assess pulse, motor, and sensory functions. Move the hand into the position of function. Place a soft roller bandage in the palm.

2. Apply a padded board splint on the palmar side with fingers exposed.

3. Secure the splint with a roller bandage. (page 832)

Chapter 19: Respiratory Emergencies

Matching

1. B	(page 860)	**13.** I	(page 864)	**25.** HH	(page 855)
2. D	(page 856)	**14.** AA	(page 859)	**26.** R	(page 862)
3. H	(page 855)	**15.** Y	(page 858)	**27.** DD	(page 851)
4. J	(page 858)	**16.** U	(page 853)	**28.** S	(page 855)
5. L	(page 863)	**17.** T	(page 853)	**29.** V	(page 851)
6. C	(page 862)	**18.** Q	(page 859	**30.** Z	(page 856)
7. G	(page 888)	**19.** EE	(page 856)	**31.** EE	(page 853)
8. E	(page 855)	**20.** P	(page 866)	**32.** W	(page 853)
9. M	(page 852)	**21.** FF	(page 851)	**33.** X	(page 860)
10. A	(page 851)	**22.** HH	(page 859)	**34.** CC	(page 855)
11. K	(page 865)	**23.** N	(page 858)	**35.** JJ	(page 864)
12. F	(page 860)	**24.** O	(page 862)		

Multiple Choice

1. D   (page 850)

2. C   (page 851)

3. D   (page 852)

4. C – This will replace the carbon dioxide content in the CSF. (page 853)

5. B – Rapid and deep breathing helps to blow off excess carbon dioxide (page 853)

6. A – Pale or cyanotic skin (B), pursed lips and nasal flaring (C) and cool, damp skin (D) are signs of inadequate breathing. (page 853)

7. D   (page 853)

8. B   (page 853)

9. B   (page 853)

10. A   (page 853)

11. B – Epiglottitis (A) and colds (C) create obstruction·of the flow of air in the major passages. (page 854)

12. C   (page 853)

13. B   (page 853)

14. A   (page 856)

15. D   (page 856)

16. D   (page 857-858)

17. C   (page 857-858)

18. D   (page 857-858)

19. D   (page 857-858

20. A   (page 858)

21. D   (page 859)

22. B – Blood pressure (A) of COPD patients is normal. The pulse (C) of COPD patients is rapid and occasionally irregular. (page 859)

23. C   (page 861)

24. D   (page 861

25. C   (page 862)

26. C   (page 860)

27. B   (page 860)

28. D   (page 861)

29. C   (page 863)

30. A   (page 863)

31. D   (page 864-865)

32. B   (page 865)

33. B   (page 866-867)

34. C   (page 868)

35. D   (page 868-869)

36. D   (page 869-870)

37. C – Ventolin (A) and Metaprel (B) are trade names. (page 871)

38. D   (page 872)

39. D   (page 861)

40. C   (page 860)

Labeling

Upper Airway (page 850)

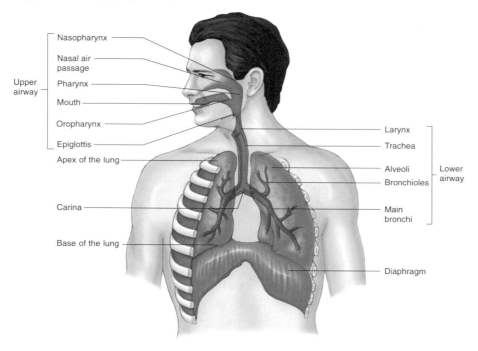

Vocabulary

1. Stridor: High-pitched, rough barking inspiratory sound often heard with upper airway obstruction. (page 856)
2. Croup: Inflammation and swelling of the lining of the larynx. (page 856)
3. Rales: Cracking, rattling breath sounds. (page 859)
4. Rhonchi: Coarse, gravelly breath sounds. (page 859)
5. Diphtheria: An infectious disease in which a membrane lining the pharynx is formed that can severely obstruct passage of air into the larynx. (page 855)
6. Chronic Obstructive Pulmonary Disease (COPD): A slow process of dilation and disruption of the airways and alveoli caused by chronic bronchial obstruction. (page 858)

Fill-in

1. carbon dioxide (page 853)
2. oxygen (page 853)
3. Carbon dioxide, oxygen (page 851)
4. alveoli (page 851)
5. Pulmonary edema (page 857)
6. 8, 24 (page 853)
7. carbon dioxide (page 853)
8. extrinsic, intrinsic (page 860)
9. spontaneous pneumothorax (page 862)
10. capnometry (page 870)

True/False

1. F (page 858)
2. T (page 862)
3. F (page 861)
4. F (page 860)
5. T (page 864)
6. T (page 865 to866)
7. F (pages 865 to 866)
8. T (page 858)
9. T (page 854)
10. T (page 856)

Short Answer

1. 1. Normal rate and depth

2. Regular pattern of inhalation and exhalation

3. Good audible breath sounds on both sides of the chest

4. Regular rise and fall on both sides of the chest

5. Pink, warm, dry skin (page 853)

2. 1. Rales: fine crackling sounds

2. Rhonchi: coarse tattling sounds

3. Wheezing: whistling sound typically heard on expiration (page 859)

3. 1. Patient is unable to coordinate administration and inhalation.

2. Inhaler is not prescribed for patient.

3. You did not obtain permission from medical control or local protocol.

4. Patient has already met maximum prescribed dose before your arrival. (page 872)

4. An ongoing irritation of the respiratory tract; excess mucus production obstructs small airways and alveoli. Protective mechanisms are impaired. Repeated episodes of irritation and pneumonia can cause scarring and alveolar damage, leading to COPD. (page 855)

5. -Respiratory rate of slower than 12 breaths/min or faster than 20 breaths/min

-Reduced flow of expired air at the nose and mouth

-Muscle retractions above the clavicles, between ribs, and below rib cage, especially in children

-Diminished, noisy, or absent breath sounds

-Unequal chest wall movement

-Pale or cyanotic skin

-Cool damp (clammy) skin

-Shallow respirations

-Pursed lips

-Nasal flaring (page 853)

6. A condition characterized by a chronically high blood level of carbon dioxide in which the respiratory center no longer responds to high blood levels of carbon dioxide. In these patients, low blood oxygen causes the respiratory center to respond and stimulate respiration. If the arterial level of oxygen is then raised, as happens when the patient is given additional oxygen, there is no longer any stimulus to breathe; both the high carbon dioxide and low oxygen drives are lost. (page 853)

Word Fun

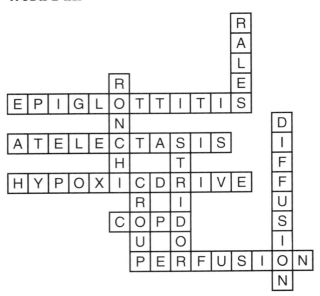

Ambulance Calls

1. -Maintain a clear airway as needed

   -Use high-flow oxygen and assist ventilations as needed

   -Transport in position of comfort

   -Rapid transport

   -Establish IV of isotonic crystalloid solution

   -Give fluid hydration based on clinical symptoms

   -Consider intubation and cardiac monitoring

   -Consider pharmacological interventions as per protocol (page 865)

2. -Place patient in position of comfort

   -Administer high-flow oxygen

   -Try to calm the patient and talk her into slowing respirations. Have her mimic your respiratory rate.

   -Monitor vital signs

   -Patient's condition dictates the transport mode (page 866)

3. -Make scene safe by having patient put out the cigarette

   -Monitor airway, assist ventilations as necessary

   -Discontinue home oxygen support and place high-flow oxygen via nonrebreathing mask

   -Place patient in position of comfort

   -Establish IV hydrate as necessary

   -Assist with metered-dose inhaler as necessary

   -Consider intubation and cardiac monitoring

   -Consider beta agonists (albuterol or epinephrine) as per protocol

   -Monitor vital signs

   -Rapid transport (page 861)

Skill Drills

Skill Drill 19-1: Assisting a Patient with a Metered-Dose Inhaler

1. warmer
2. lip seal, spacer
3. breath holding
4. oxygen, breaths, dose (page 873)

Chapter 20: Cardiovascular Emergencies

Matching

1. D	(page 893)	**11.** K	(page 892)	**21.** S	(page 893)			
2. B	(page 899)	**12.** M	(page 905)	**22.** V	(page 951)			
3. E	(page 900)	**13.** I	(page 895)	**23.** Y	(page 888)			
4. G	(page 891)	**14.** P	(page 899)	**24.** Z	(page 940)			
5. C	(page 888)	**15.** M	(page 952)	**25.** CC	(page 939)			
6. F	(page 897)	**16.** Q	(page 884)	**26.** W	(page 947)			
7. A	(page 962)	**17.** O	(page 926)	**27.** X	(page 961)			
8. H	(page 939)	**18.** T	(page 962)	**28.** DD	(page 902)			
9. J	(page 895)	**19.** U	(page 892)	**29.** AA	(page 967)			
10. L	(page 891)	**20.** R	(page 896)	**30.** BB	(page 913)			

Multiple Choice

1. D (page 886)

2. D (page 886)

3. A (page 886)

4. B – Pulmonary veins transport blood from the lungs, where it has picked up oxygen. (page 886)

5. A (page 888)

6. A (page 886)

7. B (page 887)

8. C (page 896)

9. A (page 889)

10. C – Diastolic blood pressure is the resting phase of the ventricles. (pages 895 to 896)

11. A (page 899)

12. C (page 891)

13. B (page 899)

14. D (page 902)

15. B (page 900)

16. D – It is usually felt in the mid-chest, under the sternum, but may radiate. (page 900)

17. D (page 900)

18. D (page 905)

19. C (page 901)

20. C (page 901)

21. B – Nitroglycerin acts as a smooth-muscle relaxant. When it is given to a patient with cardiac-related chest pain, the coronary arteries dilate, which increases oxygen supply to the myocardium. (page 910)

22. D (page 902)

23. D (page 902)

24. A – Asystole (B) is absence of electrical activity. Ventricular stand still (C) is the same thing as asystole. Ventricular tachycardia (D) is a rapid heart rate greater than 100 beats/min. (page 352)

25. B (page 903)

26. A (page 903)

27. D (page 905)

28. B (page 905)

29. A (page 905)

30. C (page 907)

31. D (page 914)

32. B – AVPU (A) is used to assess level of consciousness. SAMPLE (B) is used to assess history. CHART (D) is used for documentation. (page 908)

33. D (page 912)

34. D (page 910)

35. C (page 909)

36. B (page 912)

37. D (page 913)

38. C (page 916)

39. C (page 917)

40. B (page 917)

41. C (page 917)

42. D (page 917)

Labeling

Blood flow through the heart (page 886)

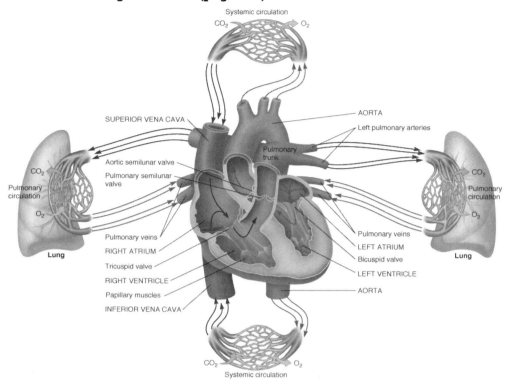

Systemic circulation
CO_2 O_2

SUPERIOR VENA CAVA

AORTA

Left pulmonary arteries

Pulmonary trunk

CO_2

Pulmonary circulation

Lung

O_2

Aortic semilunar valve

Pulmonary semilunar valve

Pulmonary veins

RIGHT ATRIUM

Tricuspid valve

RIGHT VENTRICLE

Papillary muscles

INFERIOR VENA CAVA

CO_2

Pulmonary circulation

Lung

O_2

Pulmonary veins

LEFT ATRIUM

Bicuspid valve

LEFT VENTRICLE

AORTA

CO_2 O_2

Systemic circulation

The coronary arteries (page 898)

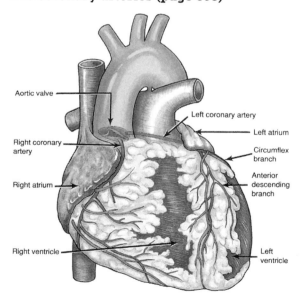

Aortic valve

Right coronary artery

Right atrium

Right ventricle

Left coronary artery

Left atrium

Circumflex branch

Anterior descending branch

Left ventricle

The cardiovascular system (page 898)

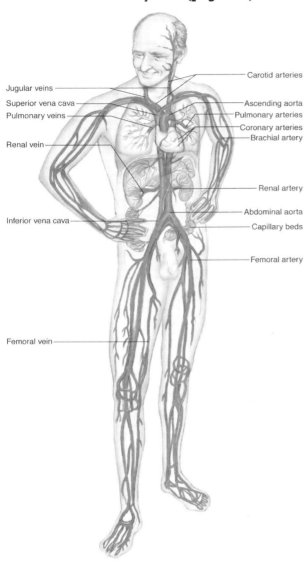

Jugular veins

Superior vena cava

Pulmonary veins

Renal vein

Inferior vena cava

Femoral vein

Carotid arteries

Ascending aorta

Pulmonary arteries

Coronary arteries

Brachial artery

Renal artery

Abdominal aorta

Capillary beds

Femoral artery

Vocabulary EMT-I vocab explorer web

1. Angina pectoris: Transient chest discomfort caused by partial or temporary blockage of blood flow to heart muscle (page 900)

2. Ventricular fibrillation: Disorganized, ineffective twitching of the ventricles, resulting in no blood flow to the heart (page 902)

3. Cardiogenic shock: Body tissues do not get enough oxygen because the heart lacks enough power to force the proper volume of blood through the circulatory system. (page 903)

4. Acute myocardial infarction (AMI): Heart attack; death of myocardium following obstruction of blood flow to the heart muscle (page 901)

5. Cardiac arrest: A state in which the heart fails to generate an effective and detectable blood flow (page 902)

6. Syncope: Fainting spell or transient loss of consciousness (page 913)

7. Congestive heart failure (CHF): A disorder in which the heart loses part of its ability to effectively pump blood, usually as a result of damage to the heart muscle and usually resulting in a backup of fluid into the lungs (page 905)

Fill-in

1. interatrial septum (page 885)
2. aorta (page 885)
3. right (page 898)
4. AV (page 889)
5. Red blood (pages 885-886)
6. four (page 885)

7. left (page 885)
8. Leads (page 925)
9. 1/25th or 0.04 (page 933)
10. less than 0.12 seconds (page 931)
11. SA node, normal sinus rhythm (page 940)
12. Artifact (page 937)

True/False

1. F   (page 886)
2. F   (page 896)
3. T   (page 899)
4. F   (page 899)
5. T   (page 900)
6. F   (page 901)
7. F   (page 902)
8. F   (page 925)

9. T   (page 900)
10. F   (page 180)
11. T   (page 903)
12. T   (page 905)
13. T   (page 906)
14. T   (page 884)
15. F   (page 899)

Short Answer

1. Automated: Operator needs only to apply pads and turn on the machine. It performs all functions for analyzing and shocking. This type of defibrillator often has a computer voice synthesizer to advise the EMT which steps to take.

   Semi-automated: Operator applies pads, turns on the machine, and pushes button to shock. (page 916)

2. 1. Not having a charged battery
   2. Applying the AED to a patient who is moving
   3. Applying the AED to a responsive patient with a rapid heart rate (pages 916 to 917)

3. 1. If the patient regains a pulse
   2. After six to nine shocks have been delivered
   3. If the machine gives three consecutive "no shock" messages (page 918)

4. 1. Place pads correctly.
   2. Make sure no one is touching the patient.
   3. Do not defibrillate a patient who is in pooled water.
   4. Dry the chest before defibrillating a wet patient.
   5. Do not defibrillate a patient who is touching metal that others are touching.
   6. Remove nitroglycerin patches and wipe the area with a dry towel before defibrillation. (page 923)

5. 1. Obtain an order from medical direction.
   2. Take the patient's blood pressure; continue with administration only if the systolic blood pressure is greater than 100 mm Hg.
   3. Check that you have the right medication, patient, and delivery route.
   4. Check the expiration date of the nitroglycerin.
   5. Question the patient about the last dose he or she took and its effects.
   6. Be prepared to have the patient lie down.
   7. Give the medication sublingually.
   8. Advise the patient to keep his or her mouth closed to allow the medication to dissolve.
   9. Recheck blood pressure within 5 minutes.
   10. Record each medication and the time of administration.
   11. Perform continued assessment. (pages 910 to 912)

6. 1. It may or may not be caused by exertion but can occur at any time.

2. It does not resolve in a few minutes.

3. It may or may not be relieved by rest or nitroglycerin. (pages 902-903)

7. 1. Sudden death

2. Cardiogenic shock

3. Congestive heart failure (pages 902 to 903)

8. 1. Sudden onset of weakness, nausea, or sweating without an obvious cause

2. Chest pain/discomfort that does not change with each breath

3. Pain in lower jaw, arms, or neck

4. Sudden arrhythmia with syncope

5. Pulmonary edema

6. Sudden death

7. Increased and/or irregular pulse

8. Normal, increased, or decreased blood pressure

9. Normal or labored respirations

10. Pale or gray skin

11. Feelings of apprehension (page 902)

9. Remove clothing from the patient's chest area. Apply the pads to the chest: one just to the right of the sternum, just below the clavicle, the other on the left chest with the top of the pad 2 to 3 inches below the armpit. Ensure that the pads are attached to the patient cables (and that they are attached to the AED in some models). (page 918)

10. SA node   60-100 BPM
Atrial cells   55-60 BPM
AV node   45-50 BPM
His bundle   40-45 BPM
Bundle branch   40-45 BPM
Purkinje cells   35-40 BPM
Myocardial cells   30-35 BPM (page 889)

11. Sometimes a patient has heart rhythms that should not be shocked but are fast enough to confuse the computer. (page 917)

Rhythm Recognition

1. Rate: About 33 BPM
Regularity: Regular
P Waves: None
P:QRS Ratio: None

P-R Intervals: None
QRS Width: Normal
Grouping: None
Dropped Beats: None
Rhythm: Junctional rhythm

2. Rate: About 135 BPM
Regularity: Regular
P Waves: Present
P:QRS Ratio: 1:1

P-R Intervals: Normal, consistent
QRS Width: Normal
Grouping: None
Dropped Beats: None
Rhythm: Sinus tachycardia

3. Rate: About 55 BPM
Regularity: Regularly irregular
P Waves: Variable
P:QRS Ratio: 1:1

P-R Intervals: Variable
QRS Width: Normal
Grouping: None
Dropped Beats: None
Rhythm: Wandering atrial pacemaker

4. Rate: About 95 BPM   P-R Intervals: None
  Regularity: Irregularly irregular   QRS Width: Wide
  P Waves: None   Grouping: None
  P:QRS Ratio: None   Dropped Beats: None
                                           Rhythm: Atrial fibrillation

5. Rate: Atrial: 350 BPM   P-R Intervals: None
                      Ventricular: 135 BPM
  Regularity: Regular   QRS Width: Unable to tell by this strip. Should refer
                                                              to additional leads or full 12-lead ECG.
  P Waves: None, F waves are present Grouping: None
  F:QRS Ratio: 2:1   Dropped Beats: None
                                           Rhythm: Atrial flutter

6. Rate: About 110 BPM   P-R Intervals: Normal, except in events
  Regularity: Regularly irregular   QRS Width: Normal, except in events
  P Waves: Present   Grouping: None
  P:QRS Ratio: 1:1   Dropped Beats: None
                                           Rhythm: Sinus tachycardia with multiple PACs
                                                              and a PJC

7. Rate: About 51 BPM   P-R Intervals: None
  Regularity: Regular   QRS Width: Normal
  P Waves: None   Grouping: None
  P:QRS Ratio: None   Dropped Beats: None
                                           Rhythm: Junctional rhythm

8. Rate: About 95 BPM   P-R Intervals: None
  Regularity: Irregularly irregular   QRS Width: Normal
  P Waves: None   Grouping: None
  P:QRS Ratio: None   Dropped Beats: None
                                           Rhythm: Atrial fibrillation

9. Rate: Atrial: 300 BPM   P-R Intervals: Not applicable
                      Ventricular: 150 BPM
  Regularity: Regular   QRS Width: Normal
  P Waves: F waves   Grouping: None
  F:QRS Ratio: 2:1   Dropped Beats: None
                                           Rhythm: Atrial flutter

10. Rate: Atrial: 300 BPM   P-R Intervals: Not applicable
                      Ventricular: 150 BPM
  Regularity: Regularly irregular   QRS Width: Normal
  P Waves: Present   Grouping: None
  F:QRS Ratio: 2:1   Dropped Beats: None
                                           Rhythm: Atrial flutter

11. Rate: About 128 BPM   P-R Intervals: Not applicable
  Regularity: Regular   QRS Width: Normal
  P Waves: Pseudo-S   Grouping: None
  P:QRS Ratio: 1:1   Dropped Beats: None
                                           Rhythm: Junctional tachycardia

12. Rate: Atrial: 300 BPM   P-R Intervals: Not applicable
                      Ventricular: 70 BPM
  Regularity: Regularly irregular   QRS Width: Normal
  P Waves: F waves   Grouping: None
  F:QRS Ratio: 5:1   Dropped Beats: None
                                           Rhythm: Atrial flutter

13. Rate: Not applicable
    Regularity: None
    P Waves: None
    P:QRS Ratio: None

P-R Intervals: None
QRS Width: None
Grouping: None
Dropped Beats: None
Rhythm: Ventricular fibrillation

14. Rate: About 60 BPM
    Regularity: Regular with event
    P Waves: None
    P:QRS Ratio: None

P-R Intervals: None
QRS Width: Wide
Grouping: None
Dropped Beats: None
Rhythm: Accelerated idioventricular rhythm

15. Rate: About 110 BPM
    Regularity: Regularly irregular
    P Waves: Present
    P:QRS Ratio: 4:3

P-R Intervals: Variable
QRS Width: Normal
Grouping: Yes
Dropped Beats: Yes
Rhythm: Mobitz I second-degree AV block

16. Rate: About 70 BPM
    Regularity: Regularly irregular
    P Waves: Present
    P:QRS Ratio: 3:2

P-R Intervals: Variable
QRS Width: Normal
Grouping: Yes
Dropped Beats: Yes
Rhythm: Mobitz I second-degree AV block

17. Rate: About 50 BPM
    Regularity: Regular
    P Waves: Present
    P:QRS Ratio: 1:1

P-R Intervals: None (R-P interval)
QRS Width: Wide
Grouping: None
Dropped Beats: None
Rhythm: Accelerated idioventricular rhythm

18. Rate: Atrial: 51 BPM
                Ventricular: 61 BPM
    Regularity: Regular
    P Waves: Present
    P:QRS Ratio: Not applicable

P-R Intervals: Not applicable

QRS Width: Normal
Grouping: None
Dropped Beats: None
Rhythm: Third-degree AV block

19. Rate: About 66 BPM
    Regularity: Regular with an event
    P Waves: None
    P:QRS Ratio: None

P-R Intervals: None
QRS Width: Normal
Grouping: None
Dropped Beats: None
Rhythm: Accelerated junctional rhythm
           with a PVC

20. Rate: Atrial: 300 BPM
                Ventricular: 150 BPM
    Regularity: Regular

    P Waves: F waves
    F:QRS Ratio: 2:1

P-R Intervals: Not applicable

QRS Width: Appears to be wide, but this could be an illusion caused by a fusion of the F wave with the overlying QRS in this lead. Should refer to a 12-lead ECG.

Grouping: None
Dropped Beats: None
Rhythm: Atrial flutter

21. Rate: None
    Regularity: None
    P Waves: None
    P:QRS Ratio: None

P-R Intervals: None
QRS Width: None
Grouping: None
Dropped Beats: None
Rhythm: Ventricular fibrillation

22. Rate: About 220 BPM
Regularity: Irregularly irregular
P Waves: None
P:QRS Ratio: None

P-R Intervals: None
QRS Width: Wide
Grouping: None
Dropped Beats: None
Rhythm: Atrial fibrillation

23. Rate: About 70 BPM
Regularity: Regularly irregular
P Waves: Present
P:QRS Ratio: 1:1

P-R Intervals: Variable
QRS Width: Normal
Grouping: Yes
Dropped Beats: None
Rhythm: Supraventricular bigeminy

24. Rate: About 300 BPM
Regularity: Irregularly irregular
P Waves: None
P:QRS Ratio: None

P-R Intervals: None
QRS Width: Wide
Grouping: None
Dropped Beats: None
Rhythm: Atrial fibrillation in a patient with
Wolff-Parkinson-White

Word Fun

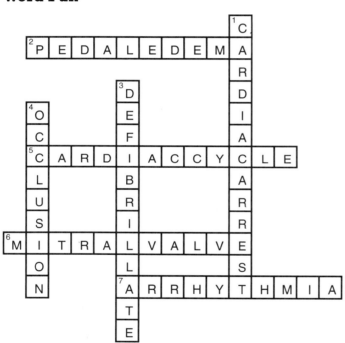

Ambulance Calls

1. -Place patient in the position of comfort.

-Administer high-flow oxygen via nonrebreathing mask.

-Monitor vital signs and ECG tracing.

-Gain IV access, fluid bolus of 20mL/kg if hypotensive.

-Consider nitroglycerin as per protocol if systolic is appropriate.

-Provide normal transport.

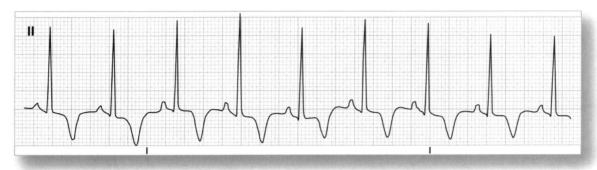

Rate:	Slightly under 100 BPM		P-R intervals:	Normal, consistant
Regularity:	Regular		QRS width:	Normal
P waves:	Present		Rhythm:	Normal sinus rhythm

Discussion: This ECG shows some pretty tall QRS complexes and some deep, inverted T waves. The rhythm, however, is NSR. Don't let the size of he complexes or any other pathology steer you from making the correct call on the rhythm. Remember, to really talk about cardiac pathology, you need a full 12-lead ECG and not just a rhythm strip.

2. -Explain the need for seeking medical attention.

-Place patient in position of comfort.

-Administer high-flow oxygen via nonrebreathing mask.

-Monitor vital signs and ECG tracing.

-Gain IV access, fluid bolus of 20mL/kg if hypotensive.

-Check a SAMPLE history and assist patient with nitroglycerin after contacting medical control if he currently has a prescription.

-Provide rapid transport.

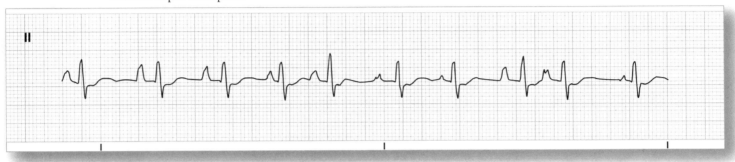

Rate:	About 90 BPM		P-R intervals:	Variable
Regularity:	Irregularly irregular		QRS width:	Normal
P waves:	Present		Grouping:	None
Morphology	Variable		Dropped beats:	None
Axis:	Variable			
P:QRS ratio:	1:1		Rhythm:	Wandering atrial pacemaker

Discussion: This ECG shows an irregularly irregular rhythm with P waves of at least three different morphologies. The rate is mostly within the normal range, with a few complexes occurring more rapidly. These criteria are consistent with wandering atrial pacemaker. The slight discrepancies in the morphologies of the QRS complexes is consistent with the fusion and abberrancy that is commonly seen in both irregularly irregular and multifocal atrial tachycardia. A 12-lead ECG should be obtained to evaluate the slight ST depression that is evident throughout the strip.

3. -Sit the patient upright with legs down.

-Administer high-flow oxygen and be prepared to ventilate with BVM if needed.

-High-flow oxygen via nonrebreathing mask

-Monitor vital signs and ECG tracing.

-Gain IV access, fluid bolus of 20mL/kg if hypotensive.

-Check a SAMPLE history and assist patient with nitroglycerin after contacting medical control if she currently has a prescription.

-Provide rapid transport.

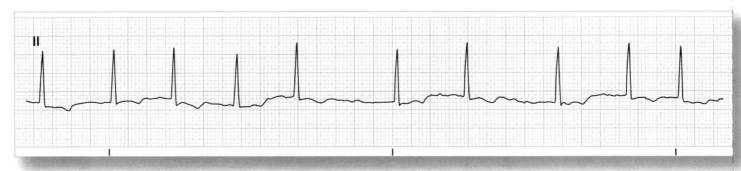

Rate:	About 80 BPM		P-R intervals:	None
Regularity:	Irregularly irregular		QRS width:	Normal
P waves:	None		Grouping:	None
Morphology	None		Dropped beats:	None
Axis:	None			
P:QRS ratio:	None		Rhythm:	Atrial fibrillation

Discussion: This ECG shows an irregularly irregular rhythm occurring at a rate of about 80 BPM. There are no visible P waves anywhere on the strip. Remember the three main irregularly irregular rhythms are atrial fibrillation, wandering atrial pacemaker, and multifocal atrial tachycardia. WAP and MAT both have P waves. By a process of elimination, the answer is controlled atrial fibrillation, Other possibilities for irregularly irregular rhythms exist, but are not commonly found. These include variable conduction atrial flutter, very frequent premature complexes (usually regularly irregular), and the initial period at the onset of many tachycardias.

Skill Drills

Skill Drill 20-3: Caring for a Conscious Patient with Chest Discomfort

1. Reassure, oxygen.
2. cardiac moniter, dysrhythmias
3. Position, vital signs, IV
4. focused history, chest discomfort
5. nitroglycerin, expiration date
6. nitroglycerin
7. Transport (page 910)

Skill Drill 20-4: AED and CPR

1. Stop CPR if in progress. Assess responsiveness. Check breathing and pulse.
2. If pulseless, begin CPR. Remove sufficient clothing to gain access to the patient's chest. Prepare the AED pads.
3. Turn on the AED; begin narrative if needed. Apply AED pads. Stop CPR.
4. Verbally and visually clear the patient. Push the analyze button if there is one. Wait for the AED to analyze the rhythm. If no shock advised, perform CPR for 1 minute. If a shock is advised, recheck that all are clear, and push the shock button. Check pulse. Push the analyze button, if needed, to analyze the rhythm again. Press shock if advised (second shock). Check pulse. Push the analyze button, if needed, to analyze the rhythm again. Press shock if advised (third shock).
5. Check pulse. If pulse is present, check breathing.
6. If breathing adequately, give 100% oxygen and transport. If apneic or breathing inadequately, ensure an open airway, ventilate, and transport. If no pulse, perform CPR for 1 minute. Clear the patient, and analyze again. If necessary, repeat one cycle of up to three shocks, checking for a pulse after each shock. Transport the patient, and contact medical control. Continue to support breathing or perform CPR, as needed. (pages 920–921)

Skill Drill 20-6: Defibrillation

1. cardiac rhythm
2. defibrillation pads, paddles, gel
3. CPR
4. rhythm, shock
5. 5 cycles (2 minutes) (page 966)

Skill Drill 20-7: Transcutaneous Pacing

1. Determine the need for pacing. Attach the three-lead cables.
2. Apply the pacing electrodes.
3. Connect the electrodes to the cardiac monitor, and select desired heart rate. Slowly adjust the electrical current setting until electrical capture is obtained.
4. Assess the patient's pulse to ensure mechanical capture. (page 968)

Chapter 21: Diabetic Emergencies

Matching

1. H	(page 986)	**9.** G	(page 987)	**17.** U	(page 987)
2. F	(page 988)	**10.** C	(page 988)	**18.** T	(page 987)
3. I	(page 987)	**11.** A	(page 991)	**19.** Q	(page 988)
4. B	(page 986)	**12.** N	(page 986)	**20.** S	(page 987)
5. L	(page 988)	**13.** D	(page 988)	**21.** P	(page 988)
6. M	(page 986)	**14.** K	(page 990)	**22.** V	(page 989)
7. O	(page 991)	**15.** J	(page 986)		
8. E	(page 988)	**16.** R	(page 987)		

Multiple Choice

1. B – Type II diabetes usually appears later in life (page 987)

2. A   (page 988)

3. D – Diabetes mellitus is considered a metabolic disorder in which the body cannot metabolize glucose, usually because of the lack of insulin; the result is a wasting of glucose in the urine. (page 988)

4. C – Kussmaul respirations. With metabolic acidosis, the compensatory mechanism is the respiratory system. Because carbon dioxide is an acid, an increase in the rate an depth of respirations (Kussmaul respirations) will attempt to decrease the amount of acid in the body. (page 988)

5. D   (page 992)

6. A – When fat is used as an immediate energy source, chemicals called ketones and fatty acids are formed as waste products. As they accumulate in the blood and tissue, they can produce the dangerous form of acidosis seen in uncontrolled diabetes called diabetic ketoacidosis. (page 986)

7. C – Diabetic ketoacidosis (page 988)

8. C – Polyphagia is excessive eating as a result of cellular hunger or starvation.

9. D – Insulin is a hormone that is normally produced by the pancreas that enables glucose to enter the cells. (page 987)

10. D – Diabetic coma occurs in the patient who is not under medical treatment, who takes insufficient insulin, who markedly overeats, or who is undergoing some sort of stress, such as infection, illness, overexertion, fatigue, or drinking alcohol. (page 991)

11. B – With the exception of the brain, insulin is needed to allow glucose to enter individual body cells to fuel their functioning. (page 997)

12. B – A sweet or fruity (acetone) odor on the breath caused by the unusual waste products in the blood (ketones). (page 991)

13. B   (page 988)

14. D   (page 987)

15. A – Glucose, or dextrose, is one of the basic sugars in the body. (page 986)

16. A   (page 987)

17. A   (page 988)

18. C – When fat is used as an immediate energy source, chemicals called ketones and fatty acids are formed as waste products and are hard for the body to excrete. (page 988)

19. A   (pages 987 to 988)

20. B – Insulin shock develops much more quickly than diabetic coma. In some instances it can occur in a matter of minutes. (page 991)

21. D – Glucose is the major source of energy for the body, and all cells need it to function properly. A constant supply to the brain is as important as oxygen. (page 991)

22. C – Although brief seizures are not harmful, they may indicate a more dangerous and potentially life-threatening underlying condition. Kussmaul respirations and polydipsia (A, D) are signs of diabetic ketoacidosis. (pages 997 to 998)

23. B – A bolus of 20 mL/kg. (page 993)

24. A – Diabetic coma occurs in the patient who takes insufficient insulin. Too much insulin (B) results in insulin shock. (page 991)

25. B – If unable to perform a blood glucose test, you must always suspect hypoglycemia in any patient with altered mental status. (page 992)

26. C – The first step in caring for any patient is to perform an initial assessment to verify that the airway is open. All the others (A, B, D) are secondary to airway. (page 992)

27. D – You must use your knowledge of the signs and symptoms to decide whether the problem is diabetic coma or insulin shock when dealing with an unresponsive diabetic patient. However, this assessment should not prevent you from providing prompt treatment and transport (A, B, C). (page 991)

28. A – Do not treat the patient as if he/she is intoxicated. Confinement by police in a "drunk tank" because a person is thought to be intoxicated puts the hypoglycemic patient at risk of dying. Therefore, assume the patient is hypoglycemic until proven otherwise. Giving glucose to a patient who is hyperglycemic (B) or intoxicated (C) will not cause harm to the patient. However, lack of glucose to the brain can be fatal. (page 998)

29. A – The only contraindications to glucose are an inability to swallow or unconsciousness because aspiration can occur. (page 992)

30. D (page 996)

31. D – All of the others (A, B, C) are signs of diabetic ketoacidosis. (page 990)

32. B – In insulin shock, the problem is hypoglycemia. The others (A, C, D) all equate to high glucose levels. (page 991)

33. C – Dehydration can be indicated by sunken eyes. Good skin turgor (A) would indicate sufficient hydration, and elevated blood pressure (B) could indicate overhydration. (page 991)

34. A – Diabetes may mask signs and symptoms of other problems. All diabetics complaining of not feeling well, with no mechanism of injury, should have their glucose level evaluated to rule out hypo- or hyperglycemia, followed by the appropriate medical assessment (B). As long as the mental status is intact, oral glucose (D) is not immediately indicated, nor is rapid transport to the closest facility (C). Transport, whether slow or rapid, should always be to the closest, most appropriate facility. (page 992)

35. D (page 991)

36. A – Because of high energy levels and difficulty in keeping them on a strict schedule of medication and eating, management of children with diabetes poses a particularly troublesome task. (page 991)

37. C – Oral glucose (A) and a reduction in insulin (D) will cause an increase in glucose levels. Treatment includes a reversal of the condition under closely monitored conditions that may take many hours. (page 991)

38. C – If the patient has an altered mental status, a glucose test should be performed to rule out possible diabetic complications. (page 992-993)

39. D – You should NOT attempt to give anything by mouth to unconscious patients. The risk of choking or aspirating liquid into the lungs outweighs the benefits of the small amount of glucose they would receive. (page 992)

40. D – Do not be afraid to give too much sugar. An entire candy bar or a full glass of sweetened juice is often needed. (page 995)

Labeling

TABLE 21-1	Characteristics of Diabetic Emergencies	
	Hyperglycemia	**Hypoglycemia**
History		
Food intake	Excessive	Insufficient
Insulin dose	Insufficient	Excessive
Onset	Gradual	Rapid, within minutes
Skin	Warm and dry	Pale and moist
Infection	Common	Uncommon
Gastrointestinal Tract		
Thirst	Intense	Absent
Hunger	Absent	Intense
Vomiting	Common	Uncommon
Respiratory System		
Breathing	Rapid, deep (Kussmaul respirations)	Normal or rapid
Odor of breath	Sweet, fruity	Normal
Cardiovascular System		
Blood pressure	Normal to low	Low
Pulse	Tachycardia	Rapid, weak
Nervous System		
Consciousness	Ranging from restlessness to coma	Irritability, confusion, seizures, or coma
Urine		
Sugar	Present	Absent
Acetone	Present	Absent
Treatment		
Response	Gradual, within 6 to 12 hours following medication and fluid	Immediately after administration of glucose

Vocabulary

1. Diabetes mellitus: A metabolic disorder in which the body cannot metabolize glucose, usually because of the lack of insulin. (page 986)
2. Kussmaul respirations: Deep, rapid breathing that results from accumulation of certain acids when insulin is not available in the body. (page 1001)
3. Glucagon: The hormone released from the alpha cells in the islets of Langerhans that converts glycogen to glucose when the body's blood glucose level drops. (page 987)
4. Insulin: A hormone produced by the islets of Langerhans that enables sugar in the blood to enter the cells of the body. (page 986)
5. Ketoacidosis: The form of acidosis seen in uncontrolled diabetes; byproduct of the burning of fatty tissue. (page 988)

Fill-in

1. diabetes mellitus (page 986)
2. metabolic disorder (page 986)
3. ineffective (page 987)
4. diabetic coma (page 991)
5. sugar, insulin (page 992)
6. blood glucose test (page 998)

True/False

1. T	(page 988)	**9.** F	(page 986)
2. T	(page 987)	**10.** F	(page 996)
3. T	(page 988)	**11.** T	(page 986)
4. T	(page 991)	**12.** F	(page 992)
5. T	(page 990)	**13.** F	(page 993)
6. T	(page 990)	**14.** T	(page 993 to 994)
7. T	(page 988)	**15.** T	(page 998, 992)
8. F	(page 986)		

Short Answer

1. Insulin is a hormone that enables glucose to enter body cells. (page 986)
2. 1. Glucose
   2. Insta-Glucose (page 993)
   3. A patient who is unconscious or not able to swallow should not be given oral glucose. (page 993)
4. -Diabinase
   -Orinase
   -Micronase
   -Glucotrol (page 987)
5. 1. Ketoacidosis
   2. Dehydration
   3. Hyperglycemia (page 991)
6. -Kussmaul respirations
   -dehydration
   -fruity odor on breath
   -rapid weak pulse
   -normal or slightly low blood pressure
   -varying degrees of unresponsiveness (page 991)
7. You should suspect insulin shock, which develops rapidly, as opposed to diabetic coma, which takes longer to develop. (pages 990 to 991)

8. It will immediately benefit the patient in insulin shock and is unlikely to worsen the condition of the patient in a diabetic coma. (pages 992 to 993)

9. -Major trauma to the head unequal pupil

-Battle's sign

-blood

-cerebrospinal fluid coming from the ears, nose, and mouth (page 996)

Word Fun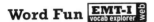

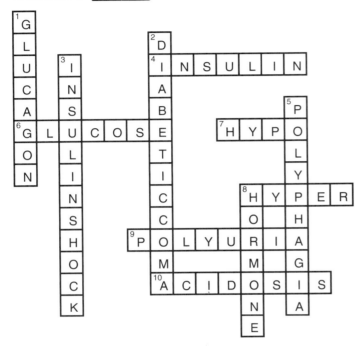

Ambulance Calls

1. Turn the patient on her side immediately or use suction to clear the airway.

   Insert an oral or nasal airway; consider intubation, and apply high-flow oxygen.

   Perform a focused physical exam.

   Attempt to obtain a blood glucose level.

   Establish IV access and cardiac monitoring following ACLS protocols.

   Administer IV bolus and/or dextrose as per protocol.

   Transport patient rapidly.

   Monitor the patient closely.

2. Consider cervical spine immobilization.

   Apply high-flow oxygen.

   Try to obtain a SAMPLE history, but do not delay treatment or transport.

   Perform a detailed physical exam.

   Attempt to obtain a blood glucose level.

   Gain IV access.

   With permission from medical control, administer oral glucose/D_5W.

   Employ cardiac monitoring per ACLS protocols.

   Monitor the patient closely for any changes.

3. Apply high-flow oxygen and maintain the airway.

   Obtain a SAMPLE history from the staff while loading the patient.

   Attempt a blood glucose level.

Give an IV bolus 20 mL of isotonic crystalloid.

Employ cardiac monitoring per ACLS protocols.

Transport in a semi-Fowler's position.

Support vital signs and monitor the patient en route to the hospital.

Skill Drills

Skill Drill 21-1: Administering Glucose

1. Make sure that the tube of glucose is intact and has not expired.

2. Squeeze the entire tube of oral glucose onto the bottom third of a bite stick or tongue depressor.

3. Open the patient's mouth. Place the tongue depressor on the mucous membranes between the cheek and the gum with the gel side next to the cheek. (page 994)

Skill Drill 21-2: Administration of D_{50}

1. blood

2. proximal, slowly

3. half, blood return

4. Flush (page 997)

Chapter 22: Allergic Reactions and Envenomations

Matching

1. E   (page 1006)
2. B   (page 1006)
3. I   (page 1006)
4. J   (page 1006)
5. F   (page 1006)
6. C   (page 1011)
7. H   (page 1007)
8. D   (page 1009)

9. A   (page 1017)
10. G   (page 1009)
11. P   (page 1006)
12. O   (page 1012)
13. N   (page 1006)
14. L   (page 1024)
15. K   (page 1011)
16. M   (page 1007)

Multiple Choice

1. C – (A) Epinephrine can be given repeatedly. (B) The patient cannot be given too much oxygen. (page 1012)
2. D – Side effects may also include increased blood pressure, pallor, dizziness, headache, vomiting, and anxiety. (page 1012)
3. D – Black widows prefer dry, dim places and are found in every state except Alaska. (page 1017)
4. A – (B) The tip is placed against the lateral thigh. (C) Needles are never to be recapped. (page 1013)
5. A – Coral snakes live primarily in Florida and in the desert Southwest. (page 1022)
6. B – Cytotoxins cause local tissue damage, whereas neurotoxins affect the nervous system. (page 1018)
7. B – Ticks are only a fraction of an inch long and can easily be mistaken for a freckle due to their brown color, small size, and round shape. (page 1023)
8. A – Rocky Mountain spotted fever and Lyme disease are both spread through the tick's saliva, which is injected into the skin when the tick attaches itself. (page 1023)
9. D – Additional signs, which may or may not occur, include weakness, sweating, fainting, and shock. (page 1020)
10. C – (A) Suffocating it with gasoline or (B) trying to burn it with a lighted match will only succeed in burning the patient. (C) Pulling it straight out will usually remove the whole tick. (page 1023)
11. D – Almost any substance can trigger the body's immune system and cause an allergic reaction: animal bites, food, latex gloves, or even semen can be an allergen. (page 1007)
12. B – The wasp's stinger is unbarbed, meaning that it can inflict multiple stings. (page 1009)
13. A – Severe cases can rapidly result in death. (page 1006)
14. D – The patient may also experience sudden pain, redness, and itching. (page 1007)
15. C – The patient becomes tachycardic because of the body's attempt to circulate the decreased oxygen supply to the brain and other vital organs. (page 1006)
16. B – More than two thirds of patients who die of anaphylaxis do so within the first half hour, so speed on your part is essential. (page 1007)
17. D – It is also important to determine what the effects of the exposure have been and how they have progressed, what interventions have been completed, and if the patient has been prescribed medication for allergic reactions. (page 1010)
18. D – Symptoms may also include fainting. (page 1025)
19. D – Maintaining the ABCs is essential for all patients. (page 1017)
20. D   (page 1021)
21. C – 0.15 mg (B) is the pediatric dose. (page 1016)
22. D – Epinephrine constricts the blood vessels, which raises blood pressure. Epinephrine also raises the pulse rate, inhibits allergic reactions, and dilates the bronchioles. (page 1016)
23. A – In some cases, a bite on the abdomen causes muscle spasms so severe that the patient may be thought to have an acute abdomen, possibly peritonitis. (page 1017)

24. B – Epinephrine (C) should only be administered in extreme reaction cases, and the patient with no signs or symptoms should be placed in the position of comfort (A). (page 1016)

25. C – Localized swelling and ecchymosis (A, B) are local signs, not systemic. (page 1020)

26. B – Systemic signs of envenomation by a coral snake include (A, C, D) respiratory problems, bizarre behavior, and paralysis of the nervous system. (page 1022)

27. C – Because the stinger of the honeybee remains in the wound, it can continue to inject venom for up to 20 minutes following the sting. (page 1009)

28. A – Generally, you should not use tweezers or forceps because squeezing may cause the stinger to inject still more venom into the wound. (page 1009)

29. D – Any patient experiencing an allergic reaction should receive a complete assessment after maintaining the ABCs. Be sure to assess mental status as well. (page 1010)

30. C – By going through the digestive tract it takes longer to get into the system. The person may also be unaware of the exposure or inciting agent. (page 1007)

31. C – Certain allergens may cause swelling of the airway resulting in partial or complete obstruction. (page 1006)

32. A – Wheezing occurs because excessive fluid and mucus are secreted into the bronchial passages, and muscles around these passages tighten in reaction to the allergen. (page 1010)

33. D – This will improve perfusion to the brain while easing respiratory effort. (page 1011)

Vocabulary

1. Anaphylaxis: An extreme, possibly life-threatening systemic allergic reaction that may include shock and respiratory failure. (page 1006)

2. Histamine: A substance released by the immune system in allergic reactions that is responsible for many of the symptoms of anaphylaxis. (page 1006)

3. Epinephrine: A substance produced by the body (adrenaline) and a drug produced by pharmaceutical companies that increases pulse rate and blood pressure; the drug of choice for an anaphylactic reaction. (page 1012)

4. Envenomation: When an insect or snake bites and injects the bite with its venom. (page 1007)

5. Rabies: An acute, fatal viral infection of the central nervous system that can affect all warm-blooded animals. (page 1024)

Fill-in

1. bronchial passages (page 1006)
2. urticaria (page 1006)
3. barbed (page 1008)
4. systemic (page 1007)
5. hypoperfusion (page 1011)
6. supine (page 1011)
7. bronchioles (page 1012)
8. imminent death (page 1006)
9. rabid (page 1024)
10. wheezing, urticaria (page 1006)

True/False

1. F (page 1011)
2. F (page 1019)
3. T (page 1019)
4. F (page 1023)
5. F (page 1025)
6. T (page 1006)
7. T (page 1006)
8. T (page 1006)
9. F (page 1011)
10. F (page 1025)
11. T (page 1024)
12. T (page 1021)

Short Answer

1. -Increased blood pressure
   -tachycardia, pallor
   -dizziness
   -chest pain
   -headache
   -nausea
   -vomiting (page 1012)

2. 1. Insect bites/stings
   2. Medications
   3. Plants
   4. Food
   5. Chemicals (page 1010)

3. 1. Obtain order from medical control
   2. Follow BSI techniques
   3. Make sure medication was prescribed for that patient
   4. Check for discoloration or expiration of medications
   5. Remove cap
   6. Wipe thigh with alcohol if possible
   7. Place tip against lateral mid-thigh
   8. Push firmly until activation
   9. Hold in place until medication is injected
   10. Remove and dispose
   11. Record the time and dose
   12. Reassess and record patient's vital signs (pages 1013 to 1014)

4. Respiratory: Sneezing or itchy, runny nose; chest or throat tightness; dry cough; hoarseness; rapid, noisy, or labored respirations; wheezing and/or stridor
   Circulatory: Decreased blood pressure, increased pulse (initially), pale skin and dizziness, loss of consciousness and coma (page 1006)

5. 1. Have the patient lie flat and stay quiet.
   2. Wash the bite area with soapy water.
   3. Splint the extremity.
   4. Mark the skin with a pen to monitor advancing swelling. (page 1021)

6. Black widow: Bite has a systemic effect (venom is neurotoxic)
   Brown recluse: Bite destroys tissue locally (venom is cytotoxic) (pages 1017 to 1018)

7. Because dog and human mouths contain virulent bacteria (page 1024)

8. 1. Limit further discharge of nematocysts.
   2. Keep the patient calm.
   3. Reduce motion of the extremity.
   4. Apply alcohol (isopropyl, rubbing, or any kind available).
   4. Remove remaining tentacles by carefully scraping.
   6. If necessary, immerse injury in hot water for 30 minutes.
   7. Transport. (page 1026)

9. Adult weighing more than 50kg: 0.3 to 0.5 mg of 1:1,000; 0.1 to 0.03 mg of 1:1,000 for children, depending on weight (page 1016)

Word Fun

```
          ¹U                ²W
           R                 H
           T                 A
   ³A N G I O E D E M A
           C                 A
       ⁴A N A P ⁵H Y L ⁶A X I S
        L   R   I     N
        L   I   S     T
        E   A   ⁷T O X I N
        R       A     V
        G       M     E
        E       I     N
        N       N     I
          ⁸W H E E Z I N G
               S
```

Ambulance Calls

1. -Scene safety
   -Immobilize with splint or bandage
   -Control bleeding and cover the bites with dry sterile dressings
   -Prompt transport
   -Monitor vital signs and cardiac rhythms
   -Gain IV access per protocol
   -Reassure the patient (page 1025)

2. -Scene safety
   -Assure ABCs
   -Limit further discharge of nematocysts
   -As per protocol, 0.3 mg of 1:1,000 epinephrine
   -Monitor vitals and cardiac rhythm
   -Inactivate the nematocysts by applying alcohol
   -Remove remaining tentacles by scraping them off
   -Reassess patient at least every 5 minutes
   -Place patient in supine position with head and shoulders up
   -Gain IV access
   -Rapid transport (page 1026)

3. -Check the EpiPen for clarity, expiration date, etc.
   -Obtain a physician's order to administer the EpiPen to the patient
   -Administer the EpiPen and promptly dispose of auto-injector
   -Apply high-flow oxygen
   -Initiate IV, maintain adequate perfusion
   -Rapid transport, cardiac monitoring
   -Monitor the patient and assess vital signs frequently
   -Use follow-up epinephrine as needed and per protocol
   -Consider early intubation if patient's status warrants it (page 1016)

Skill Drills

Skill Drill 22-1: Using an Auto-Injector

1. safety cap, antiseptic
2. lateral
3. injector, thigh (page 1013)

Skill Drill 22-2: Using an AnaKit

1. Prepare the injection site with antiseptic and remove the needle cover.
2. Hold the syringe upright and carefully use the plunger to remove air.
3. Turn the plunger one-quarter turn.
4. Quickly insert the needle into the muscle.
5. Hold the syringe steady and push the plunger until it stops.
6. Have the patient take the Chlo-Amine tablets provided in the kit
7. If available, apply a cold pack to the sting site. (page 1014)

Chapter 23: Poisonings and Overdose Emergencies

Matching

1. G (page 1035)
2. I (page 1035)
3. H (page 1036)
4. E (page 1041)
5. K (page 1041)
6. J (page 1035)
7. L (page 1041)
8. F (page 1045)
9. B (page 1035)
10. A (page 1041)
11. D (page 1046)
12. C (page 1040)
13. N (page 1037)
14. O (page 1042)
15. M (page 1041)

Multiple Choice

1. B (page 1040)
2. B – The presence of such injuries at the mouth strongly suggests the swallowing of a poison, such as lye. (page 1035)
3. D – Assess ABCs (A) in all patients. Take the plant with you (B) for identification of the poison, and always provide prompt transport (C) for suspected or known poisonings. (page 1038)
4. C – You cannot treat the patient if you become a victim. Maintaining the airway (A) and applying oxygen (B) come after scene safety. (page 1048)
5. D – In addition to these, clues to help determine the nature of the poison include an overturned bottle, an overturned or damaged plant, the remains of any food or drink found nearby, and any containers such as pill bottles. (page 1035)
6. C – You can administer oxygen for inhaled poisons (B) and give activated charcoal for ingested poisons (A). You can also flush the skin/eyes for absorbed poisons (D), but it is very difficult to remove or dilute injected poisons (C). (page 1037)
7. C – It may also cause nausea and vomiting. (page 1041)
8. B – Alcohol dulls the sense of awareness (A) and decreases reaction time (C). (page 1041)
9. C – Heroin (A) and morphine (B) are natural, not synthetic. (page 1042)
10. D – Maintain the ABCs of all patients and provide rapid transport (C) for any respiratory problem. (page 1043)
11. A – Anticholinergics are antagonists to the parasympathetic (A) division of the autonomic nervous system. (page 1047)
12. C – In the smoked (C) form, crack reaches the capillary network of the lungs and can be absorbed into the body in seconds. (page 1046)
13. D (page 1048)
14. D (page 1036)
15. B – (A) and (C) are symptoms of poisoning by botulism. (page 1050)
16. A (pages 1044 to 1045)
17. D (page 1045)
18. D – Almost any substance can be abused. (page 1041)
19. D – Patients who are unable to swallow (C) or have a decreased LOC (B) may aspirate the charcoal into their lungs. (page 1040)
20. D – These would be unusual responses to the drug and require assessment in an emergency department. (page 1046)
21. C – Adrenalin causes an increase in the heart's rate, automaticity, contractility, and conductivity, thereby significantly increasing the workload and oxygen demand. (page 1044)
22. B – (A and C) are signs seen with depressant use. (pages 1045 to 1046)
23. D – Carbon monoxide is odorless and can produce severe hypoxia without damaging the lungs. (page 1045)
24. C – Chlorine is very irritating and can cause airway obstruction as well as pulmonary edema. (page 1038)
25. B – (A) is not a sign or symptom but part of the interview process. (C) Dyspnea is a systemic rather than localized problem. (page 1039)

26. C – (page 1039)

27. D – Do not use water to flush the skin as it will ignite these substances and cause severe burns. (page 1040)

28. A (page 1039)

29. D – Many injuries and illnesses cause the patient to have an altered mental status. Remember to do a thorough assessment on each patient, including checking glucose levels (C) and the mechanism of injury (A) and obtaining a complete history of the illness (B) when possible. (page 1041)

30. D – Also confusion, disorientation, delusions, and hallucinations. (page 1042)

31. A – Move the patient into fresh air (A) immediately. Rescuers should wear SCBAs (B) if the situation indicates. (page 1039)

32. D – They may also present with burning eyes, sore throat, hoarseness, headache, respiratory distress, dizziness, confusion, stridor, seizures, or an altered mental status. (pages 1038 to 1039)

33. D (page 1037)

34. A – Accounts for approximately 80%. (page 1037)

35. D (page 1038)

36. A – Venom (B) is injected, and dieffenbachia (C) is ingested. (page 1038)

37. A (page 1040)

38. C – Most poisons do not have a specific antidote (A). Syrup of ipecac (D) is only used for specific instances. Oxygen (B) is never contraindicated, but it will not solve the problem this patient is experiencing. (page 1039)

39. C (page 1042)

40. B (page 1042)

41. A (page 1045)

42. C (page 1048)

43. D (page 1048)

Vocabulary

1. Sedative-hypnotic: A drug class that produces CNS depression and an altered level of consciousness with effects similar to those of alcohol. (page 1043)

2. Anticholinergic: Drug that blocks the parasympathetic nerves, such as atropine, Benadryl, jimsonweed, and certain cyclic antidepressants. (page 1047)

3. Delirium tremens: Syndrome seen with alcohol withdrawal, characterized by restlessness, fever, sweating, disorientation, agitation, and convulsions. (page 1042)

4. Hallucinogen: An agent that produces false perceptions in any one of the five senses. (page 1046)

5. Addiction: An overwhelming desire or need to continue using a drug or agent. (page 1041)

6. Substance abuse: The knowing misuse of any substance to produce a desired effect. (page 1035)

7. Hypnotic: A sleep-inducing effect or agent. (page 1041)

Fill-in

1. ABCs (page 1038)

2. alcohol (page 1041)

3. adsorbing (page 1040)

4. 5 to 10 minutes, 15 to 20 minutes (pages 1039 to 1040)

5. respiratory depression (page 1042)

6. hypoglycemia (pages 1041 to 1042)

7. recognize (page 1035)

8. 1 gram, kilogram (page 1040)

9. outward (pages 1039 to 1040)

10. ingestion (page 1037)

11. delirium tremens (DTs) (page 1042)

12. ignite (page 1040)

13. addiction (page 1041)

14. Hypovolemia (page 1042)

15. poisonous substance (page 1035)

16. monitoring, arrhythmias (page 1046)

17. atropine (page 1048)

18. ACLS (page 1045)

True/False

1. T   (page 1040)
2. F   (pages 1038, 1040)
3. F   (pages 1037 to 1038)
4. F   (page 1038)
5. F   (page 1040)
6. T   (page 1042)
7. T   (page 1048)
8. F   (page 1041)
9. T   (page 1042)
10. T   (page 1045)
11. T   (page 1036)
12. T   (page 1038)
13. T   (page 1041)
14. F   (page 1042)
15. T   (page 1045)

Short Answer

1. Activated charcoal adsorbs (binds to) the toxin and keeps it from being absorbed in the gastrointestinal tract. (page 1040)

2. 1. Ingestion
2. Inhalation
3. Injection
4. Absorption (page 1037)

3. Hypertension, tachycardia, dilated pupils, and agitation/seizures (page 1045)

4. 1. The organism itself causes the disease.
2. The organism produces toxins that cause disease. (page 1049)

5. Symptoms of acetaminophen overdose do not appear until the damage is irreversible, up to a week later. Finding evidence at the scene can save a patient's life. (page 1048)

6. They describe patient presentation in cholinergic poisoning (organophosphate insecticides, wild mushrooms).
DUMBELS: Defecation, Urination, Miosis, Bronchorrhea, Emesis, Lacrimation, Salivation
SLUDGE: Salivation, Lacrimation, Urination, Defecation, Gastrointestinal irritation, Eye constriction/emesis (page 1048)

7. 1. Opioid analgesics (page 1042)
2. Sedative-hypnotics (page 1043)
3. Inhalants (page 1044)
4. Sympathomimetics (page 1045)
5. Hallucinogens (page 1046)
6. Anticholinergic agents (page 1047)
7. Cholinergic agents (page 1048)

8. 1. What substance did you take?
2. When did you take it or become exposed to it?
3. How much did you ingest?
4. What actions have been taken?
4. How much do you weigh? (page 1035-1036)

9. Because they ignite when they come into contact with water. (page 1040)

10. Adverse side effects to be alert for are:
-dysrhythmias
-combativeness
-increased blood pressure
-tremors
-nausea and vomiting
-V-fib
-sweating and tachycardia (pages 1042 to 1043)

Word Fun

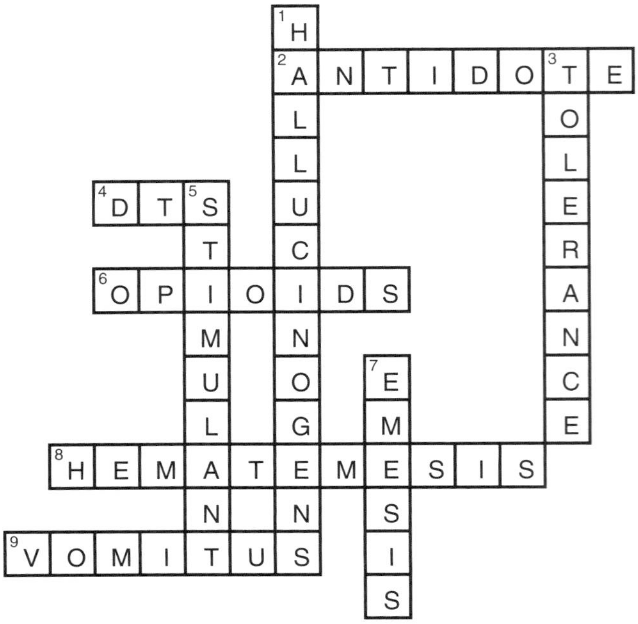

The completed crossword puzzle reads:

2 Across: ANTIDOTE
4 Across: DTS
6 Across: OPIOIDS
8 Across: HEMATEMESIS
9 Across: VOMITUS

1 Down: HALLUCINOGEN
3 Down: TOLERANCE
5 Down: STIMULANT
6 Down: OMNIBUS (OMULN...)
7 Down: EMESIS

Ambulance Calls

1. Maintain c-spine control.

Assess ABCs and provide support.

Control bleeding if necessary.

Check glucose level.

Establish an IV, give 20 mL/kg bolus of isotonic crystalloid solution.

Monitor cardiac rhythm.

Monitor vital signs.

Place in Trendelenburg's position.

Transport patient promptly because of alteration in mental status.

2. Assess the ABCs.

Make sure the mouth is free of all plant material.

Keep the patient as calm as possible.

Learn when the incident first took place.

Take the plant, or at least part of it, with you for identification.

Monitor the vital signs and provide support en route.

Rapid transport

3. Maintain the airway with an adjunct and high-flow oxygen via BVM or nonrebreathing mask with 100% oxygen.

Remove any remaining pills from the mouth.

Monitor vital signs and provide supportive measures.

Monitor cardiac rhythm.

Establish IV, consider 20 mL/kg bolus

Rapid transport.

Take the pill bottle along to the emergency department.

Be alert for possible vomiting.

Monitor patient closely and be prepared for the possible need for CPR.

Chapter 24: Neurologic Emergencies

Matching

1. D (page 1073)	**10.** H (page 1066)	**19.** P (page 1065)
2. G (page 1066)	**11.** L (page 1068)	**20.** V (page 1062)
3. E (page 1064)	**12.** K (page 1064)	**21.** Q (page 1062)
4. B (page 1062)	**13.** A (page 1068)	**22.** N (page 1061)
5. I (page 1064)	**14.** R (page 1062)	**23.** T (page 1064)
6. F (page 1063)	**15.** X (page 1062)	**24.** O (page 1064)
7. J (page 1061)	**16.** U (page 1065)	**25.** Y (page 1062)
8. C (page 1064)	**17.** S (page 1062)	
9. M (page 1064)	**18.** W (page 1061)	

Multiple Choice

1. D   (page 1060)

2. A – The cerebellum (B) controls muscle and body coordination. The cerebrum (C) controls emotion, thought, touch, movement, and sight. (page 1060)

3. A   (page 1060)

4. C   (page 1060)

5. C – A hemorrhagic stroke (A) is bleeding in the brain. Atherosclerosis (B) is usually the cause of the blockage. A cerebral embolism (D) may be the cause of the blockage. (pages 1061 to 1062)

6. A – (B and C) may also result in a hemorrhagic stroke, but (D) leads to ischemic stroke. (page 1062)

7. B   (page 1062)

8. B   (page 1062)

9. D   (page 1063)

10. A   (page 1064)

11. D – Epilepsy (A) is congenital in origin. A brain tumor (B) is a structural cause. A seizure due to a fever (C) is a febrile seizure. (page 1064)

12. D   (page 1065)

13. D   (page 1065)

14. C – Unequal pupils may be seen in conjunction with a head injury, but they are not the cause of the altered mental status. (page 1066)

15. B – A patient who has had a stroke may be alert and attempting to communicate normally, whereas a patient with hypoglycemia almost always has an altered or decreased level of consciousness. (page 1066)

16. C   (page 1066)

17. D   (page 1067)

18. D   (page 1067)

19. B – Aphasia (A) is an inability to produce or understand speech. With expressive aphasia (C), the patient will be able to understand the question but cannot produce the right sounds in order to answer. With dysarthria (D), they will understand language and be able to speak, but their words may be slurred and hard to understand. (page 1068)

20. D   (page 1070 to 1071)

21. A   (page 1069)

22. B – The airway is assessed first with any patient. (page 1069)

23. D   (page 1070)

24. A – Key physical tests for patients suspected of having a stroke include tests of speech, facial movement, and arm movement. (page 1071)

25. C – A score of 11 to 13 indicates moderate to severe dysfunction. A score of 14 to 15 indicates mild dysfunction (B). A score of 10 or less indicates severe dysfunction (D). (page 1071)

26. C   (page 1072)

27. B – The body is attempting to rid itself of an excessive buildup of acid. (page 1072)

28. C   (page 1073)

29. D   (page 1075)

30. B   (page 1062)

31. A   (page 1063)

32. A   (page 1066)

33. D   (page 1067)

Labeling

Brain (page 1061)

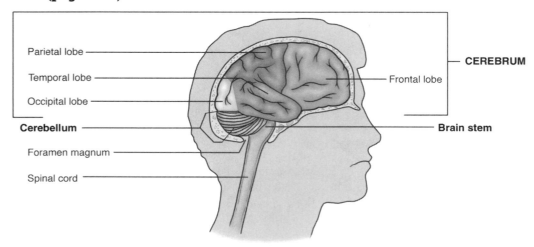

Parietal lobe

Temporal lobe

Occipital lobe

Cerebellum

Foramen magnum

Spinal cord

CEREBRUM

Frontal lobe

Brain stem

Spinal Cord (page 1061)

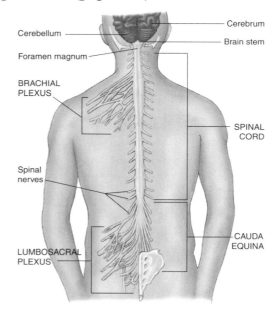

Cerebellum

Foramen magnum

BRACHIAL PLEXUS

Spinal nerves

LUMBOSACRAL PLEXUS

Cerebrum

Brain stem

SPINAL CORD

CAUDA EQUINA

Vocabulary

1. Cerebrovascular accident (CVA): An interruption of blood flow to the brain that results in the loss of brain function. (page 1061)

2. Ischemic stroke: Occurs when blood flow to a particular part of the brain is cut off by blockage inside a blood vessel. (page 1062)

3. Transient ischemic attack (TIA): Stroke symptoms that resolve spontaneously within 24 hours. (page 1063)
4. Hemorrhagic stroke: Occurs as a result of bleeding inside the brain. (page 1062)
5. Generalized seizure: Neurologic emergency characterized by unconsciousness and a generalized twitching of all the body's muscles that lasts several minutes or longer. (page 1064)
6. Absence seizure: Seizure characterized by a brief lapse of attention during which the patient simply stares or does not respond to anyone. (page 1064)
7. Atherosclerosis: A disorder in which cholesterol and calcium buildup inside the walls of blood vessels, forming plaque, which eventually leads to partial or complete blockage of blood flow. (page 1062)
8. Cerebral embolism: Obstruction of a cerebral artery caused by a clot that was formed elsewhere in the body and traveled to the brain. (page 1062)
9. Febrile seizures: Convulsions that result from sudden high fevers, particularly in children. (page 1065)
10. Thrombosis: Clotting of the cerebral arteries that may result in the interruption of cerebral blood flow and subsequent stroke. (page 1062)

Fill-in

1. 12 (page 1060)
2. cerebellum (page 1060)
3. emotion, thought (page 1060)
4. head (page 1060)
5. three (page 1060)
6. nerves (page 1060)
7. opposite, same (page 1060)
8. cerebrum (page 1060)
9. Incontinence (page 1065)
10. brain (page 1060)
11. epidural (page 1069)
12. hemiparesis (page 1066)
13. altered mental status (page 1067)
14. Fibrinolytic drugs, 3 hours (page 1062)
15. "normal" (page 1070)
16. anticonvulsants, muscle relaxers (page 1076)

True/False

1. F (page 1064)
2. F (page 1064)
3. T (page 1065)
4. F (page 1066)
5. T (page 1069)
6. F (page 1070)
7. F (page 1071)
8. T (page 1060)
9. F – Hypertensive patients are (page 1062)
10. T (page 1068)
11. T (page 1069)

Short Answer

1. 1. Facial droop; ask patient to show teeth or smile.
   2. Arm drift; ask patient to close eyes and hold arms out with palms up.
   3. Speech; ask patient to say, "The sky is blue in Cincinnati." (page 1071)
2. Newer clot-busting therapies may be helpful in reversing damage in certain kinds of strokes, but treatment must be started within 3 hours after onset of the event. (page 1075)
3. -Remove clothing.
   -Spray/wipe with tepid water, particularly about the head/neck.
   -Fan moistened areas. (page 1075)
4. A period of time after a seizure, generally lasting from 5 to 30 minutes, that is characterized by some degree of altered mental status and labored respirations. (page 1064)
5. Infarcted cells are dead. Ischemic cells are still alive, although they are not functioning properly because of hypoxia. (pages 1061 to 1062)
6. 1. Hypoglycemia
   2. Postictal state
   3. Subdural or epidural bleeding (page 1069)

Word Fun

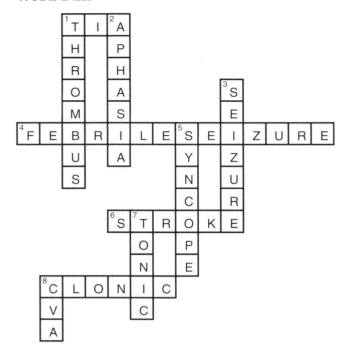

Ambulance Calls

1. High-flow oxygen

   Cool the patient by removing clothing and covering with wet towels and fanning

   Obtain glucose reading

   Establish IV access

   Monitor vital signs

   Transport

2. Maintain the airway; high-flow oxygen

   Suction if necessary or put patient in lateral recumbent position to clear secretions

   Check glucose level and consider 50% dextrose per protocol

   Initiate IV access, consider fluid bolus of 20 mL/kg

   Monitor cardiac rhythm

   Consider intubation

   Rapid transport (pages 1064, 1072, 1074)

3. High-flow oxygen

   Check LOC; obtain current history

   Perform Cincinnati Stroke Scale/Glasgow Coma Scale and notify hospital of results

   Check glucose level

   Initiate IV access and consider fluid bolus of 20 mL/kg

   Position of comfort, probably left side with the head elevated

   Protect the airway from secretions

   Monitor vital signs

   Monitor cardiac rhythm

   Rapid transport

Chapter 25: Nontraumatic Abdominal Emergencies

Matching

1. I	(page 1090)	**10.** B	(page 1084)
2. D	(page 1084)	**11.** G	(page 1084)
3. E	(page 1084)	**12.** N	(page 1086)
4. M	(page 1088)	**13.** L	(page 1091)
5. K	(page 1090)	**14.** O	(page 1084)
6. A	(page 1084)	**15.** H	(page 1084)
7. C	(page 1086)	**16.** P	(page 1085)
8. J	(page 1085)	**17.** R	(page 1085)
9. F	(page 1084)		

Multiple Choice

1. C – Loss of body fluid into the abdominal cavity decreases the volume of circulating blood and may eventually cause hypovolemic shock. (page 1085)

2. A – To gauge the degree of distention, simply look at the patient's abdomen. (page 1086)

3. A – The mass or lump, at times, will disappear back into the body cavity in which it belongs. If so, it is said to be reducible. If it cannot be pushed back within the body, it is said to be incarcerated. (page 1091)

4. A – The spinal cord supplies sensory nerves to the skin and muscles; these nerves are called the somatic nervous system. The autonomic nervous system controls the abdominal organs and the blood vessels. (page 1084)

5. D – Occasionally, an organ within the abdomen will be enlarged (swollen) and very fragile. The abdomen may be distended because of the swelling. Rough palpation could cause further damage and possibly rupture the organ. (page 1088)

6. A – The aorta lies immediately behind the peritoneum on the spinal column. The patient may experience severe back pain because of the peritoneum being rapidly stripped away from the wall of the main abdominal cavity by the hemorrhage or the pressure of blood on the back itself. (page 1090)

7. B – The kidneys, genitourinary structures, and large vessels (inferior vena cava, abdominal aorta) are found in the retroperitoneal space. The stomach, gall bladder, liver, pancreas, and uterus (answers A, C, D) are all found within the peritoneum. The adrenal glands (D) sit atop the kidneys in the retroperitoneal space. (page 1088)

8. C – A hernia may result from a surgical wound that has failed to heal properly, a congenital defect, or a natural weakness in an area such as the groin. (page 1090)

9. B – The parietal peritoneum is supplied by the same nerves from the spinal cord that supply the skin of the abdomen. Therefore, it can perceive many of the same sensations: pain, touch, pressure, heat, and cold. The visceral peritoneum is supplied by the autonomic nervous system, and the nerves are far less able to localize sensation. (page 1084)

10. D – All of these conditions (A, B, C) may cause severe abdominal pain. (page 1089)

11. C – The patient with peritonitis usually has abdominal pain, even when lying quietly. The patient may have difficulty breathing and may take rapid, shallow breaths because of the pain. (page 1085)

12. C – Rebound tenderness and fever are signs and symptoms associated with inflammation of the peritoneum. The patient usually has abdominal pain, even when resting (A), and will present with hypotension and tachycardia (B) if associated with shock/fluid loss. (page 1087)

13. C – Fever and distention (A, B) are common signs of peritonitis, but the degree of pain and tenderness is usually related directly to the severity of peritoneal inflammation. (page 1086)

14. D – Pain associated with diverticulitis is usually felt in the left lower quadrant. (page 1089)

15. C – The acute abdomen is associated with possible fluid loss and bleeding. You should anticipate the possible development of hypovolemic shock and be prepared to provide prompt treatment. (page 1085)

16. B – The loss of body fluid into the abdominal cavity usually results from abnormal shifts of fluid from the bloodstream into body tissues. (page 1085)

17. D – Pain medications should be avoided because they may mask the patient's signs and symptoms, making the physician's examination more difficult. (page 1092)

18. D   (page 1089)

Labeling

Solid Organs (page 1088)

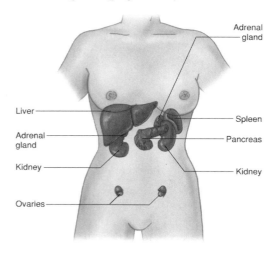

Hollow Organs (page 1088)

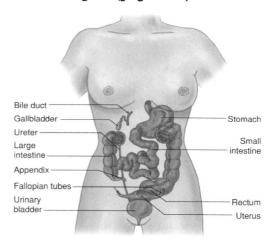

Vocabulary

1. Acute abdomen: Sudden onset of abdominal pain indicating an irritation of the peritoneum. (page 1084)

2. Diverticulitis: An inflammation of small pockets in the colon. (page 1085)

3. Ectopic pregnancy: A fertilized egg implanted outside the uterus. (page 1089)

4. Cholecystitis: Inflammation of the gall bladder. (page 1085)

5. Mittelschmertz: Common lower abdominal pain associated with the release of the egg from the ovary, characteristically occurring in the middle of the menstrual cycle. (page 1089)

True/False

1. F   (page 1084)   **7.** F   (page 1087)

2. F   (page 1089)   **8.** T   (page 1090)

3. F   (page 1089)   **9.** T   (page 1090)

4. F   (page 1084)   **10.** T   (page 293)

5. T   (page 1084)   **11.** T   (page 1092)

6. F   (page 1085)

Short Answer

1. Referred pain occurs because of connections between the body's two nervous systems. The abdominal organs are supplied by autonomic nerves, which, when irritated, stimulate close-lying sensory (somatic) nerves. (page 1084)

2. No. It is too complex and treatment is the same. (page 1084)

3. Paralysis of muscular contractions in the bowel results in retained gas and feces. Nothing can pass through. (page 1084)

4. -Bleeding

   -Fluid shifts (page 1085)

5. -Do not attempt to diagnose the cause.

   -Clear and maintain the airway.

   -Anticipate vomiting.

   -Administer 100% oxygen.

   -Give nothing by mouth.

   -Document pertinent information.

   -Avoid analgesics.

   -Anticipate hypovolemic shock.

   -Establish IV access and give a 20-mL/kg bolus of isotonic crystalloid if appropriate.

   -Keep the patient comfortable.

   -Monitor vital signs. (pages 1091 to 1092)

Word Fun

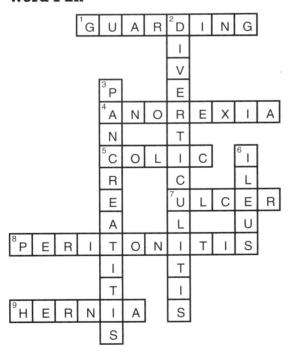

Ambulance Calls

1. Maintain airway.

   Anticipate hypovolemic shock.

   Anticipate vomiting.

   Establish IV access and give 20-mL/kg fluid bolus

   Place patient in the position of comfort.

   Apply high-flow oxygen.

Keep the patient warm.

Provide rapid transport.

Document information from the school nurse and try to obtain a SAMPLE/OPQRST-I history.

Monitor cardiac rhythm.

Monitor vital signs and the patient closely.

2. This is possible appendicitis or ectopic pregnancy, but it is necessary to diagnose.

-Maintain the airway.

-Anticipate hypovolemic shock.

-Anticipate vomiting.

-Establish IV access; consider 20-mL/kg fluid bolus.

-Place patient in the position of comfort.

-Apply high-flow oxygen.

-Keep the patient warm.

-Try to obtain a SAMPLE/OPQRST-I history.

-Document information from patient/family/friends.

-Provide rapid transport.

-Monitor cardiac rhythm.

-Monitor vital signs and the patient closely.

3. Place patient in a position of comfort.

Apply high-flow oxygen.

Establish IV access and consider 20-mL/kg fluid bolus

Lock up the house.

Provide normal transport.

Obtain a SAMPLE/OPQRST-I history.

Monitor cardiac rhythm.

Monitor vital signs and the patient.

Chapter 26: Environmental Emergencies

Matching

1. J	(page 1024).	**11.** G	(page 1022)	**21.** T	(page 1124)
2. H	(page 1023)	**12.** M	(page 1111)	**22.** Y	(page 1117)
3. K	(page 1021)	**13.** L	(page 1111)	**23.** Q	(page 1121)
4. F	(page 1111)	**14.** D	(page 1117)	**24.** W	(page 1122)
5. A	(page 1122)	**15.** Z	(page 1124)	**25.** P	(page 1108)
6. N	(page 1022)	**16.** CC	(page 1113)	**26.** U	(page 1117)
7. I	(page 1021)	**17.** X	(page 1122)	**27.** O	(page 1111)
8. C	(page 1118)	**18.** BB	(page 1115)	**28.** S	(page 1122)
9. B	(page 1112)	**19.** V	(page 1124)	**29.** R	(page 1102)
10. E	(page 1022)	**20.** AA	(page 1124)		

Multiple Choice

1. D – With convection (A), heat is transferred directly to circulating air. Conduction (B) is the direct transfer of heat from the body to a colder object by touch. Radiation (C) is the loss of body heat directly to colder objects in the environment. (page 1102)

2. A   (page 1102)

3. D   (page 1103)

4. C – Venous blood is naturally low in oxygen (A). Frostbite (B) causes a white, waxy appearance. (page 1103)

5. C – Confusion is seen in moderate hypothermia. (pages 1104)

6. D   (page 1104)

7. A – It is necessary to assess the trunk of the body to get a true feel for the extent of the cold emergency. The cooler the core temperature, the more serious the emergency. (page 1104)

8. B   (page 1103)

9. D   (page 1105)

10. B – The patient could be bradycardic, and initiating chest compressions could cause cardiac arrhythmias. (page 1105)

11. D   (page 1108)

12. B   (page 1108)

13. C – (A), (B), and (D) are all localized signs and symptoms. (page 1104)

14. A – (B), (C), and (D) are conditions that result from hyperthermia. (page 1111)

15. D   (page 1111)

16. D   (page 1111)

17. A   (pages 1111 to 1112)

18. D   (page 1113)

19. A – The patient should also be transported if the level of consciousness decreases; if the temperature remains elevated; or if the person is very young, elderly, or has any underlying medical condition such as diabetes, cardiovascular disease, or another worrisome condition. (page 1113)

20. A   (page 1115)

21. D   (page 1115)

22. B   (page 1118)

23. D   (page 1118)

24. A – Take care to stabilize and protect the patient's spine because associated cervical spine injuries are possible. (page 1118)

25. C   (page 1122)

26. D   (page 1118)

27. B   (page 1105)

28. B – (A) Heat is transferred from the body to the water, resulting in hypothermia. (C) Hypothermia lowers the metabolic rate in an effort to preserve body heat. (page 1122)

29. D   Half of all teenage and adult drownings are associated with alcohol. (page 1125)

30. A – The skin, joints, and vision are areas with signs and symptoms of air embolism. (page 1122)

31. D   (page 1123)

32. A – The brain and spinal cord require a constant supply of oxygen. (page 1123)

33. B   (page 1107)

34. D – They all have the same meaning: heat exhaustion. (page 1113) Don't you hate these types of questions?

35. D   (page 1113)

Vocabulary

1. Hyperbaric chamber: A chamber pressurized to more than atmospheric pressure for the treatment of diving injuries. (page 1124)

2. Decompression sickness: Condition seen in divers in which gas, usually nitrogen, forms bubbles that obstruct blood vessels. (page 1124)

3. Heat exhaustion: The result of the body losing so much water and so many electrolytes through very heavy sweating that hypovolemia occurs. (page 1113)

4. Frostbite: The most serious local cold injury. Because the tissues are actually frozen, the freezing permanently damages the cells. (page 1108)

5. Near drowning: Survival, at least temporarily, after suffocation in water. (page 1117)

6. Pneumomediastinum: Air entering the mediastinum and resulting in pain and severe dyspnea. (page 1123)

Fill-in

1. moderate, severe (page 1106)
2. ascent (page 1123)
3. rewarming (page 1109)
4. self-protection (page 1110)
5. Shivering (page 1104)
6. diving reflex (page 1122)
7. mild (pages 1105 to 1106)
8. taping hot packs (page 1107)
9. taping cold packs (page 1107)
10. Cardiac medications, metabolic rate (page 1107)
11. dysrhythmias (page 1117)
12. regurgitation, aspiration (page 1118)
13. give up (page 1123)

True/False

1. T   (page 1111)
2. T   (pages 1104)
3. F   (page 1104)
4. T   (page 1111)
5. T   (page 1111)
6. T   (page 1111)
7. F   (page 1125)
8. T   (page 1122)
9. T   (page 1113)
10. T   (page 1108)
11. T   (page 1111)
12. T   (page 1112)
13. T   (page 1113)
14. T   (page 1117)
15. T   (page 1123)
16. T   (page 1124)
17. T   (page 1124)

Short Answer

1. 1. Increase heat production: shiver, jump, walk around, etc.
   2. Move to another area where heat loss decreases: out of wind, into sun, etc.
   3. Wear insulated clothing: layer with wool, down, synthetics, etc. (page 1103)

2. 1. Move the patient out of the hot environment and into the ambulance.
   2. Set air conditioning to maximum cooling.
   3. Remove patient's clothing.
   4. Administer high-flow oxygen.

5. Apply cool packs to patient's neck, groin, and armpits.

6. Cover patient with wet towels or spray with cool water and fan.

7. Keep fanning.

8. Transport immediately.

9. Notify the hospital. (page 1115)

3. An air embolism is a bubble of air in the blood vessels caused by breathholding during rapid ascent. The resulting high pressure in the lungs causes alveolar rupture. (page 1123)

4. Treatment of air embolism and decompression sickness (page 1124)

5. 1. Remove the patient from the cold.

2. Handle injured part gently and protect from further injury.

3. Administer oxygen.

4. Remove wet or restricting clothing. (page 1110)

6. 1. Do not break blisters.

2. Do not rub or massage area.

3. Do not apply heat or rewarm unless instructed by medical control.

4. Do not allow patient to stand or walk on a frostbitten foot. (page 1110)

7. Blotching; froth at the nose and mouth; severe pain in muscles, joints, abdomen; dyspnea and/or chest pain; dizziness; nausea; vomiting; dysphasia; difficulty with vision; paralysis and/or coma; and irregular pulse with possible cardiac arrest. (page 1123)

8. Inhaling very small amounts of water can severly irritate the larynx, sending muscles of the larynx into spasm. It is the body's attempt to prevent water from getting into the lungs. Too much laryngospasm, however, will make ventilating the patient difficult until he or she becomes unconscious and the spasm stops. (page 1118)

Word Fun

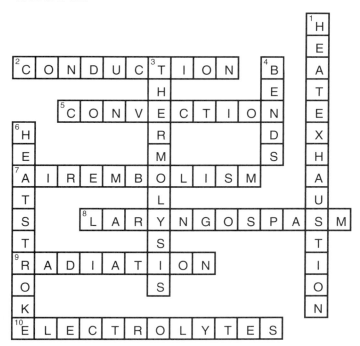

Ambulance Calls

1. -Provide BLS.

-Administer oxygen.

-Transport the patient in the left lateral recumbent position with the head down.

-Transport to a facility with hyperbaric chamber access.

-Consider endotracheal intubation if needed. Place on cardiac monitor and treat any dysrhythmias according to local and ACLS protocols. (page 1124)

2. -Don't allow the patient to walk, and handle her gently.

-Assess pulse for 30 to 45 seconds.

-Wrap patient in blankets.

-Apply heat packs to the groin, axillary, and neck regions.

-Turn the heat up in the ambulance.

-Administer warmed/humidified oxygen.

-Monitor cardiac rhythm.

-Monitor vital signs and core temperature. (pages 1124 to 1123)

3. -Remove the patient from the hot environment, preferably into an air-conditioned office.

-Rest: have the patient lie down with knees pulled up to relieve pressure on the abdomen.

-Replace fluid loss with water, diluted Gatorade, etc. If cramps continue, start an IV.

-Transport if patient still complains of cramps after this treatment or if IV was initiated.

-Monitor cardiac rhythm.

-Monitor vital signs. (pages 1112 and 1113)

4. -Take measure to protect self, crew, and bystanders from being struck by lightning.

-Using rapid extraction technique, protect the c-spine and move patient to shelter.

-Check pulse, monitor cardiac rhythm, and treat arrhythmias according to local and ACLS/CPR protocols.

-Secure the airway as needed, considering intubation.

-Monitor ABCs; give oxygen 15 L/min via nonrebreather or BVM.

-Initiate at least one large-bore IV of isotonic solution.

-Give a fluid bolus of 20mL/kg.

-If patient presents with seizure, consider diazepam as directed by local protocol.

-Locate entrance and exit wounds and treat appropriately.

-Provide rapid transport.

-Monitor vital signs. (page 1117)

Skill Drills

Skill Drill 26-1: Treating for Heat Exhaustion

1. extra clothing.

2. cooler environment, oxygen, supine, fan

3. fully alert

4. transport (page 1114)

Skill Drill 26-2: Stabilizing a Suspected Spinal Injury in the Water

1. Turn the patient to a supine position by rotating the entire upper half of the body as a single unit.

2. As soon as the patient is turned, begin artificial ventilation using the mouth-to-mouth method or a pocket mask.

3. Float a buoyant backboard under the patient.

4. Secure the patient to the backboard.

5. Remove the patient from the water.

6. Cover the patient with a blanket and apply oxygen if breathing. Begin CPR if breathing and pulse are absent. (page 1121)

Chapter 27: Behavioral Emergencies

Matching

1. C (page 1133)
2. F (page 1137)
3. B (page 1134)
4. D (page 1133)
5. E (page 1134)
6. A (page 1132)
7. I (page 1147)
8. G (page 1134)
9. H (page 1133)

Multiple Choice

1. D (page 1134)
2. B – (A) and (C) are both indications that the patient may indeed have a behavioral problem. (page 1132)
3. D (page 1134)
4. D (page 1134)
5. A (page 1132)
6. B (page 1133)
7. A (page 1133)
8. D (page 1134)
9. C – (A), (B), and (D) would have no influence on mental status because they are all normal measures. (page 1134)
10. D – All are correct because anything that creates a temporary or permanent dysfunction of the brain may cause OBS. (page 1134)
11. A – (B) and (C) are both diseases or dysfunctions of the brain. Schizophrenia (A) cannot be identified as a problem with the brain itself. (page 1134)
12. B – (A) All findings should be documented objectively; (C) Quote the patient's own words using quotation marks. (page 1134)
13. D – (A) Scene safety is top priority on any call; (B) It may take longer to assess, listen to, and prepare the patient for transport; (C) Help the patient to prepare by dressing and gathering appropriate belongings to take to the hospital. (page 1134)
14. B – (A), (C), and (D) are all important aspects of the assessment, but scene safety (B) is first on any call. (page 1134)
15. D (page 1137)
16. C – (A) Substance abuse and (B) divorce may be considered risk factors. (page 1138)
17. A – Suicidal patients may have no qualms about taking others with them who try to interfere with their plans. (page 1138)
18. D – All of these as well as heat- and cold-related illnesses, poisoning or overdose, TIAs, and infection may cause altered behavior. (page 1140)
19. D – Ordinarily, a restraint of a person must be ordered by a physician, a court order, or a law enforcement officer. (page 1141)
20. C – Legal actions may involve charges of assault, battery, false imprisonment, and violation of civil rights. (page 1141 to 1142)
21. B – The airway (B) must be assessed frequently due to the possibility of obstruction from vomit or the patient's inability to maintain his or her own airway because of mental status or positioning. (page 1142)
22. C – Not all mentally unstable patients are violent (A), and because they are in an altered mental state, they cannot refuse treatment.(page 1140)
23. D (page 1142)
24. D (page 1136)

Vocabulary

1. Mental disorder: An illness with psychological or behavioral symptoms that may result in an impairment in functioning, caused by a social, psychological, genetic, physical, chemical, or biologic disturbance. (page 1133)

2. Activities of daily living (ADL): The basic activities a person usually accomplishes during the normal day. (page 1133)

3. Altered mental status: A change in the way a person thinks or behaves. (page 1134)

4. Implied consent: The law assumes that there is implied consent when a patient is not mentally competent to grant consent for emergency medical care. (page 1141)

Fill-in

1. Behavior (page 1132)

2. behavioral crisis (page 1133)

3. depression (page 1133)

4. Organic brain syndrome (page 1134)

5. Family, friends, and observers (page 1137)

6. suicide (page 1138)

7. mental disorder (page 1133)

8. limit (1138)

True/False

1. T (page 1133)

2. F (page 1134)

3. F (page 1133)

4. F (page 1141)

5. F (page 1142)

6. F (page 1136)

7. F (page 1138)

8. T (page 1140)

9. F (page 1132)

10. F (page 1133)

11. T (page 1142)

12. F – your safety (page 1134)

13. T (page 1141)

14. T (page 1143)

Short Answer

1. A behavioral crisis is a temporary change in behavior that interferes with ADL or that is unacceptable to the patient or others. A mental health problem is this kind of behavioral change recurring on a regular basis. (page 1133)

2. 1. Improper functioning of the central nervous system

2. Drugs or alcohol

3. Psychogenic circumstances (page 1137 to 1138)

3. 1. The degree of force necessary to keep the patient from injuring self or others

2. Patient's gender, size, strength, and mental status

3. The type of abnormal behavior the patient is exhibiting (page 1141)

4. 1. Be prepared to spend extra time.

2. Have a definite plan of action.

3. Identify yourself calmly.

4. Be direct.

5. Assess the scene.

6. Stay with the patient.

7. Encourage purposeful movement.

8. Express interest in the patient's story.

9. Do not get too close to the patient.

10. Avoid fighting with the patient.

11. Be honest and reassuring.

12. Do not judge. (page 1135)

5. 1. Depression at any age

2. Previous suicide attempt

3. Current expression of wanting to commit suicide or sense of hopelessness

4. Family history of suicide

5. Age greater than 40 years, particularly for single, widowed, divorced, alcoholic, or depressed individuals

6. Recent loss of spouse, significant other, family member, or support system

7. Chronic debilitating illness or recent diagnosis of serious illness

8. Holidays

9. Financial setback, loss of job, police arrest, imprisonment, or some sort of social embarrassment

10. Substance abuse, particularly with increasing usage

11. Children of an alcoholic parent

12. Severe mental illness

13. Anniversary of death of loved one, job loss, marriage, etc.

14. Unusual gathering or new acquisition of things that can cause death, such as purchase of a gun, a large volume of pills, or increased use of alcohol (page 1138)

6. Public misconceptions concerning mental disorders include the mistaken belief that the patient's behavior is bizarre, and that the patient is always dangerous or unstable. There is also the misconception that mental disorders are incurable or uncontrollable. Finally, many believe that having a mental disorder is a cause for embarrassment and shame. Education of the public is crucial to removing these doubts and to ensuring that people with mental illness can lead productive and happy lives. (page 1134)

Word Fun

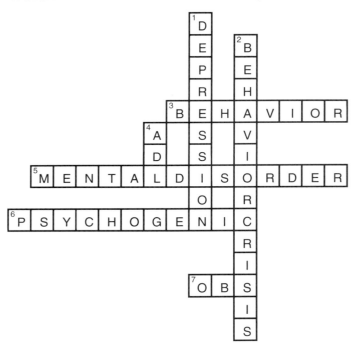

Ambulance Calls

1. -Call for police, and wait for their arrival before approaching the scene.

-Use direct eye contact and practice "reflective listening."

-Keep between the patient and the door.

-Calmly speak to the patient without being judgmental.

-Stay out of his "personal space;" leave yourself an out.

-Try to obtain the patient's consent for treatment and transport.

2. -Apply high-flow oxygen via a nonrebreathing mask for possible hypoxia.

-Attempt to obtain a blood glucose level to rule out hypoglycemia.

-Obtain vital signs.

- Monitor airway and vital signs en route.

3. - Be understanding and listen.

- Explain to the patient that she needs medical care.

- Monitor vital signs and reassure patient en route.

Chapter 28: Gynecologic Emergencies

Matching

1. D (page 1152)
2. C (page 1152)
3. L (page 1152)
4. B (page 1152)
5. N (page 1152)
6. H (page 1152)
7. M (page 1152)
8. E (page 1158)
9. F (page 1152)
10. O (page 1152)

11. K (page 1154)
12. I (page 1152)
13. A (page 1152)
14. G (page 1154)
15. J (page 1152)
16. CC (page 1158)
17. S (page 1159)
18. R (page 1158)
19. V (page 1152)
20. P (page 1152)

21. W (page 1152)
22. Q (page 1152)
23. Y (page 1152)
24. T (page 1152)
25. Z (page 1152)
26. U (page 1152)
27. AA (page 1154)
28. X (page 1152)
29. BB (page 1154)

Multiple Choice

1. A – After scene safety, airway is the first priority for every patient. (page 509)
2. B (page 494)
3. D (page 1152)
4. D (page 1154)
5. D – They are all true statements. (A: page 1155), (B: page 1152), (C: page 1152)
6. D (page 1158)
7. D (page 1159)

Labeling

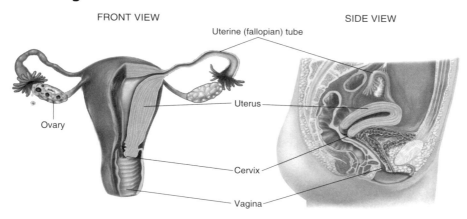

FRONT VIEW · SIDE VIEW

Uterine (fallopian) tube

Ovary

Uterus

Cervix

Vagina

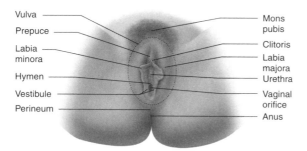

Vulva

Prepuce

Labia minora

Hymen

Vestibule

Perineum

Mons pubis

Clitoris

Labia majora

Urethra

Vaginal orifice

Anus

Vocabulary

1. Ectopic pregnancy: A pregnancy that develops outside the uterus, typically in a fallopian tube (page 1158)
2. Pelvic Inflammatory Disease: Acute or chronic infection in the organs of the female pelvic cavity (page 1157)
3. Fallopian tubes: Tubes or ducts that extend from near the ovaries and terminate at the uterus (page 1152)
4. Placenta abruptio: Premature separation of the placenta from the wall of the uterus (page 1159)
5. Placenta previa: A condition in which the placenta develops over and partially or completely covers the cervix (page 1158)

Fill-in

1. infections (page 1155)
2. estimate (page 1152)
3. clots, tissue (page 1156)
4. rhythm disturbances (page 1157)
5. Analgesics (page 1157)

True/False

1. T (page 1157)
2. F (page 1158)
3. T (page 1158)
4. T (page 1158)
5. T (page 1159)
6. T (page 1160)

Short Answer

1. When the patient demonstrates signs of shock or has excessive vaginal bleeding. (page 1156)
2. Establish at least one IV line using a large-bore (14- or 16-gauge) IV catheter in a large vein. Use an isotonic crystalloid solution and titrate as necessary. (page 1156)
3. Straddle injury, blows to the perineum, blunt force to the lower abdomen, foreign bodies inserted into the vagina, abortion attempt, soft-tissue injury (page 1159)

Word Fun

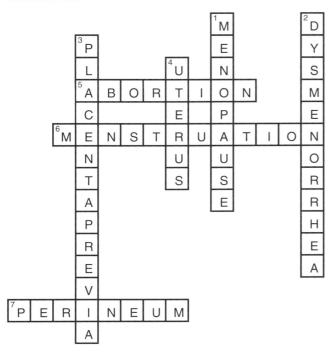

Ambulance Calls

1. -Provide privacy by clearing everyone out of the restroom.

-If possible, have an EMT-I of the same sex provide patient care.

-Provide compassion without judgment, being sure not to touch her without permission.

-Provide high-flow oxygen.

-Monitor vital signs.

-Place her on cot and get her into the ambulance.

-Do a focused assessment only as necessary, explaining each step.

-Discourage her from washing, douching, urinating, or defecating.

-Transport. (page 1159)

2. -Determine her LOC and ability to refuse care.

-Try and gain her confidence, and be aware of your own feelings and prejudices.

-Offer to call the local rape crisis center for her.

-Provide reassurance.

-Document in detail and obtain appropriate signatures. (pages 1159 to 1160)

Chapter 29: Obstetric Emergencies

Matching

1. D	(page 1168)	**13.** A	(page 1186)	**25.** AA	(page 1172)
2. C	(page 1170)	**14.** G	(page 1189)	**26.** HH	(page 1173)
3. L	(page 1171)	**15.** J	(page 1178)	**27.** V	(page 1172)
4. P	(page 1172)	**16.** T	(page 1168)	**28.** DD	(page 1172)
5. N	(page 1171)	**17.** S	(page 1175)	**29.** JJ	(page 1179)
6. H	(page 1177)	**18.** B	(page 1172)	**30.** W	(page 1174)
7. M	(page 1168)	**19.** Q	(page1179)	**31.** X	(page 1172)
8. E	(page 1172)	**20.** R	(page 1176)	**32.** Z	(page 1172)
9. F	(page 1169)	**21.** JJ	(page1171)	**33.** BB	(page 1177)
10. O	(page 1189)	**22.** CC	(page 1176)	**34.** GG	(page 1173)
11. K	(page 1189)	**23.** U	(page 1177)	**35.** FF	(page 1175)
12. I	(page 1172)	**24.** Y	(page 1179)	**36.** EE	(page 1189)

Multiple Choice

1. D   (page 1186)

2. B   (pages 1179–1180)

3. B – Aggressive suctioning of the baby's mouth and oropharynx before delivery of the body may prevent meconium aspirations and respiratory distress. (pages 1185–1186)

4. B   (page 1188)

5. A   (page 1189

6. D   (page 1190)

7. D   (pages 1179–1180)

8. B   (page 1179)

9. D   (page 1179)

10. A   (page 1179)

11. C   (page 1179)

12. B – (A), (C), and (D) are signs of preeclampsia. (page 1176)

13. B   (page 1175)

14. A   (page 1176)

15. D   (page 1177)

16. D   (page 1190)

17. C   (page 1178)

18. B   (page 1177)

19. A   (page 1176)

20. B   (page 1171)

21. D – The umbilical cord contains two arteries and one vein. The umbilical arteries carry deoxygenated blood and waste away from the fetus, and the umbilical vein carries oxygenated blood and nutrients to the fetus. Therefore, you would infuse the infant through the single vein. (page 1172)

22. B   (page 1173)

23. D   (page 1175)

24. A   (page 1175)

25. D   (page 1176)

Labeling

The Female Reproductive Tract (page 1167)

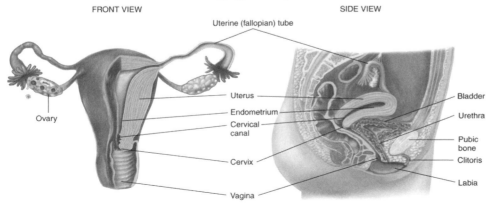

FRONT VIEW   SIDE VIEW

Uterine (fallopian) tube

Ovary

Uterus

Endometrium

Cervical canal

Cervix

Vagina

Bladder

Urethra

Pubic bone

Clitoris

Labia

The Female External Genitalia (page 1170)

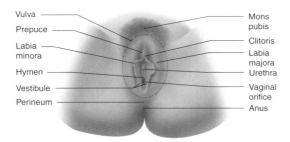

Vulva
Prepuce
Labia minora
Hymen
Vestibule
Perineum

Mons pubis
Clitoris
Labia majora
Urethra
Vaginal orifice
Anus

Anatomic Structures of the Pregnant Woman (page 1172)

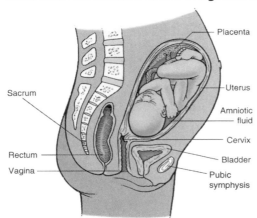

Sacrum
Rectum
Vagina

Placenta
Uterus
Amniotic fluid
Cervix
Bladder
Pubic symphysis

Vocabulary

1. Primigravida: A woman who is experiencing her first pregnancy. (page 1172)
2. Multigravida: A woman who has had previous pregnancies. (page 1172)
3. Ectopic pregnancy: A pregnancy that develops outside the uterus, typically in a fallopian tube. (page 1175)
4. Crowning: The appearance of the top of the infant's head at the vaginal opening during labor. (page 1179)
5. Eclampsia: A seizure in a pregnant woman who has preeclampsia and no other cause for the seizure. (page 1176)
6. Uterine rupture: Rupture of the uterus usually by trauma that can result in life-threatening hemorrhage in the woman's fetus. (page 1179)
7. Supine hypotensive syndrome: Low blood pressure resulting from compression of the inferior vena cava by the weight of the gravid uterus when the mother is supine. (page 1177)

Fill-in

1. placenta (page 1171)
2. arteries, vein (page 1172)
3. 500 to 1000 mL (page 1172)
4. 36, 40 (page 1173)
5. trimesters (page 1173)
6. ectopic pregnancy (page 1175)
7. fontanelles (page 1184)
8. 50% (page 1173)
9. 10, 20 (page 1173)
10. 30%, growth, fetus (page 1173, 1174)
11. 10, 15 mm Hg (page 1174)

True/False

1. F (page 1179)
2. F (page 1179)
3. F (page 1172)
4. F (page 1182)
5. T (page 1189)
6. F (page 1188)
7. T (page 1189)
8. T (page 1174)
9. T (page 1175)
10. T (page 1175)
11. T (page 1176)
12. T (page 1191)

Short Answer

1. -Early: spontaneous abortion (miscarriage) or ectopic pregnancy (page 1175)

-Later: Placenta previa or abruptio placentae (page 1177–1178)

2. On the left side, to prevent supine hypotensive syndrome (low blood pressure resulting from the weight of the fetus compressing the inferior vena cava) (page 1177)

3. 1. Uterine contractions

2. Bloody show

3. Rupture of amniotic sac (page 1180)

4. 1. When delivery can be expected in a few minutes

2. When some natural disaster or catastrophe makes it impossible to reach the hospital

3. When no transportation is available (page 1180)

5. The brain is covered by only skin and membrane at the fontanelles. (page 1184)

6. Exerting gentle pressure horizontally across the perineum with a sterile gauze pad may reduce the risk of perineal tearing. (page 1184)

7. 1. During a breech delivery to protect the infant's airway

2. When the umbilical cord is prolapsed (page 1191)

Word Fun

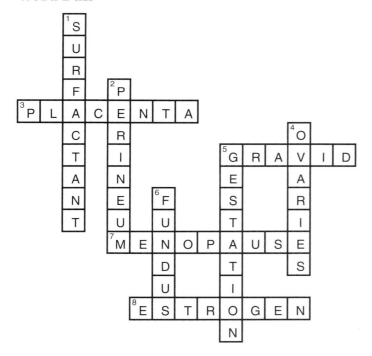

Ambulance Calls

1. -Place the mother on her left side.

-Maintain the airway, suctioning as needed.

-Consider intubation.

-Provide high-flow oxygen.

-Monitor vital signs.

-Protect the mother from harm if seizing starts again.

-Place patient on cardiac monitor.

-Consider magnesium sulfate (2–4 g diluted in 50–100 mL of normal saline IV bolus over slow 5 minute push).

-Consider diazepam if seizure still hasn't terminated.

-Provide rapid transport. (page 1176)

2. -Place patient on her left side.

-Provide high-flow oxygen. The baby needs extra oxygen if the placenta is abruptio or if there are other serious conditions.

-Estimate blood loss and place a sterile pad or sanitary napkin over the vagina.

-Large-bore IV line of isotonic crystalloid

-Take any clots to the hospital.

-Do not offer her false reassurance that everything will be okay or that the baby is fine.

-Transport promptly. (page 1175)

3. -Position the mother for delivery and administer high-flow oxygen.

-As crowning occurs, use a clamp to puncture the sac away from the infant's face.

-Push the ruptured sac away from the infant's face as the head is delivered.

-Clear the infant's mouth and nose immediately.

-Continue with the delivery as normal. (page 1184)

Skill Drills

Skill Drill 29-1: Delivering the Infant

1. Support the bony parts of the head with your hands as it emerges. Suction fluid from the mouth, then the nostrils.

2. As the upper shoulder appears, guide the head down slightly, if needed, to help deliver the shoulder.

3. Support the head and upper body as the shoulders deliver. Guide the head up slightly if needed to deliver the lower shoulder.

4. Handle the slippery delivered infant firmly but gently, keeping the neck in neutral position to maintain the airway.

5. Place the first clamp 7″ from the infant's body and the second 3″ farther and cut between them.

6. Allow the placenta to deliver itself. Never pull on the cord to speed up placental delivery. (page 1185)

Chapter 30: Neonatal Resuscitation

Matching

1. A (page 1206)	**11.** G (page 1213)	**21.** L (page 1204)
2. F (page 1212)	**12.** K (page 1205)	**22.** O (page 1206)
3. J (page 1221)	**13.** N (page 1204)	**23.** R (page 1204)
4. M (page 1221)	**14.** Q (page 1219)	**24.** W (page 1221)
5. P (page 1219)	**15.** T (page 1214)	**25.** AA (page 1207)
6. S (page 1204)	**16.** V (page 1217)	**26.** D (page 1210)
7. U (page 1214)	**17.** Z (page 1210)	**27.** I (page 1204)
8. Y (page 1211)	**18.** CC (page 1216)	**28.** X (page 1211)
9. BB (page 1209)	**19.** C (page 1206)	**29.** E (page 1212)
10. B (page 1214)	**20.** H (page 1220)	

Multiple Choice

1. D (page 1205)	**8.** B (page 1210)	**15.** B (page 1214)
2. B (page 1026)	**9.** B (page 1210)	**16.** D (page 1214)
3. D (page 1207)	**10.** A (page 1210)	**17.** D (page 1215)
4. B (page 1207)	**11.** D (page 1211)	**18.** C (page 1215)
5. A (page 1209)	**12.** C (page 1211)	**19.** D (page 1216)
6. D (page 1209)	**13.** C (page 1211)	**20.** D (page 1216)
7. A (page 1210)	**14.** C (page 1214)	

Vocabulary

1. Acrocyanosis: Cyanosis of the hands and feet (page 1224)

2. Meconium aspirator: A device used in conjunction with an ET tube to suction meconium from the newborn's airway (page 1219)

3. Neonate: The phase from the first few minutes to the first hours after birth (page 1204)

4. Peripheral cyanosis: Cyanosis of the hands and feet (page 1214)

5. Primary apnea: Apnea that is not reversed with tactile stimulation and suctioning (page 1211)

6. Secondary apnea: Apnea that is not reversed with tactile stimulation and suctioning; requires positive pressure ventilation. (page 1211)

7. Umbilical vein catheterization: Inserting a UVC into the umbilical vein; an alternate route for administering drugs and IV fluids to the newborn. (page 1207)

Fill-in

1. 10% (page 1204)	**7.** 30 seconds (page 1212)
2. 28 (page 1204)	**8.** Perform endotracheal intubation (page 1212)
3. Foramen ovale (page 1204)	**9.** 10 mL/kg, 5, 10 (page 217)
4. Heater, turned on (page 1209)	**10.** meconium staining (page 1219)
5. folded towel (page 1209)	**11.** meconium aspirator (page 1219)
6. both sides,chest rise (page 1212)	**12.** hostile (page 1222)

True/False

1. T (page 1205)	**7.** T (page 1212)
2. T (page 1205)	**8.** T (page 1213)
3. T (page 1205)	**9.** T (page 1217)
4. F (page 1208)	**10.** T (page 1217)
5. T (page 1212)	**11.** F (page 1217)
6. T (page 1212)	**12.** T (page 1218)

Short Answer

1. Persistent cyanosis and/or bradycardia secondary to hypoxia (page 1206)
2. 1. What is your due date or how many weeks pregnant are you?
   2. How many infants are you expecting?
   3. Has your amniotic sac ruptured? If so, what was the color and consistency of the fluid? Did it smell?
   4. Have you had any depressant drugs or alcohol within the last four hours? (page 1206)
3. 1. Diabetes
   2. Cardiac disease
   3. Hypertension
   4. Preeclampsia or eclampsia
   5. Multiple gestation
   6. Mother's age less than 16 years or greater than 35 years
   7. Inadequate or no prenatal care
   8. Postterm gestation (longer than 40 weeks)
   9. History of perinatal morbidity or mortality
   10. Use of illicit drugs, certain medications, alcohol, or cigarettes (page 1206)
4. 1. Is the amniotic fluid clear of meconium?
   2. Is the infant breathing or crying?
   3. Does the newborn have good muscle tone?
   4. Is the skin color pink?
   5. Is this a term gestation? (page 1208)
5. The danger in going too far is that the catheter may go into the portal venous system and allow certain drugs to enter the liver. (page 1217)
6. If the mother is addicted, so is her infant; giving naloxone under these circumstances can precipitate an acute withdrawal seizure in the newborn. (page 1218)
7. It is attached to a standard 15/22-mm fitting on the proximal end of the endotracheal tube: the ribbed end attaches to suction machine. While visualizing the vocal cords, insert the ET tube in between the vocal cords. Then, while applying you thumb to the open port on the meconium aspirator, suction the hypopharynx while withdrawing the ET tube. (pages 1219–1220)

Word Fun

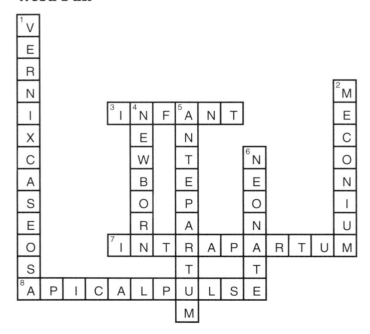

Ambulance Calls

1. -Turn on the heater in the ambulance on the way there.

-Dry and warm the newborn.

-Position the newborn.

-Suction the airway.

-Use tactile stimulation if necessary.

-Clamp and cut umbilical cord.

-Assess respiratory effort.

-Assess heart rate.

-Assess color.

-Note APGAR scale at both 1 minute and 5 minute mark.

-Provide rapid transport. (pages 1209-1214)

2. -If there are signs of decomposition, make no resuscitative efforts.

-Allow parents to see the fetus if desired.

-Provide emotional support.

-Be aware of hostility.

-Provide normal care for the mother, delivering placenta and taking it with you to the hospital.

-Provide rapid transport.

-Consider CISD. (page 1222)

3. -Keep the newborn warm.

-Keep the mouth and nose clear of mucus.

-Carefully observe the cut end of the cord for bleeding.

-Give oxygen, being careful of the eyes.

-Notify the hospital.

-Provide rapid transport. (page 1221–1222)

Skill Drills

Skill Drill 30-1: Giving Chest Compressions to a Newborn

1. Find the proper position: just below the nipple line, middle of the lower third of the sternum.

2. Wrap your hands around the body, with your thumbs resting at that position.

3. Press your thumbs gently against the sternum, compressing to a depth that is approximately one third the anteroposterior diameter of the chest. (page 1213)

Skill Drill 30-2: Inserting an Orogastric Tube in the Newborn

1. tip, nose, earlobe, earlobe, xiphoid process

2. tube, nose, ventilations

3. gastric, 20, tube, air, cheek (page 1215)

Chapter 31: Pediatric Emergencies

Matching

1. O (page 1236)
2. G (page 1237)
3. T (page 1237)
4. A (page 1236)
5. K (page 1236)
6. C (page 1238)
7. M (page 1286)

8. B (page 1287)
9. Q (page 1288)
10. I (page 1291)
11. S (page 1249)
12. F (page 1240)
13. J (page 1303)
14. R (page 1300)

15. D (page 1279)
16. H (page 1321)
17. P (page 1234)
18. E (page 1235)
19. L (page 1316)
20. N (page 1247)

Multiple Choice

1. C (page 1234)
2. D (page 1235)
3. C – Physical stimuli include light, warmth, cold, hunger, sound, and taste. (page 1236)
4. B (page 1236)
5. C (page 1237)
6. D (page 1240)
7. A (page 1240)
8. C – Infants have very little use of their chest muscles to make their chests expand during inspiration, so they depend on the diaphragm. (page 1240)
9. B (page 1241)
10. C (page 1238)
11. D (page 1239)
12. A – The ribs (B) are lifted by the intercostal muscles. (page 1239)
13. D (page 1244)
14. D (page 1245)
15. C (page 1244)
16. D (page 1247)
17. D (page 1249)
18. D – Signs of complete airway obstruction also include an ineffective cough (no sound) and/or loss of consciousness. (page 1254)
19. B (page 1259)
20. B – Using a nasal airway with a possible basilar skull fracture may result in the adjunct being pushed into the brain. It may also increase intracranial pressure in patients with head trauma. (page 1261)
21. D (page 1264)
22. D (page 1265)
23. D (page 1266)
24. C (page 1266)
25. B (page 1268)
26. B (page 1265)
27. D (page 1269)

28. B (page 1272)
29. C (page 1272)
30. B (page 1273)
31. A (page 1274)
32. B (page 1274)
33. A (page 1279)
34. B (page 1279)
35. A (page 1281)
36. A (page 1282)
37. D (page 1282)
38. D (page 1284)
39. C (page 1285)
40. D (page 1285)
41. C (page 1286)
42. A (page 1286)
43. B (page 1288)
44. C (page 1290)
45. D (page 1290)
46. D (page 1291)
47. D (page 1291)
48. A (page 1292)
49. D (page 1292)
50. B (page 1292)
51. A (page 1294)
52. D (page 1295)
53. A (page 1295)
54. B (page 1295)
55. C (page 1296)
56. C (page 1297)
57. C (page 1297)
58. C (page 1297)
59. D (page 1297)
60. B (page 1298)
61. B (page 1299)
62. B (page 1299)
63. D (page 1299)

64. B   (page 1300)

65. C   (page 1301)

66. D   (page 1301)

67. D   (page 1302)

68. C   (page 1303)

69. D   (page 1303)

70. D   (page 1304)

71. B   (page 1304)

72. A   (page 1307)

73. D – When dealing with the death of an infant, your assessment of the scene should also include any signs of illness, including medications, humidifiers, thermometers, etc. (page 1308)

74. D – A classic apparent life-threatening event (ALTE) is also characterized by cyanosis and apnea. (page1308)

75. D – In dealing with the family after the death of a child, also:
  -speak to the family members at eye level
  -use the word "dead" or "died" instead of euphemisms
  -offer to call other family members or clergy
  -ask each adult family member individually whether or not he or she wants to hold the child
  -wrap the dead child in a blanket
  -stay with the family while they hold the child
  -ask them not to remove equipment that was used in attempted resuscitation (page 1309)

76. D   (page 1310)

77. C – Elevate (A) only injured extremities if needed. Only assist ventilations (B) if needed. Remove helmets (D) as called for by the situation or local protocols. (page 1313)

78. D   (page 1316)

79. C   (page 1316)

80. D   (page 1316)

81. C   (page 1318)

82. A   (page 1318)

83. D – Child abuse also includes sexual abuse and any improper or excessive action that injures or otherwise harms a child or infant. (page 1321)

84. B   (page 1321)

85. C   (page 1325)

Vocabulary

1. Acrocyanosis: Cyanosis of the hands and feet in newborns and infants younger than 2 months. This occurs when the infant is cold and is a normal finding. (page 1246)

2. Apical pulse: Obtained by auscultating heart tones over the chest with a stethoscope. (page 1249)

3. Apparent life-threatening event: An event that causes unresponsiveness, cyanosis, and apnea in an infant who then resumes breathing with stimulation. (page 1308)

4. Bronchiolitis: A viral infection that results in inflammation and constriction of the bronchioles; seen most commonly in children younger than 2 years. (page 1290)

5. Child abuse: Any improper or excessive action that injures or otherwise harms a child or infant; includes physical abuse, sexual abuse, neglect and emotional abuse. (page 1321)

6. Croup: Infection of the airway below the level of the vocal cords, Usually caused by a virus; also referred to as laryngotracheobronchitis. (page 1286)

7. Epiglottitis: An acute bacterial infection that results in rapid swelling of the epiglottis and surrounding tissues; also referred to as acute supraglottic laryngitis. (page 1287)

8. Epiphyseal plate: The growth plate of the bone; responsible for normal bone growth and development. (page 1240)

9. Fontanelles: Areas where the infant's skull has not fused together; usually disappear at approximately 18 months of age. (page 1238)

10. Greenstick fracture: An incomplete fracture of a bone seen in children, whose bones are pliable and may not completely fracture. (page 1240)

11. Grunting: An "uh" sound heard during exhalation that reflects the child's attempt to keep the alveoli open; a sign of increased work of breathing. (page 1247)

12. Medullary canal: The space within the bone that contains bone marrow. (page 1278)

13. Nebulizer: A device that aerosolizes medications for inhalation into the lungs. (page 1289)

14. Nuchal rigidity: A stiff or painful neck; commonly associated with meningitis. (page 1304)

15. Osteomyelitis: Infection of the bone and muscle; a potential complication of intraosseous infusion. (page 1279)

16. Pediatric assessment triangle: A structured assessment tool that allows you to rapidly form a general impression of the infant or child without touching him or her; consists of assessing appearance, work of breathing and circulation of the skin. (page 1244)

17. Reactive airway disease: A term used to describe any condition that causes hyperactive bronchioles and bronchospasm. (page 1289)
18. Separation anxiety: Fear of being separated from a parent or caregiver; common in young children. (page 1284)
19. Tenting: A condition where the skin remains depressed after you remove your finger; indicates overhydration. (page 1251)
20. Volutrol: A special type of microdrip set that allows you to fill a large drip chamber with a specific amount of fluid to avoid fluid overload. (page 1277)

Fill-in

1. Trauma (page 1234)
2. adolescents (page 1237)
3. fontanelles (page 1238)
4. tongue (page 1239)
5. trachea (page 1239)
6. ribs (page 1239)
7. 200 (page 1241)
8. epiphyseal (growth) plates (page 1240)
9. pediatric assessment triangle (page 1244)
10. apical pulse (page 1249)
11. Tidal volume (page 1263)
12. Volutrol (page 1277)
13. Jamshedi (page 1278)
14. oxygen (page 1280)
15. Respiratory failure (page 1285)
16. albuterol (page 1289)
17. Septic shock (page 1294)
18. Status epilepticus (page 1299)
19. Fever (page 1303)
20. Meningitis (page 1303)
21. vomiting, diarrhea (page 1304)
22. administer glucose (page 1307)
23. stressful (page 1310)
24. abdominal (page 1312)
25. Drowning (page 1318)

True/False

1. T (page 1236)
2. T (page 1240)
3. F (page 1235)
4. F (page 1236)
5. T (page 1237)
6. F (page 1240)
7. T (page 1248)
8. F (page 1251)
9. T (page 1264)
10. F (page 1300)
11. T (page 1304)
12. F (page 1310)
13. T (page 1310)
14. T (page 1312)
15. F (page 1315)
16. T (page 1241)
17. T (page 1316)
18. F (page 1321)
19. T (page 1324)
20. T (page 1324)

Short Answer

1. 1. Appearance (muscle tone and mental status)
   2. Work of breathing
   3. Circulation to the skin (page 1244)
2. 1. Hold the laryngoscope handle with your left hand.
   2. Open the mouth
   3. Insert a pediatric straight blade into the mouth.
   4. Exert gentle traction upward along the axis of the laryngoscope blade.
   5. Watch the tip until the foreign body is visible.
   6. Use suction to improve visibility.
   7. Insert the Magill forceps into the mouth with tips closed.
   8. Grasp the foreign body and remove it.
   9. Look to make sure the airway is clear of debris. (pages 1257 to 1258)
3. 1. Clinical assessment (assessing breath sounds and oxygen saturation)
   2. End-tidal carbon dioxide detectors
   3. Esophageal detector bulbs or syringes (page 1269)

4. 1. Insert the tube gently through the nostril, directing the tube straight back. Do not angle the tube superiorly.

2. If the tube does not pass easily, try the opposite nostril or a smaller tube. Never force the tube.

3. If NG passage is unsuccessful, use the OG approach. (page 1273)

5. 1. Ensure the airway is open.

2. Assess breathing adequacy.

3. Control bleeding if present.

4. Administer 100% oxygen.

5. Position the patient.

6. Keep the patient warm.

7. Provide immediate transport.

8. Initiate IV of isotonic crystalloid solution.

9. Continue monitoring vital signs.

10. Allow caregiver to accompany child when possible. (pages 1292 to 1293)

6. -mother younger than 20 years

-mother smoked during pregnancy

-low birth weight

-baby placed on his or her stomach in a crib (page 1307)

7. C: consistency of the injury with the child's developmental age

H: history inconsistent with injury

I: inappropriate parental concerns

L: lack of supervision

D: delay in seeking care

A: affect

B: bruises of varying ages

U: unusual injury pattern

S: suspicious circumstances

E: environmental clues

Word Fun

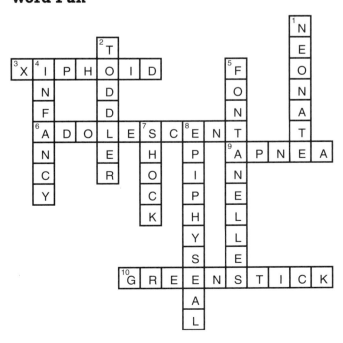

Ambulance Calls

1. -Talk to the child directly.

-Explain that you need to check for a pedal pulse before touching the child

-Once equipment is prepared, show it to the child and explain how it will work.

-Explain that moving the injured leg will be painful and ask the mother to help by allowing the child to squeeze her hand, etc.

-Manipulate the leg as little as possible, but be expedient.

-Transport in the position of comfort, allowing the child to dictate movement, within reason.

2. -Position the child with the airway in a neutral sniffing position.

-Insert a nasopharyngeal airway.

-Assist ventilations with a BVM and 100% oxygen.

-Apply the cardiac monitor and pulse oximeter.

-If respiratory status deteriorates further, intubate.

-Rapid transport, continuing assessment en route.

-Obtain SAMPLE history from staff en route.

3. -Immediately apply oxygen

-Place the child on the cardiac monitor and pulse oximeter.

-Administer nebulized albuterol.

-Rapid transport, continuing assessment en route.

-Establish IV access en route.

-Monitor for deterioration and possible need for intubation.

Skills Drills

Skill Drill 31-1: Positioning the Airway in a Child

1. firm

2. folded, 1, shoulders, back

3. Immobilize, movement (page 1253)

Skill Drill 31-2: Removing a Foreign Body Airway Obstruction in an Unresponsive Child

1. firm, flat

2. Inspect, Remove

3. rescue breathing, head

4. chest compressions

5. Open, obstruction

6. rescue breathing, reposition, chest compressions (pages 1256 to 1257)

Skill Drill 31-3: Inserting an Oropharyngeal Airway in a Child

1. Determine the appropriately sized airway by visualizing the device next to the patient's face.

2. Position the child's airway with the appropriate method.

3. Open the mouth. Insert the airway until the flange rests against the lips. Reassess the airway. (page 1261)

Skill Drill 31-6: Performing Pediatric Endotracheal Intubation

1. BSI
2. Check, prepare, assemble
3. adjunct
4. Preoxygenate, 30
5. right, left, teeth, gums, fulcrum
6. vocal cords, cricoid pressure
7. right
8. vocal cords
9. end-tidal carbon dioxide detector
10. BVM, axillae, abdomen
11. teeth, gums (pages 1270 to 1271)

Skill Drill 31-11: Immobilizing a Child

1. Use a towel under the shoulders to maintain the head in the neutral position.
2. Apply an appropriately sized cervical collar.
3. Log roll the child onto the immobilization device.
4. Secure the torso first.
5. Secure the head.
6. Ensure that the child is strapped properly.

Chapter 32: Geriatric Emergencies

Matching

1. E   (page 1345)
2. C   (page 1343)
3. G   (page 1360)
4. I   (page 1360)
5. K   (page 1358)
6. F   (page 1359)
7. D   (page 1359)
8. H   (page 1359)
9. A   (page 1343)
10. J   (page 1345)
11. B   (page 1345)

Multiple Choice

1. B – Leading causes of death in the elderly also include stroke and trauma. (page 1342)
2. D   (page 1339)
3. D   (page 1339)
4. A   (page 1342)
5. C   (page 1342)
6. D   (page 1343)
7. B   (page 1343)
8. C   (page 1344)
9. B   (page 1344)
10. D   (page 1344)
11. A   (page 1345)
12. C   (page 1345)
13. A – Kidney function in the elderly declines and they are unable to effectively eliminate medications, which causes a buildup that equates to a drug overdose. (page 1345)
14. D – The 10% reduction in brain weight can also result in a decrease in the ability to perform psychomotor skills. (page 1345)
15. B – This decrease in bone density is also known as osteoporosis. (page 1346)
16. D   (page 1348)
17. B   (page 1348)
18. A   (page 1352)
19. D   (page 1353)
20. C   (page 1354)
21. B   (page 1355)
22. D   (page 1356)
23. A   (page 1357)
24. D – Although an injury may be considered isolated and not alarming in most adults, an elderly patient's overall physical condition may lessen the body's ability to compensate for the effects of even simple injuries. (page 1357)
25. D   (page 1357)
26. A   (page 1357)
27. D   (page 1359)
28. C – Delirium has an acute or recent onset. (page 1360)
29. D   (page 1347)
30. B   (page 1348)
31. B   (page 1361)
32. D – Poor temperature regulation is also a sign of neglect. (page 1362)
33. B   (page 1344)
34. D   (page 1349)
35. D   (page 1350)
36. D   (page 1350)
37. A   (page 1352)

Vocabulary

1. Advance directives: Written document that specifies medical treatment for a competent patient should he or she become unable to make decisions (page 1346)
2. Atherosclerosis: The most common form of arteriosclerosis, in which fatty material is deposited and accumulates in the innermost layer of medium- and large-sized arteries (page 1345)
3. Arteriosclerosis: A disease that is characterized by hardening, thickening, and calcification of the arterial walls (page 1345)
4. Elder abuse: Any action on the part of an elderly individual's family member, caretaker, or other associated person that takes advantage of the elderly individual's person, property, or emotional state; also called granny battering or parent battering (page 1360)
5. Osteoporosis: A generalized bone disease, commonly associated with postmenopausal women, in which there is a reduction in the amount of bone mass, leading to fractures after minimal trauma in either sex (page 1358)
6. Macular degeneration: A disease that reduces the center of vision (page 1343)

Fill-in

1. 65 (page 1338)
2. mask (page 1338)
3. stereotypes (page 1342)
4. sweat glands (page 1343)
5. Cardiac output (page 1344)
6. aneurysm (page 1345)
7. kyphosis (page 1346)
8. Polypharmacy (page 1354)
9. macular degeneration (page 1343)
10. Activities of daily living (page 1341)
11. Septic shock (page 1346)
12. fever (page 1350)
13. weather (page 1351)
14. dehydration (page 1352)
15. sensory (page 1352)

True/False

1. F   (page 1345)
2. T   (page 1342)
3. T   (page 1342)
4. F   (page 1353)
5. T   (page 1355)
6. T   (page 1355)
7. T   (page 1356)
8. T   (page 1358)
9. F   (page 1360)
10. F   (page 1342)
11. T   (page 1340)
12. F   (page 1344)
13. F   (page 1344)
14. T   (page 1350)
15. T   (page 1351)

Short Answer

1. 1. Physical
    2. Psychological
    3. Financial (page 1362)

2. 1. Cardiac dysrhythmias/myocardial infarction: The heart is beating too fast or too slowly, the cardiac output drops, and blood flow to the brain is interrupted. A heart attack can also cause syncope.
    2. Vascular and volume: Medication interactions can cause venous pooling, and vasodilation, widening of the blood vessel, results in a drop in blood pressure and inadequate blood flow to the brain. Another cause of syncope can be a drop in blood volume because of hidden bleeding from a condition such as an aneurysm.
    3. Neurologic: A transient ischemic attack (TIA) or "brain attack" can sometimes mimic syncope. (page 1359)

3. 1. Repeated visits to the emergency department or clinic
    2. A history of being "accident prone"
    3. Soft-tissue injuries
    4. Unbelievable or vague explanations of injuries
    5. Psychosomatic complaints
    6. Chronic pain
    7. Self-destructive behavior
    8. Eating and sleep disorders
    9. Depression or lack of energy
    10. Substance and/or sexual abuse (page 1361)

4. 1. Dyspnea
    2. Weak feeling
    3. Syncope/confusion/altered mental status (page 1359)

5. G – Geriatric patients
   E – Environmental assessment
   M – Medical assessment
   S – Social assessment (Page 1339 – See table for explanation)

Word Fun

The completed crossword puzzle:

- 4 Across: DYSPNEA
- 6 Across: COLLAGEN
- 7 Across: MELENA
- 9 Across: ATHEROSCLEROSIS
- 10 Across: OSTEOPOROSIS
- 1 Down: COMPENSATED
- 2 Down: HEMATEMESIS
- 3 Down: DECOMPENSATED
- 4 Down: DEMENTIA
- 5 Down: CONTRACTED
- 8 Down: CEREBRUM

Ambulance Calls

1. -Survey the scene for any signs of or clues to the patient's care.
   -Ask about the patient's normal mental status.
   -Apply high-flow oxygen.
   -Obtain the patient's medications to take to the hospital.
   -Place the patient supine on stretcher with legs elevated.
   -Keep the patient warm.
   -Check glucose level.
   -IV bolus of 20 mL/kg of an isotonic crystalloid solution
   -Provide rapid transport.
   -Monitor vital signs en route.
   -Monitor cardiac rhythm.
   -Consider the use of a vasopressor.
   -Consider endotracheal intubation.

2. -C-spine immobilization
   -Apply high-flow oxygen (especially important due to altered mental status that may have caused crash).
   -Control bleeding with direct pressure.
   -Provide rapid transport because of altered mental status.
   -Keep the patient warm.
   -Question the patient about previous medical history and medications.
   -Gain IV access and administer fluid as needed.
   -Check glucose level.
   -Monitor vital signs and continue the secondary assessment en route.
   -Monitor cardiac rhythm.

3. -Fully immobilize the patient.
   -Apply high-flow oxygen and keep the patient warm.
   -Treat for possible shock in case of bleeding from possible hip fracture.
   -Provide rapid transport and continue a complete assessment en route.
   -Gain IV access and administer 20 mL/kg bolus of an isotonic crystalloid solution as needed.
   -Monitor vital signs.
   -Accurately document all findings and alert the proper authorities at the receiving facility or your department (according to local protocols) to the possibility of elder abuse.
   -Monitor cardiac rhythm.

Chapter 33: Ambulance Operations

Matching

1. B (page 1386)
2. E (page 1387)
3. G (page 1386)
4. I (page 1395)
5. A (page 1387)
6. H (page 1374)
7. D (page 1395)
8. F (page 1387)
9. C (page 1395)

Multiple Choice

1. C (page 1374)
2. A (page 1374)
3. A (page 1376)
4. B (page 1375)
5. D (page 1376)
6. D (page 1377)
7. A (page 1377)
8. D (page 1377)
9. D (page 1377)
10. B (page 1379)
11. D (page 1381)
12. B (page 1381)
13. A (page 1382)
14. D (page 1383)
15. D (page 1383)
16. C (page 1384)
17. C (page 1385)
18. D – You should not be driving if you are taking medications that may cause drowsiness or slow reaction times. Emotional stability is closely related to the ability to operate under stress. (page 1385)
19. B (page 1385)
20. D (page 1385)
21. B (page 1386)
22. A (page 1386)
23. A (page 1386)
24. D (page 1387)
25. A (page 1387)
26. C (page 1387)
27. D (page 1389)
28. B (page 1390)
29. C (page 1390)
30. C (page 1390)
31. B (page 1390)
32. D – Guidelines for sizing up the scene also include determining the nature of the illness for a medical patient, determining the mechanism of injury in a trauma patient, and taking BSI precautions. (page 1391)
33. D (page 1392)
34. C (page 1393)
35. D (page 1394)
36. D – Air medical unit crews can also include flight nurses. (page 1395)
37. D (page 1396)
38. D (page 1396)

Vocabulary EMT-I [vocab explorer] web

1. Air ambulances: Fixed-wing aircraft and helicopters that have been modified for medical care; used to evacuate and transport patients with life-threatening injuries to treatment facilities. (page 1395)
2. Coefficient of friction: A measure of the grip of the tire on the road surface. (page 1386)
3. Decontaminate: To remove or neutralize radiation, chemical, or other hazardous material from clothing, equipment, vehicles, and personnel. (page 1377)
4. Hydroplaning: A condition in which the tires of a vehicle may be lifted off the road surface as water "piles up" under them, making the vehicle feel as though it is floating. (page 1388)
5. High-level disinfection: The killing of pathogenic agents with the use of potent means of disinfection. (page 1395)

Fill-in

1. jump kit (page 1381)
2. Star of Life (page 1374)
3. hearse (page 1374)
4. First-responder vehicles (page 1374)
5. nine (page 1375)

6. decontaminate (page 1377)
7. airway (page 1378)
8. CPR board (page 1379)
9. Friction (page 1386)
10. length, width (page 1387)

True/False

1. T (page 1376)
2. F (page 1379)
3. T (page 1376)
4. T (page 1386)
5. F (page 1385)
6. T (page 1387)

7. F (page 1390)
8. T (page 1391)
9. T (page 1396)
10. F (page 1395)
11. F (page 1397)
12. F (page 1395)

Short Answer

1. Type I: Conventional, truck cab-chassis with modular ambulance body that can be transferred to a newer chassis as needed.

   Type II: Standard van, forward-control integral cab-body ambulance

   Type III: Specialty van, forward-control integral cab-body ambulance (page 1375)

2. State motor vehicle statutes or codes often grant an emergency vehicle the right to disregard the rules of the road when responding to an emergency. In doing so, the operator of an emergency vehicle must not endanger people or property under any circumstances. (page 1390)

3. 1. Lack of experience of the dispatcher

   2. Inadequate equipment in the ambulance

   3. Inadequate training of the EMT

   4. Inadequate driving ability

   5. Siren syndrome (page 1386)

4. 1. To the best of your knowledge, the unit must be on a true emergency call.

   2. Both audible and visual warning devices must be used simultaneously.

   3. The unit must be operated with due regard for the safety of all others, on and off the roadway. (page 1390)

5. -Select the shortest and least congested route to the scene at the time of dispatch.

   -Avoid routes with heavy traffic congestion.

   -Avoid one-way streets.

   -Watch carefully for bystanders as you approach the scene.

   -Park the ambulance in a safe place once you arrive at the scene.

   -Drive within the speed limit while transporting patients except in the rare extreme emergency.

   -Go with the flow of the traffic.

   -Use the siren as little as possible en route.

   -Always drive defensively.

   -Always maintain a safe following distance.

   -Try to maintain an open space in the lane next to you as an escape route in case the vehicle in front of you stops suddenly.

   -Use your siren if you turn on the emergency lights except when you are on a freeway.

   -Always assume that other drivers will not hear the siren or see your emergency lights. (page 1391)

6. Approach from the front of the aircraft using an approach area between 9 o'clock and 3 o'clock as the pilot faces forward. (page 1396)

7. 1. A clear site that is free of loose debris, electric or telephone poles and wires, or any other hazards that might interfere with the safe operation of the helicopter.

2. A minimum of 100′ by 100′ is recommended for the landing zone. (page 1397)

8. The siren may have a psychological effect on the driver causing him/her to drive faster and faster. (page 1386)

9. When motorists see the first vehicle pass, they may assume that is the only emergency vehicle and not look for others. (page 1390)

Word Fun

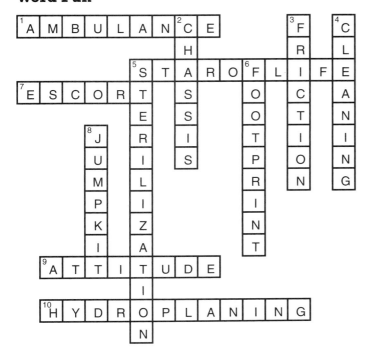

Ambulance Calls

1. -Consult your street and area maps.

-Ask the dispatcher for a cross street or reference point.

-During down time between calls, familiarize yourself with streets and alternative routes.

2. -Take your foot off the gas.

-Continue to steer, possibly shimmying the steering wheel.

-Apply a light pressure to the brakes to gradually slow down.

-Once clear of the water, lightly tap the brakes to dry them.

3. -Park your ambulance in a safe area.

-Ensure personal safety.

-Either you or your partner should handle traffic control until the police arrive.

-The person not handling traffic control should assess the patient.

-Provide patient care while ensuring personal safety and patient safety.

Chapter 34: Lifting and Moving

Matching

1. C   (page 1427)
2. G   (page 1435)
3. H   (page 1437)
4. E   (page 1437)
5. A   (page 1437)

6. I   (page 1436)
7. F   (page 1426)
8. B   (page 1435)
9. D   (page 1430)

Multiple Choice

1. D   (page 1441)
2. D   (page 1421)
3. B   (page 1405)
4. D   (page 1406)
5. D   (page 1406)
6. D   (page 1409)
7. A   (page 1408)
8. B   (page 1412)
9. B   (page 1411)
10. D   (page 1414)
11. A – The command of execution is done during each phase of moving. (pages 1414 to 1415)
12. D   (page 1415)
13. D – When carrying a patient in a stair chair, you should also bend at the knees. (page 1416)
14. D   (page 1417)
15. C – When you can move no further, stop and move back another 15 to 20 inches. (page 1417)
16. D   (page 1418)
17. B   (page 1419)
18. A   (page 1419)
19. A   (page 1421)
20. D   (page 1419)

21. D   (page 1421)
22. C   (page 1420)
23. D   (page 1421)
24. D – An urgent move may also be necessary if the patient needs immediate intervention that requires a supine position, if the patient's condition requires immediate transport to the hospital, or if there is an extreme weather condition. (page 1421)
25. D   (page 1426)
26. C   (page 1429)
27. D – To move a patient from the ground or the floor to the cot, you may also log roll the patient onto a blanket, centering the patient on the blanket and rolling up the excess material on each side. Lift the patient by the blanket, and carry him or her to the nearby cot. (page 1429)
28. B   (page 1436)
29. B   (page 1436)
30. A   (page 1437)
31. D   (page 1437)
32. D   (page 1438)
33. D   (page 1438)

Vocabulary

1. Diamond carry: A carrying technique in which one EMT-I is located at the head end, one at the foot end, and one at each side of the patient. Each of the two EMT-Is at the sides uses one hand to support the stretcher so that all are able to face forward as they walk. (page 1409)

2. Rapid extrication technique: A technique to move a patient from a sitting position inside a vehicle to supine on a backboard in less than 1 minute when conditions do not allow for standard immobilization. (page 1421)

3. Power grip: A technique in which the litter or backboard is gripped by inserting each hand under the handle with the palm facing up and the thumb extended, fully supporting the underside of the handle on the curved palm with the fingers and thumb. (page 1408)

4. Power lift: A lifting technique in which the EMT-I's back is held upright, with legs bent, and the patient is lifted when the EMT-I straightens the legs to raise the upper body and arms. (page 1406)

5. Emergency move: A move in which the patient is dragged or pulled from a dangerous scene before initial assessment and care are provided. (page 1419)

Fill-in

1. body mechanics (page 1404)
2. upright (page 1406)
3. power lift (page 1406)
4. palm (page 1408)
5. locked-in (page 1411)
6. 250 (page 1415)
7. sideways (page 1418)
8. locked (page 1418)

9. overhead (page 1419)
10. less strain (page 1419)
11. spine movement (page 1422)
12. direct ground lift (page 1426)
13. extremity lift (page 1427)
14. fluid resistant (page 1432)
15. scoop stretcher (page 1437)

True/False

1. T   (page 1438)
2. T   (page 1435)
3. T   (page 1406)
4. F   (page 1415)
5. F   (page 1429)

6. T   (page 1421)
7. F   (page 1437)
8. F   (page 1412)
9. F   (page 1421)
10. F   (page 1426)

Short Answer

1. 1. Front cradle
    2. Fire fighter's drag
    3. One-person walking assist
    4. Fire fighter's carry
    5. Pack strap (page 1422)

2. 1. The vehicle or scene is unsafe.
    2. The patient cannot be properly assessed before being removed from the car.
    3. The patient needs immediate intervention that requires a supine position.
    4. The patient's condition requires immediate transport to the hospital.
    5. The patient blocks the EMT-I's access to another seriously injured patient. (page 1421)

3. -Make sure there is sufficient lifting power.
    -Follow the manufacturer's directions for safe and proper use of the cot.
    -Make sure that all cots and patients are fully secured before you move the ambulance. (page 1435)

4. -Be sure that you know or can find out the weight to be lifted and the limitations of the team's abilities.
    -Coordinate your movements with those of the other team members while constantly communicating with them.
    -Do not twist your body as you are carrying the patient.
    -Keep the weight that you are carrying as close to your body as possible while keeping your back in a locked-in position.
    -Be sure to flex at the hips, not at the waist, and bend at the knees while making sure that you do not hyperextend your back by leaning back from your waist. (page 1409)

5. Always keep your back in a straight, upright position and lift without twisting. (page 1406)

Word Fun

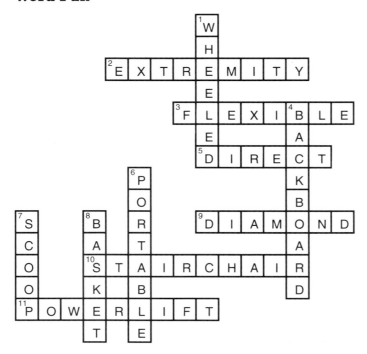

Ambulance Calls

1. -Immobilize the patient on a long spine board and apply high-flow oxygen.
   -Use four persons to carry the board back up the ledge.
   -Plan the route and brief your helpers before moving the patient.
   -Clarify whether you will move on "three" or count to three then move.
   -Coordinate the move until the patient is loaded into the ambulance.

2. -Move the patient's legs so they are clear of the pedals and are against the seat.
   -Rotate the patient so that his back is positioned facing the open car door.
   -Place your arms through the armpits and grasp either the patient's forearms or your own forearms.
   -Support the patient's head against your body.
   -While supporting the patient's weight, drag the patient from the seat.
   -Place him supine on the ground and secure the airway.
   -Assist ventilations with 100% oxygen until further help arrives.

3. -Have your partner maintain manual c-spine immobilization.
   -Apply a cervical collar.
   -Rotate the patient 90° while your partner maintains c-spine control.
   -Slide the patient out of the vehicle onto a long spine board.
   -Secure the torso, legs, then the head to the board.
   -Place the backboard on the stretcher and load into the ambulance.
   -Treat for shock and rapid transport.
   -Continue your assessment en route.

Skill Drills

Skill Drill 34-1: Performing the Power Lift

1. upright, Spread, Balance, center
2. straddle, distribute
3. Straighten (page 1407)

Skill Drill 34-2: Performing the Diamond Carry

1. Position yourselves facing the patient.

2. After the patient has been lifted, the EMT-I at the foot turns to face forward.

3. EMT-Is at the sides each turn the head-end hand palm down and release the other hand.

4. EMT-Is at the side turn toward the foot end. (page 1410)

Skill Drill 34-3: Performing the One-Handed Carrying Technique

1. Face, hands

2. carrying height

3. Turn, switch (page 1411)

Skill Drill 34-4: Carrying a Patient on Stairs

1. Strap

2. foot, head

3. head (page 1413)

Skill Drill 34-5: Using a Stair Chair

1. chair

2. head, foot

3. rescuer, foot

4. Lower (page 1416)

Skill Drill 34-6: Performing Rapid Extrication Technique

1. First EMT-I provides in-line manual support of the head and cervical spine.

2. Second EMT-I gives commands, applies a cervical collar, and performs the initial assessment.

3. Second EMT-I supports the torso. Third EMT-I frees the patient's legs from the pedals and moves the legs together, without moving pelvis or spine.

4. Second and Third EMT-Is rotate the patient as a unit in several short coordinated moves. First EMT-I (relieved by Fourth EMT-I or bystander as needed) supports the head and neck during rotation (and later steps).

5. First (or Fourth) EMT-I places the backboard on the seat against patient's buttocks. Second and Third EMT-Is lower the patient onto the long spine board.

6. Third EMT-I moves to an effective position for sliding the patient. Second and Third EMT-Is slide the patient along the backboard in coordinated, 8″ to 12″ moves until the hips rest on the backboard.

7. Third EMT-I exits the vehicle, moves to the backboard opposite Second EMT-I, and they continue to slide the patient until patient is fully on the board.

8. First (or Fourth) EMT-I continues to stabilize the head and neck while Second and Third EMT-Is carry the patient away from the vehicle. (pages 1424 to 1425)

Skill Drill 34-7: Extremity Lift

1. crossed, forearms, sitting

2. armpits, forearms, wrists, legs, knees

3. crouching, command (page 1428)

Skill Drill 34-8: Scoop Stretcher

1. length

2. Lift, slide

3. Lock, pinching

4. Secure, transfer (page 1430)

Skill Drill 34-9: Loading a Cot into an Ambulance

1. Tilt the head of the cot upward, and place it into the patient compartment with the wheels on the floor.

2. Second rescuer on the side of the cot releases the undercarriage lock and lifts the undercarriage.

3. Roll the cot into the back of the ambulance.

4. Secure the cot to the brackets mounted in the ambulance. (page 1434)

Chapter 35: Gaining Access

Matching

1. E (page 1446)
2. A (page 1450)
3. D (page 1450)
4. F (page 1446)
5. B (page 1452)
6. G (page 1454)
7. C (page 1454)

Multiple Choice

1. D (page 1446)
2. B (page 1446)
3. C (page 1446)
4. A (page 1446)
5. D (page 1447)
6. A – You have no control over the patient's level of consciousness (B). The patient may be unconscious and the person holding the head is responsible for immobilization (C). (page 1448)
7. B – You must triage when multiple patients are involved to ensure that as many patients as possible receive optimal care. (page 1449)
8. D (page 1450)
9. D (page 1451)
10. C (page 1452)
11. D (page 1453)
12. B (page 1453)

Vocabulary

1. Entrapment: To be caught (trapped) within a vehicle, room, or container with no way out or to have a limb or other body part trapped. (page 1446)
2. Technical rescue situation: A rescue that requires special technical skills and equipment in one of many specialized rescue areas. (page 1452)
3. Danger zone: An area where individuals can be exposed to sharp metal edges, broken glass, toxic substances, lethal rays, or ignition or explosion of hazardous materials. (page 1448)
4. Tactical situation: A hostage, robbery, or other situation in which armed conflict is threatened or shots have been fired and the threat of violence remains. (page 1453)
5. Technical rescue group: A team of individuals from one or more departments in a region that is trained and on call for certain types of technical rescue. (page 1452)

Fill-in

1. Removal (page 1446)
2. safety (page 1446)
3. communication (page 1446)
4. stable (page 1447)
5. safest (page 1449)
6. harm (page 1451)
7. self-contained breathing apparatus (page 1454)

True/False

1. F (page 1446)
2. T (page 1447)
3. T (page 1447)
4. F (page 1449)
5. F (page 1450)
6. T (page 1449)

Short Answer

1. 1. Fire fighters: Responsible for extinguishing any fire, preventing additional ignition, ensuring that the scene is safe, and washing down spilled fuel.
   2. Law enforcement: Responsible for traffic control and direction, maintaining order at the scene, investigating the crash or crime scene, and establishing and maintaining lines so that bystanders are kept at a safe distance and out of the way of rescuers.

3. Rescue group: Responsible for properly securing and stabilizing the vehicle, providing safe entrance and access to patients, extricating any patients, ensuring that patients are properly protected during extrication or other rescue activities, and providing adequate room so that patients can be removed properly.

4. EMS personnel: Responsible for assessing and providing immediate medical care, triage and assigning priority to patients, packaging the patient, providing additional assessment and care as needed once the patient has been removed, and providing transport to the emergency department. (page 1446)

2. -Is the patient in a vehicle or in some other structure?

-Is the vehicle or structure severely damaged?

-What hazards exist that pose risk to the patient and rescuers?

-In what position is the vehicle? On what type of surface? Is the vehicle stable or is it apt to roll or tip? (page 1449)

3. 1. Provide manual stabilization to protect c-spine as needed.

2. Open the airway.

3. Provide high-flow oxygen

4. Assist with or provide adequate ventilation.

4. Control any significant external bleeding.

6. Treat all critical injuries. (page 1450)

4. Assess the extent of injury and whether there is a possibility of hidden bleeding; evaluate sensation in the trapped area to discover if an object is pressing on or impaled in the patient. (page 1450)

5. -Ensure that each EMT-I can be positioned so that he/she can lift and carry at all times.

-Move the patient in a series of smooth, slow, controlled steps, with stops designed between to allow for repositioning and adjustments.

-Plan the exact steps and pathway that you will follow.

-Choose a path that requires the least manipulation of the patient or equipment.

-Make sure that sufficient personnel are available.

-Make sure that you move the patient as a unit.

-While moving the patient, continue to protect him/her from any hazards. (page 1451)

Word Fun

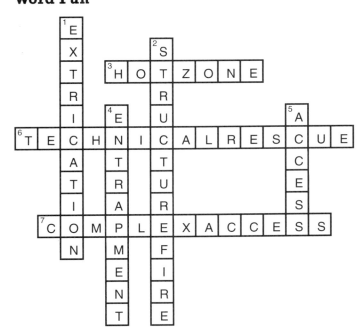

Ambulance Calls

1. -Prepare all equipment that may be required to immobilize the patient if he has fallen as well as any other equipment you may need

   -Leave all equipment in the back of the unit in case you need to drive to the site where the patient is found

   -Question family members about further history

   -Advise medical control as soon as possible and be prepared for a patient that may be hypothermic

2. -Have someone assume c-spine control.

   -Apply high-flow oxygen via nonrebreathing mask

   -Examine as much of the patient as is physically possible and control any bleeding.

   -Attempt to gain IV access if possible

   -Have someone prepare the stretcher with the backboard and PASG to use as soon as the patient is free

   -Continue to talk to the patient and try to obtain any history

   -Protect patient from debris as extrication is carried out

   -Advise medical control as soon as possible

   -Rapid transport with treatment for shock as soon as patient is disentangled

3. -Try to learn as much about the chemical as possible by having the dispatcher contact CHEMTREC or another agency to find out about possible effects to the patient

   -Prepare necessary equipment to manage the airway and ventilation

   -Be prepared to do CPR if necessary

   -Have all equipment within reach

   -Once patient is brought to you, rapidly begin to manage the ABCs and prepare for rapid transport

Chapter 36: Special Operations

Matching

1. J   (page 1473)
2. K   (page 1462)
3. L   (page 1470)
4. D   (page 1473)
5. H   (page 1471)
6. E   (page 1471)
7. B   (page 1478)
8. I   (page 1477)
9. A   (page 1465)
10. F   (page 1475)
11. G   (page 1475)
12. C   (page 1475)

Multiple Choice

1. D   (page 1462)
2. D – Extended operations also have finance and administrative sectors as part of their typical incident command structure. (page 1463)
3. C   (page 1463)
4. A   (page 1475)
5. D   (page 1475)
6. C   (page 1475)
7. D   (page 1476)
8. B   (page 1475)
9. D – Bus crashes are also an example of a mass-casualty incident. (page 1473)
10. D   (page 1470)
11. B   (page 1469-1470)
12. D   (pages 1469)
13. A   (page 1469)
14. D   (page 1468)
15. B   (page 1467)
16. D   (page 1467)
17. D   (page 1467)
18. D   (page 1466)
19. D   (page 1467)
20. B   (page 1467)
21. D   (page 1465)
22. D   (page 1464)
23. D   (page 1480)
24. C   (page 1483)
25. C   (page 1484)
26. A   (page 1474)
27. B   (page 1474)
28. D   (page 1474)
29. C   (page 1474)
30. A   (page 1474)
31. D   (page 1474)
32. A   (page 1474)
33. B   (page 1474)
34. D   (page 1474)
35. C   (page 1474)

Vocabulary

1. Command post: The designated field command center where the incident commander and support personnel are located (page 1462)
2. Danger zone: An area where individuals can be exposed to toxic substances, lethal rays, or ignition or explosion of hazardous materials (page 1467)
3. Hazardous material: Any substance that is toxic, poisonous, radioactive, flammable, or explosive and causes injury or death with exposure (page 1465)
4. Incident commander: The individual who has overall command of the scene in the field (page 1462)
5. Sector commander: The individual delegated to oversee and coordinate activity in an incident command sector (page 1463)

Fill-in

1. incident command system (page 1462)
2. command post (page 1462)
3. safety officer (page 1463)
4. hazardous materials incident (page 1465)
5. extrication (page 1474)
6. disaster (page 1477)
7. Triage (page 1473)
8. triage area, triage officer (page 1475)
9. contaminated (page 1470)
10. airway, breathing (page 1469)
11. Decontamination (page 1468-1469)
12. relocate (page 1467)
13. transportation officer (page 1475)
14. toxic (page 1466)
15. high-school chemistry (page 1481)
16. placard (page 1466)
17. contaminated (page 1481)
18. cold (page 1482)
19. decontaminated (page 1482)
20. downwind (page 1483)
21. hot zone (page 1483)
22. Methamphetamine (page 1484)

True/False

1. T   (page 1465)
2. F   (page 1468)
3. F   (page 1470)
4. F   (page 1471)
5. T   (page 1474)
6. F   (page 1474)
7. T   (page 1466–1467)
8. F   (page 1469)
9. F   (page 1469)
10. F   (page 1478)
11. T   (page 1477)
12. T   (page 1479)
13. F   (page 1468)
14. T   (page 1481)
15. F   (page 1482)
16. T   (page 1484)

Short Answer

1. Level 0: Materials that would cause little, if any, health hazard if you came into contact with them

    Level 1: Materials that would cause irritation on contact, but only mild residual injury, even without treatment

    Level 2: Materials that could cause temporary damage or residual injury unless prompt medical treatment is provided

    Level 3: Materials that are extremely hazardous to health

    Level 4: Materials that are so hazardous that minimal contact will cause death (page 1470)

2. Level A: Fully encapsulated, chemical-resistant protective clothing; SCBA; special, sealed equipment

    Level B: Nonencapsulated protective clothing, or clothing designed to protect against a particular hazard; SCBA; eye protection

    Level C: Nonpermeable clothing; eye protection; facemasks

    Level D: Work uniform (page 1471)

3. 1. Command
    2. Staging
    3. Extrication
    4. Triage
    5. Treatment
    6. Supply
    7. Transportation
    8. Rehabilitation (page 1475)

4. First priority (red): Patients who need immediate care and transport

    Second priority (yellow): Patients whose treatment and transportation can be temporarily delayed

    Third priority (green): Patients whose treatment and transportation can be delayed until last

    Fourth priority (black): Patients who are already dead or have little chance for survival (page 1474)

5.

Class	Type
Class 1	Explosives
Class 2	Gases
Class 3	Flammable liquids
Class 4	Flammable solids
Class 5	Oxidizers
Class 6	Poisons
Class 7	Radioactive
Class 8	Corrosives
Class 9	Miscellaneous (page 1468)

6. Decontamination is the process of removing or neutralizing and properly disposing of hazardous materials from equipment, patients, and rescue personnel. The decontamination area is the designated area where contaminants are removed before an individual can go to another area. (pages 1468-1469)

7. -Command and management

-Preparedness

-Resource management

-Communications and information management

-Supporting technologies

-Ongoing management and maintenance (page 1464)

8. Outside: fragmentation and incendiary devices (hand grenades and claymore mines), animal traps, and impaling stakes

Inside: vicious dogs, poisonous snakes, fishhooks hung at eye level, explosives connected to heating elements and electrical switches, and weapons such as crossbows and spear guns that discharge when the trigger mechanism is disturbed (page 1481)

9. -Nausea

-Vomiting

-Sharp headache

-Reddened face

-Burning sensation in the nose, throat, or lungs

-Drowsiness

-Numb lips

-Tingling teeth

-Unfocused eyes (page 1484)

Word Fun

Ambulance Calls

1. -The 4-year-old should be triaged as first priority (red).

    -The 27-year-old should be triaged as third priority (green).

    -The 42-year-old should be triaged as fourth priority (black).

2. -Move upwind at least 100 feet.

    -Call for a HazMat response.

    -Try to keep others out of the scene.

    -Call for help from law enforcement.

    -Have the tag number of the vehicle traced to possibly call the company for identification.

    -Do not provide any patient care until the scene is safe.

3. -The EMT riding in the patient compartment should wear goggles, a mask, a gown, two pairs of gloves, a respirator, a HazMat suit, etc.

    -Cabinet doors should be taped shut.

    -All unneeded equipment should be stored in the front of the vehicle or in outside compartments.

    -Turn on the power vent ceiling fan and the patient compartment air-conditioning unit fan.

    -Open the windows in the driver's area and sliding side windows in the patient compartment.

4. -Establish a preliminary HazMat hot zone.

    -Include the lab, surrounding area, and all personnel and equipment, as well as anything removed from the lab.

    -Notify your dispatcher and request the following agencies:

    - •Drug Enforcement Administration
    - •Environmental Protection Agency
    - •HazMat response team
    - •Additional EMS unit
    - •Bomb squad
    - •Local health department
    - •EMS supervisor
    - •Fire department

Chapter 37: Response to Terrorism and Weapons of Mass Destruction

Matching

1. H   (page 1492)
2. I   (page 1498)
3. Q   (page 1494)
4. K   (page 1494)
5. N   (page 1499)
6. G   (page 1496)
7. O   (page 1498)
8. R   (page 1500)
9. E   (page 1493)
10. S   (page 1504)
11. P   (page 1497)
12. L   (page 1498)
13. C   (page 1498)
14. B   (page 1506)
15. A   (page 1494)
16. D   (page 1507)
17. T   (page 1505)
18. M   (page 1494)
19. J   (page 1505)
20. F   (page 1505)

Multiple Choice

1. D   (page 1493)
2. C – Vesicants are blister agents designed to affect the skin. (page 1498)
3. B   (page 1498)
4. C   (page 1498)
5. D   (page 1498)
6. A   (page 1499)
7. B   (page 1499)
8. B – The patient must be decontaminated before ABCs are performed to prevent further contamination. (page 1499)
9. D   (page 1499)
10. D   (page 1500)
11. C   (page 1500)
12. A – Sarin is a nerve agent that turns from liquid to gas within seconds. (page 1500)
13. B   (page 1500)
14. D   (page 1501)
15. D – DUMBELS stands for: Diarrhea, Urination, Miosis, Bradycardia, Bronchospasm, Emesis, Lacrimation, and Seizures, Sweating, and Salivation. (page 1502)
16. C   (page 1508)
17. A   (page 1511)
18. B   (page 1511)
19. C   (page 1511)
20. D   (page 1511)
21. D   (pages 1513 to 1514)

Vocabulary

1. Weapon of mass destruction: Any agent or device designed to bring about mass death, casualties, and/or massive damage or property and infrastructure. (page 1493)
2. Weaponization: The creation of a weapon from a biologic agent generally found in nature and that causes disease; the agent is cultivated, synthesized and/or mutated to maximize the target population's exposure to the germ. (page 1494)
3. Off-gassing: Vapors are continuously released over a period of time. (page 1500)
4. Dissemination: The means by which a terrorist will spread an agent. (page 1504)
5. Syndromic surveillance: Monitoring, usually by local or state health departments, of patients presenting to the emergency departments and alternative care facilities, the recording of EMS call volume, and monitoring the use of over-the-counter medications. (page 1509)
6. Points of distribution: Strategically placed facilities that have been preestablished for the mass distribution of antibiotics, antidotes, vaccinations, and with other medications and supplies. (page 1509)
7. Special Atomic Demolition Munitions: Small suitcase-sized nuclear weapons designed to destroy individual targets. (page 1513)

Fill-in

1. mentally, physically (page 1492)
2. upwind, uphill (page 1496)
3. secondary infection (page 1499)
4. Tabun or GA (page 1501)
5. death (page 1501)
6. atropine, 2-PAM chloride (page 1501)
7. Cyanide (page 1502)
8. Bubonic plague, pneumonic plague (page 1507)
9. Botulinum (page 1508)
10. explosives (page 1513)

True/False

1. T	(page 1496)	**5.** T	(page 1499)	**9.** T	(page 1503)
2. T	(page 1497)	**6.** T	(page 1500)	**10.** T	(page 1503)
3. F	(page 1498)	**7.** T	(page 1501)	**11.** T	(page 1513)
4. F	(page 1499)	**8.** F	(page 1502)	**12.** F	(page 1513)

Short Answer

1. 1. Vesicants (blister agents)

   2. Respiratory agents (choking agents)

   3. Nerve agents

   4. Metabolic agents (blood agents) (page 1494)

2. 1. Virus

   2. Bacteria

   3. Toxins (page 1494)

3. -Type of location

   -Type of call

   -Number of patients

   -Victims' statements

   -Preincident indicators

4. Low exposure: Nausea, vomiting, and diarrhea

   Moderate exposure: First-degree burns, hair loss, depletion of the immune system, and cancer

   Severe exposure: Second- and third-degree burns, cancer, and death (page 1513)

Word Fun

Ambulance Calls

1. -Back out

   -Notify dispatch to have the appropriate teams respond

   -Notify the police to have access to the mall restricted

   -Set up in the appropriate area to accept patients after decontamination

2. Because radiation is cumulative, you should not expose yourself. Explain to the nurse that you are willing to assist in the care of this patient after an apron is located for you to wear.

Chapter 38: Assessment-Based Management

Matching

1. C (page 1529)

2. D (page 1528)

3. E (page 1530)

4. A (page 1535)

5. B (page 1531)

Multiple Choice

1. D (page 1528)

2. D (page 1528)

3. D (page 1529)

4. A (page 1531)

5. C (page 1528)

6. A (page 1528)

7. D (page 1530)

8. B (page 1530)

9. D (page 1533)

10. B (page 1533)

11. D (page 1533)

12. C (page 1533)

13. A (page 1534)

14. B (page 1535)

Vocabulary

1. Being able to ask questions and do other things while listening to the answer (page 1534)

2. A – Airway control
B – Breathing
C – Circulation
D – Disability
   Dysrhythmia
E – Exposure (page 1531)

Fill-in

1. reasoning skills (page 1528)

2. scene (page 1528)

3. Assessment (page 1528)

4. medical detective (page 1528)

5. Experience (page 1529)

6. patterns (page 1529)

7. preplan (page 1530)

8. team leader (page 1530)

9. impression (page 1533)

10. people (page 1533)

11. extensions (page 1535)

True/False

1. T (page 1536)

2. F (page 1528)

3. T (page 1530)

4. T (page 1529)

5. F (page 1530)

6. T (page 1532)

7. F (page 1533)

8. T (page 1533)

Short Answer

1. Focusing on the systems associated with the complaint without being aware of the potential for other injuries or other systems that may be affected (page 1529)

2. -Manages patient care

   -Establishes contact and a dialogue with the patient

   -Obtains the patient history

   -Performs the physical exam

   -Gives the radio report

   -Completes the written documentation (page 1530)

3. -Provides scene cover and assists team leader

-Gathers scene information

-Talks to relatives and bystanders

-Obtains vital signs

-Performs interventions requested by the team leader

-In a mass-casualty incident, acts as the triage group leader (pages 1530-1531)

4. Hypoxia, hypovolemia, hypoglycemia, head injury (page 1532)

5. -Cardiac/respiratory arrest

-Respiratory distress/failure

-Unstable dysrhythmias

-Seizures

-Coma/altered mental status

-Shock/hypotension

-Major trauma

-Possible cervical spine injury (page 1533)

Word Fun

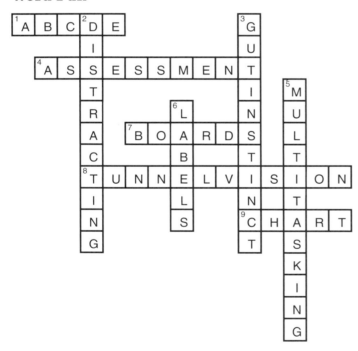

Ambulance Calls

1. Mary appears to have had a seizure based on the patterns presented. Treatment includes the following:

-C-spine control

-Assess and manage ABCs.

-Apply high-flow oxygen with an adjunct if tolerated.

-Gain IV access and assess glucose level.

-Immobilize the patient and transport monitoring vital signs en route.

-Monitor cardiac rhythm.

-Consider the administration of diazepam if seizure activity resumes or follow local protocols.</1999>

2. Do not focus on the angulated leg when your patient is unresponsive.

-C-spine control

-Assess LOC and ABCs.

-Apply high-flow oxygen with an adjunct as tolerated.

-Have your partner control bleeding if necessary.

-Immobilize the patient and provide rapid transport.

-Gain IV access and assess glucose level.

-Give a 20 mL/kg bolus of an isotonic crystalloid solution.

-Apply traction splint en route.

-Monitor cardiac rhythm.

-Consider endotracheal intubation.

3. As soon as possible, move the patient to the ambulance where you have a controlled environment in which to work without distractions. Advise family members that you will let them know something as soon as possible, but close the doors to maintain privacy.

Chapter 39: BLS Review

Matching

1. E   (pages 1546)
2. D   (page 1555)
3. B   (page 1546)
4. C   (page 1548)
5. A   (page 1546)

Multiple Choice

1. D   (page 1546)
2. C   (page 1548)
3. B   (page 1548)
4. D   (page 1548)
5. A   (page 1549)
6. D   (pages 1549 and 1570)
7. D – Causes of respiratory arrest in infants and children also include near-drowning incidents or electrocution. (page 1549)
8. D – Signs of irreversible death also include putrefaction or decomposition of the body. (pages 1549 to 1550)
9. C   (page 1550)
10. D   (page 1551)
11. A   (page 1554)
12. B – Use the jaw-thrust maneuver with head tilt if there is no suspected spinal injury. If spinal injury is suspected, use the jaw-thrust maneuver without the head tilt. (pages 1553 to 1554)
13. C   (page 1561)

14. B   (pages 1561 to 1562)
15. A   (page 1561)
16. D   (page 1564)
17. A   (page 1564)
18. D   (page 1564)
19. B   (page 1569)
20. D   (pages 1570)
21. D   (page 1572)
22. C   (page 1571)
23. D   (page 1554)
24. D   (page 1554)
25. B – The abdominal-thrust maneuver (A), also called the Heimlich maneuver (C), may injure the liver or other abdominal organs in an infant and may not be effective for an obese patient. It also may injure the fetus in a pregnant woman. (page 1556)
26. C – You should stay with the patient, give 100% oxygen via nonrebreathing mask, and provide prompt transport. (page 1558)
27. B   (page 1548)

Vocabulary

1. Gastric distention: A condition in which air fills the stomach as a result of high volume and pressure during artificial ventilation. (page 1562)
2. Head tilt–chin lift maneuver: A technique to open the airway that combines tilting back the forehead and lifting the chin. (page 1551)
3. Jaw-thrust maneuver: A technique to open the airway performed by placing the fingers behind the angles of the patient's lower jaw and forcefully moving the jaw forward; can be performed without head tilt. (page 1553)
4. Recovery position: A position that helps to maintain a clear airway in a patient with a decreased level of consciousness who has not had traumatic injuries and is breathing on his or her own. (page 1563)
5. Asynchronous CPR: The performance of CPR in which chest compressions are not paused for the delivery of a ventilation; performed after the airway has been definitively secured (for example, by intubation). (page 1567)

Fill-in

1. 4 to 6 (page 1546)
2. barrier (page 1548)
3. ABCs (page 1549)
4. airways (page 1549)
5. cardiac, respiratory (page 1549)

6. Advance directives (page 1550)
7. firm (page 1551)
8. airway (page 1551)
9. defibrillation (page 1548)

True/False

1. T (page 1549)   **8.** F (page 1567)

2. F (page 1549)   **9.** F (page 1564)

3. T (page 1549)   **10.** T (page 1562)

4. F (page 1563)   **11.** F (page 1562)

5. F (page 1552)   **12.** T (page 1548)

6. T (page 1549)   **13.** T (page 1548)

7. T (page 1566)

Short Answer

1. 1. Rigor mortis or stiffening of the body after death

2. Dependent lividity (livor mortis), a discoloration of the skin that results from pooling of blood

3. Putrefaction or decomposition of the body

4. Evidence of nonsurvivable injury, such as decapitation (pages 1549 to 1550)

2. (page 1547)

TABLE 39-1 Review of Pediatric BLS Procedures

Procedure	Infants (younger than 1 y)	Children (1 y to onset of puberty)[1]
Airway	Head tilt—chin lift; jaw thrust if spinal injury is suspected	Head tilt—chin lift; jaw thrust if spinal injury is suspected
Breathing		
Initial breaths	2 breaths with duration of 1 second each with enough volume to produce chest rise	2 breaths with duration of 1 second each with enough volume to produce chest rise
Subsequent breaths	1 breath every 3to 5 seconds; 12 to 20 breaths/min	1 breath every 3to 5 seconds; 12 to 20 breaths/min
Circulation		
Pulse check	Brachial artery	Carotid or femoral artery
Compression area	Just below the nipple line	In the center of the chest, in between the nipples
Compression width	2 fingers or 2-thumb hands-encircling technique	Heel of one or both hands
Compression depth	$\frac{1}{3}$ to $\frac{1}{2}$ the depth of the chest	$\frac{1}{3}$ to $\frac{1}{2}$ the depth of the chest
Compression rate	100/min	100/min
Ratio of compressions to ventilations	30:2 (one rescuer); 15:2 (two rescuers)[2]	30:2 (one rescuer); 15:2 (two rescuers)[2]
Foreign body obstruction	Conscious: back slaps and chest thrusts Unconscious: CPR	Conscious: abdominal thrusts Unconscious: CPR

[1] Onset of puberty is approximately 12-14 years of age, as defined by secondary characteristics (eg, breast development in girls and armpit hair in boys.

[2] Pause compressions to deliver ventilations.

3. S: The patient starts breathing and has a pulse.

T: The patient is transferred to another person who is trained in BLS or ALS or to another emergency medical responder.

O: You are out of strength or too tired to continue.

P: A physician who is present assumes responsibility for the patient. (page 1550)

4. 1. Make sure the patient is supine.

2. Place one hand on the patient's forehead, and apply firm backward pressure with your palm to tilt the head back.

3. Place the tips of your fingers of your other hand under the lower jaw near the bony part of the chin.

4. Lift the chin forward, bringing the entire lower jaw with it, helping to tilt the head back. (pages 1551 to 1552)

5. 1. Kneel above the patient's head. Place your index or middle finger behind the angle of the lower jaw on both sides. Forcefully move the jaw forward, and tilt the head back.

2. Use your thumbs to pull the patient's lower jaw down to allow breathing through the mouth and nose.

3. The nose can be sealed with your cheek. (page 1554)

6. Place both thumbs side by side over the lower half of the infant's sternum, approximately 1 fingerbreadth below an imaginary line located between the nipples. Ensure that the thumbs do not compress on or near the xiphoid process. In very small infants, you may need to overlap your thumbs. Encircle the infant's chest and support the infant's back with the fingers of both hands. With your hands encircling the chest, use both thumbs to depress the sternum approximately one third to one half the depth of the infant's chest, which will correspond to a depth of about 1/2" to 1". (page 1572)

7. Ensure that the patient is on a firm, flat surface. Place your hands in the proper position. Lock your elbows with your arms straight and your shoulders directly over your hands. Give 15 compressions at a rate of about 100 beats/minute for an adult. Using a rocking motion, apply pressure vertically from your shoulders down through both arms to depress the sternum 1 1/2" to 2" in the adult, then rise up gently. Count the compressions aloud. The ratio of compressions and relaxation should be 1:1. (page 1564)

8. 1. First EMT-I moves into position to begin chest compressions after giving a second breath.

2. Second EMT-I gives the 15th compression, then moves to the patient's head.

3. Second EMT-I checks the carotid pulse for 5 to 10 seconds. If the patient has no pulse, say, "No pulse, continue CPR." (page 1569)

9. -Standing: Stand behind the patient and wrap your arms around his or her waist. Press your fist into the patient's abdomen in a series of five quick inward and upward thrusts.

-Supine: Straddle the hips or legs. Place the heel of one hand against the patient's abdomen and the other hand on top of the first. Press your hands into the patient's abdomen in a series of five quick inward and upward thrusts. (pages 1555 to 1556)

10. -Standing: Stand behind the patient and wrap your arms under the armpits and around the patient's chest. Press your fist into the patient's chest and perform backwards thrusts until the object is expelled or the patient becomes unconscious.

-Supine: Kneel next to the patient. Place your hands as you would to deliver chest compressions. Deliver slow chest thrusts until the object is expelled. (pages 1556 to 1557)

11. 1. "Sandwich" the infant between your hands and arms.

2. Deliver five quick back slaps between the shoulder blades, using the heel of your hand.

3. Turn the infant face up.

4. Give five quick chest thrusts on the sternum at a slightly slower rate than you would give for CPR. (pages 1559 to 1560)

Word Fun

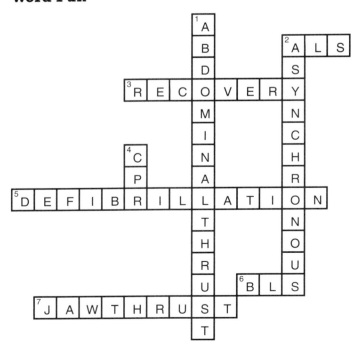

Ambulance Calls

1. -Question the family about the last time they spoke with her.

   -Explain that she has been down too long for CPR to be effective.

   -Comfort family members.

   -Notify your dispatcher to alert the supervisor and either law enforcement, the coroner, or a funeral home according to local protocols.

2. -Immediately assess the airway and apply high-flow oxygen, assisting ventilations as needed.

   -Prepare for rapid transport.

   -Obtain a SAMPLE history from co-workers if possible.

   -Continue your assessment and monitor vital signs en route.

3. -BSI precautions

   -Position the patient and begin rescue breathing with a BVM and 100% oxygen.

   -Assess circulation at the carotid artery.

   -Find proper hand positioning for chest compressions.

   -Depress sternum $1\frac{1}{2}$ to 2 inches.

   -Move patient onto stretcher on a backboard after delivering two breaths via BVM device.

   -Begin CPR again with two breaths and assessing pulse.

   -Rapid transport, if no pulse/respirations, continue CPR en route.

Skill Drills

Skill Drill 39-1: Positioning the Patient

1. Kneel beside the patient, leaving room to roll the patient toward you.
2. Grasp the patient, stabilizing the cervical spine if needed.
3. Move the head and neck as a unit with the torso as your partner pulls on the distant shoulder and hip.
4. Move the patient to a supine position with legs straight and arms at the sides. (page 1552)

Skill Drill 39-2: Performing Chest Compressions

1. index, middle, notch
2. lower portion
3. heel, index finger
4. hand
5. lock, over, $1\frac{1}{2}$, 2 (page 1565)

Skill Drill 39-3: Performing One-Rescuer Adult CPR

1. Establish unresponsiveness and call for help.
2. Open the airway.
3. Look, listen, and feel for breathing. If breathing, place in the recovery position and monitor.
4. If not breathing, give two breaths of 1 second each.
5. Check for carotid pulse.
6. If no pulse is found, apply your AED. If there is no AED, place your hands in the proper position for chest compressions.

   Give 30 compressions at about 100/min.

   Open the airway and give two ventilations of 1 second each.

   Perform five cycles of compressions.

   Stop CPR and check for return of the carotid pulse. Depending on patient condition, continue CPR, continue rescue breathing only, or place in the recovery position and monitor. (page 1568–1569)

Skill Drill 39-4: Performing Two-Rescuer Adult CPR

1. unresponsiveness
2. Open
3. recover, monitor
4. two, 1
5. carotid
6. AED, chest compressions, 100, five, condition (page 1565–1569)